WHAT SOME HEALTH EXPERTS ARE SAYING ABOUT PAUL NISON'S
RAW KNOWLEDGE

"As in the same vein as his previous book, Paul Nison in a down to earth manner, based mostly on his own experiences and corroborated by a thorough research enthusiastically conveys the importance of a raw diet and a sensible lifestyle. A book that should be on the shelves of every truth seeker."
—**Morris Krok**, Author and long time health authority

"Once again, Paul Nison has given humanity a great gift—his new book, *Raw Knowledge: Enhance the Powers of Your Mind, Body and Soul* —a great, inspiring work about nutrition and health. If one had the conviction and will power necessary to follow Nison's advice and guidelines faithfully, most certainly he/she wouldn't need the services of doctors any longer. Well done Paul."
—**Benito De Donno**, Author of *Glimpses of Reality*

"Paul Nison does it again! Using his own unique sense of wit and wisdom, he creates in his new book, *Raw Knowledge*, an adventure into a land of raw truth and freedom. Paul is so dedicated to his own lifestyle and this dedication is reflected in his books, his lectures and his relationships. I would highly recommend *Raw Knowledge* and suggest that if you ever get a chance to hear Paul in person, go see him. He is a delightful and entertaining speaker full of knowledge and caring for all of life."
—**Roe Gallo** M.A., Author of *Perfect Body*.

"In the entire health education arena, Paul Nison stands out in my mind as being in a special group of the most dynamic, truthful leaders, which I call the *"Raw Passion Gang."* Paul has joined the ranks of true health and self-empowerment teachers, carrying the torch onward. Paul exudes uncommon dedication toward helping people overcome suffering and mediocre health so that they can get their chance to enjoy life to its fullest. I endorse Paul's books, and refer health truth seekers to his lectures and seminars, because from Paul they will get a real caring person and a liberating, insight-filled, exuberant experience."

—**David Klein**, Creator of *Raw Passion Seminars*, Publisher of *Living Nutrition Magazine*, Director of *Colitis & Crohn's Health Recovery Services*, Co-founder of *Healthful Living International*.

"There will never be enough people like Paul Nison on this planet! The world needs the message from the *Raw Life*. I fully support your work and your ideas."

—**Frederic Patenaude,** Publisher of *Just Eat An Apple Magazine* and author of *Sunfood Cuisine*.

"Time's a-wasting! If you're tired of feeling tired, sick of being sick, and resist being prescribed drugs to merely treat symptoms with no attempt to get at the cause, you are ready to do what's prescribed in this book! I'm convinced that if people just knew the powerful effects in store for them with this dietary change, they'd get mad that nobody told them sooner!"

—**Ruth Heidrich**, Ph.D., Ironman Triathlete.

"*Raw Knowledge* by Paul Nison suggests a way that can make a meaningful contribution to overcoming disease, upgrading health and enjoying life more. This book testifies to the indisputable benefits of a raw diet. It is fascinating and is written with an inner conviction which will touch you. It is for everyone who wants to live a healthy and happy life."

—Professor **Célène Bernstein**, Author of *Health Seekers*.

"Paul Nison is an outstanding vibration of the emerging generation of raw and living foodists. As one who has been on the raw and living foods scene for several decades, I am personally gratified to see this young man arise from a raw and living foods student to take a strong leadership role in the growing raw and living foods move-

ment. This book is definitely key for those who are striving to gain a greater conceptual understanding of a holistic living way of life through the divine consumption of raw and living foods."
—**High Priest Kwatamani**, Author and life empowerment speaker, *www.livefoodsunchild.com*

"As Henry David Thoreau (American poet) once said, "Being is the great explainer." Paul takes these words to heart by presenting an inspiring, rare peek into the lives of fellow raw foodists. Through his signature uplifting, non-threatening manner, the reader can easily glean valuable 'Raw-Food Lifestyle' information and/or choose points which bear further personal investigation! *Rawsome!* Although Paul teaches from the heart of his own personal experience, he humbly embraces the knowledge of other raw foodists as well. His 'livi' cation and humor is beautifully reflected within, warmly inviting all to understand the beneficial truths behind raw food consumption and the many paths which lead to experiencing them."
—**Karen Fierro**, BFA, LMT, CYI, *www.GardenOfHealth.com*

"No one but Paul Nison could have written this book. His unique slant on life touches a common chord within us all. We cannot help but agreeing with him, and loving him for showing us his insights. It takes a special someone to rise up from the crowd and create something unique. Paul Nison is just such a someone. He is changing the world. With the creation of his first book, *The Raw Life*, he became a known entity in the raw world. Now, three years later, Paul Nison has shown that he is no flash in the pan, but is a leader that is here to stay. He has created another winner with his new book, *Raw Knowledge*. Like Paul himself, this book is unpretentious and worth spending time with. It is something that only Paul Nison could have created, and I am very glad he did. As you learn more of Paul's philosophy on life, you will find that succeeding on raw will become easier for you. Read the interviews with many of the world's most successful raw fooders and learn *Raw Knowledge*."
—**Dr. Douglas N. Graham**, Author of *The High Energy Diet Recipe Guide*, *Nutrition and Athletic Performance*, *Grain Damage*, *Hygienic Fasting* and *Perpetual Health*.

RAW
KNOWLEDGE

Enhance the Powers of Your Mind, Body and Soul

Paul Nison

343 Publishing Company
Brooklyn, New York

This book has been printed on recycled paper.

Art direction and design: Enrique Candioti
Cover illustration: Sunstar
All other illustrations: Tom Cushwa
Editor: Joel Brody

Library of Congress Catalog Card Number: 2001118701

ISBN # 0-9675286-1-5

343 Publishing Company
PO Box 443
Brooklyn NY 11209

Paul Nison is also the author of:

The Raw Life: Becoming Natural in an Unnatural World
Live the Raw Life Now (video)
Raw Life: Achieving Your Goals (compact disk)
The Raw Life (audio tape series)

Dedication

This book is dedicated to all the people who have found their passion in life and continue to live it every day.

Acknowledgements

I'd like to thank everyone who has helped me with this book and my raw life journey. I've made many good friends. We may not speak everyday, but you are in my mind all the time. There are too many friends to mention here, but a few of you who stand out at the time of this writing are:

First, I'd like to thank everyone who has helped me put this book together. We worked hard, and all our hard work has been rewarded, because now it's done. Thank you all so much for helping me get my message out and helping others. You are all so special to me:

Dave Norman, Fred Bisci, Tom Cushwa, Enrique Candioti, Joel Brody and an extra special thanks to Amy Yockel. Amy continues to help me realize that there are no problems in this world, only opportunities for growth. Amy is a modern day Peace Pilgrim.

Thanks to everyone I interviewed: Annette Larkins, Celene Bernstein, Rozalind Gruben, Essie Haniball, The High Priest Kofi Kwatamani and Kwatamani family community, Viktoras Kulvinskas, Youkta, Gabriel Cousens, William Esser, Renée Loux Underkoffler, Ruth Heidrich, Annie Jubb, Kathrine Clark, Karen Fierro, Rhio & Leih, Dave Klein, Arne Wingvist, John Fielder, Robert Sniadach, Arthur Andrews, and Vivian Virginia Vetrano.

Thanks to all who contributed articles: Tiffany Cole, Marion Webster, Andy and Channing Migner, Karen Ranzi, Michelle Barber, Storm & Jinjee, all the wonderful people at Health Research books.

I'd also like to thank some people very special to me, my raw family who has supported me and taught me great lessons about health, trust, life, happiness, love, freedom and success. Some of you have welcomed me into your homes when you didn't even know me, because I needed a place to stay. I will never forget your hospitality. Thank you, thank you, thank you. Once again there are far too many people to mention here, but these few stand out in my mind at the time of this writing:

Adrienne Taylor, Alissa Cohen, Anthony Paolillo, Arnold Kaufman, Benito De Donno, Charlie Mort, Cynthia Beavers, Dagger & Highvibe, Dave Norman, David Wolfe, Deborah Cox Wood, Dee Williams, Denley & Jan Fowlke, Denise Travailleur, Don at The Living Light House, Donna Perrone, Doug Graham, Frédéric Patenaude, Gil Jacobs, Gordon Kennedy, Heather Johnson, Jackie and Gindion Graft, Janice Herradora, Jason Arabach, Jo Ann Barger, Joel Brody, Joel Parker, Karen Knowler, Kyle and Jackie Zimmerman, John Bovenia, Kris Pleskey, Leigh Crizoe, Lisa Melian, Liz Johnson, Maggie Thompson, Matthew Foor, Matt Monarch, Matt Grace, Michelle Rogalin, Mike Taylor, Mike McCartney, Morris Krok, Nancy and Greg Hone, Robert Reid, Roe Gallo, Sandi Bilous, Sharon Bergida, Stacie Cohen, Stan Glaser, Shazzie, Bob and the Staff at The Raw Truth Café, Thor Blazer, Tim Trader, Todd Ewen, Tom Coviello, Robert Selby, Robin Bennett, Victoria and Igor Boutenko… The list goes on and on and on. If I didn't mention your name here, you know who you are. Thank you all.

Last but not least, I want to give special thanks to my close friends and support on my whole path towards a better life, a raw life. I could never thank you enough for your help and support in life. You are the most special, dearest people to me:

Ana Vicenti, Amy Yockel, Anthony Paolillo, Enrique Candioti, Fred Bisci, Gary Van Merit, Gina Ando, Jackie Zimmerman, Justine Allocca.

And my thanks go to everyone who has bought this book. You've given me support in continuing to help spread the message of life empowerment. You give what you get, so keep giving support and you will keep receiving support in return.

Contents

A Word from the Author

My name is Paul Nison, and I'm dedicated to getting the message out to people about how they can enhance their whole lives: mind, body and soul.

I give information to empower them in learning how to gain control of their health and how to create the possibility of achieving their goals. I want to help you learn how to help yourselves with business, health, or whatever your goals might be. The information I present will guide you toward making your dreams become reality.

I believe no one in this world is better than the next person. We are all highly talented in what we do the most. What I do the most is to make my dreams a reality, and the information I present here and in my talks is designed for all people at every level to specialize in making their dreams come true. Nothing is impossible in this world; if you dream it, you can do it! You can, no matter who you are. If someone else did it, so can you. You can become healthy, wealthy, happy and successful. There are many people who have succeeded in achieving your aims, an important sign that it's all possible.

I feel blessed to be doing what I do. I travel all the time: state after state, country after country. Sometimes I feel as if I'm walking into a building in one state, and walking out in another. Although it's fun, sometimes I wish I were at home relaxing. Being on the road all the time can be very trying. But when I give a lecture, and so many people tell me how much they were touched by my words and how much I've changed their lives, that's when I realize I've been blessed to be doing what I do. Some tell me I have a special gift. I don't believe I have a special gift or power, rather a special energy we all have. However, many of us have not yet learned to use this energy. I've learned how to work with this energy and touch people, to help them. I speak to many, and if I help one person, it's all worthwhile. This is my path and I will continue helping people, because when I help others, I help myself.

When you give, you get. In other words, when you give to the universe, you receive from the universe. The gifts I continually receive are the smiles on people's faces when they tell me how much I've helped them. I will continue to spread my knowledge and continue to receive and respond to messages. I will continue to show how to tap into this energy; and I will receive my rewards from Nature.

I'm so excited to present this information to you, and I thank you for your support in buying my book. I do what I do to get the message out, and to live in the comfort that I can afford the few things I need to pay for in life, without having to rely on anyone else. It is true that the best things in life are free. Most of the money I make from my activities goes right back into getting the word out about personal development and self-improvement to whomever cares to listen and learn. In supporting me you are also supporting this movement, so pat yourselves on the back. You've done your share. What you give, you get, and what you get, you give. Continue giving and you'll continue getting. Give support, and you'll receive support. Thanks again for your support.

When I first started on this path of personal development, I hadn't planned to do it. I was sort of forced into it. Had it not been for a deadly disease, who knows what other path I might have chosen? When others considered my disease a tragedy, I considered it my wake-up call. My story is in the back of this book in the 'About the Author' chapter. Had I not listened to my wake-up call, I would have been doomed. We are all on top of a fence, capable of falling either way. I know many people who have received their wake-up calls, but didn't recognize them. Even worse, I know many who have received their wake-up calls, but keep missing or ignoring the point. The information I present in this book will help you recognize the call, to get the point and take action. This information comes not only from me, but from many of my friends who have recognized their wake-up calls and have paved the way for me and everyone else. The information in their interviews will profoundly motivate you.

In my first book, I interviewed truth seekers who were very successful in achieving their goals in the areas of health and happiness. Many of them are long time raw food eaters for health. My readers loved hearing how they did it, and couldn't wait to read more great interviews. Many readers expressed how much knowledge they were able to get from my first book, but many others wanted more interviews. In preparing this book, I found and became friends with many more successful and happy truth seekers. I had so many interviews, I could not fit them all into one book. I've decided to put a few into this book and the rest into another book entitled: *Raw Knowledge, Part II: Interviews with Health Achievers.*

I'm so thankful for great waves of energy, happiness and love I feel for everyone and everything, and for having the opportunity to present this information to you. Thank you again for choosing this book. THANK YOU! THANK YOU! THANK YOU! Now I invite you on a quest into the *Castle of Knowledge.* Enjoy!

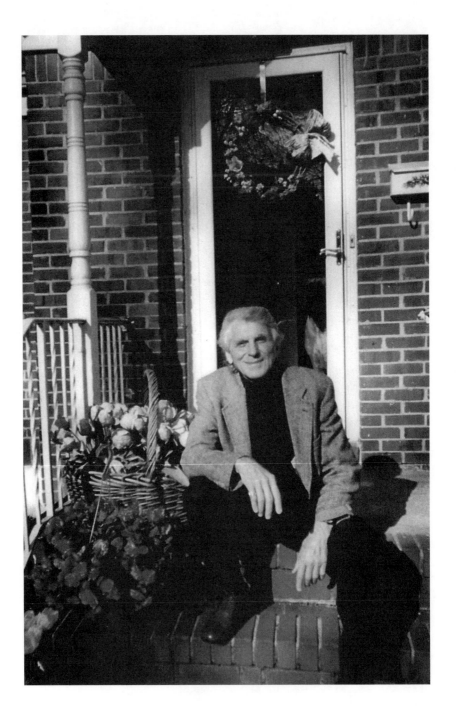

FOREWORD I
By Dr. Fred Bisci

I have been involved in the health field for close to forty years and have been a professional Nutritional Consultant for thirty years. If I were asked which is the area of greatest misunderstanding in the field of nutrition, I would immediately be forced to reply, "It is the failure to properly understand and interrupt the symptoms and changes which follow the beginning of a better nutritional program."

A good nutritional program is the introduction of foods of higher quality in place of lower quality ones. The closer food comes to the natural state in which it occurs, or the closer we come to its raw, unfired form, the higher its quality. In this condition, all the enzymes are found intact. The amino acids are in their finest form. The minerals, vitamins, trace elements, carbohydrates and "life force" are present. This life force, in turn, is capable of reproducing healthy tissue. The quality of a nutritional program is also improved by OMITTING toxic substances such as coffee, tea, chocolate, tobacco, salt, pepper, etc.

Most people do not mind making sacrifices if they feel they will be rewarded eventually for those sacrifices. People seeking health decide to sacrifice their old comfortable diet patterns and habits from a desire to be rewarded by good health. Imagine their surprise when they discover that after improving their diet, they sometimes feel much worse (for a temporary period). They feel betrayed and disappointed. "Why do I feel so terrible when I'm trying to do the right things?" is a common complaint. Most people do not understand that their recovery of health and the improvement of the diet cause unpleasant symptoms. And that good health does not happen immediately... but then again neither did poor health occur immediately. Poor health and illness are progressive, they don't occur overnight. Good health and wellbeing are also progressive; it may take weeks, months, or years. As long as you understand how your body works and allow it to perform its healthy restorative work at its own pace, the body will perform all the needed healing functions.

Your body wants to survive forever; it wants to be free from all pain and illness; it actively desires complete healing to take place within it at all times. Your body is your friend and partner in your effort to regain health. The body has the innate capacity, knowledge, and wisdom to heal itself at any time... if only it is allowed to do so.

The body possesses its own healing ability and the wisdom to desire this ability. The only thing we must do is to let the body conduct its work with as little interference as possible. We can furnish it with the highest quality food when it needs it or withhold food when not desired. We can exercise and rest the body, and give it fresh air and sunshine.

Other than that, all we can do is wait intelligently and not become alarmed by symptoms or try to suppress those symptoms. The human body has perfected itself over millions of years and through thousands of generations. It is the perfect healing system. The cellular intelligence that drives the body is infinite in its capacity. We need not have fears about its wisdom or ability to restore itself to the highest possible level of health and well-being.

It is very easy to be deceived today concerning health and well-being. The media is flooded with advertising campaigns which involve a host of health-robbing agents. This would include coffee, alcohol, cigarettes, and "junk foods." Our weapon against this misleading information is education so that we may learn the truth, so that we may know those things which destroy our health. Your health is your most valuable asset. In the world today, health is a commodity requiring a conscious effort to keep, but superior health is well within the grasp of every living being as long as the "Laws of Life" are obeyed.

Having personally experienced the quality of life that a raw food diet brings about, I can say that if this book is read and studied with an open mind, the effect it could have on one's life could be simply amazing. This belief is not simply a product of my own experience, but also of my having witnessed this change in many others. It is often so dramatic that those without knowledge and/or personal experience would say it was an exaggeration or even quackery.

Paul Nison is able to give us a second look at what and how we should be eating to achieve optimal health and well-being. He presents us with a new premise for our thinking as well as a "how" and "why" to make better choices to help us decide what we will and will not put in our bodies. The message is then confirmed by interviews with experts and others who have been following this dietary lifestyle for many years. This is a path I, myself, have chosen and have loved. I would encourage anyone to read this book to increase his or her own health and longevity and to one day be able to confirm how phenomenal this dietary lifestyle can be.

For many years, I believed we were on the verge of a new era and now that era is upon us. The raw food diet has come of age.

Many new books on nutrition are becoming available everyday. Most of them are redundant in their information but simply worded differently. This book is different. By presenting his book in parable form, Paul had my complete attention.

—Alfred Bisci, Ph.D.

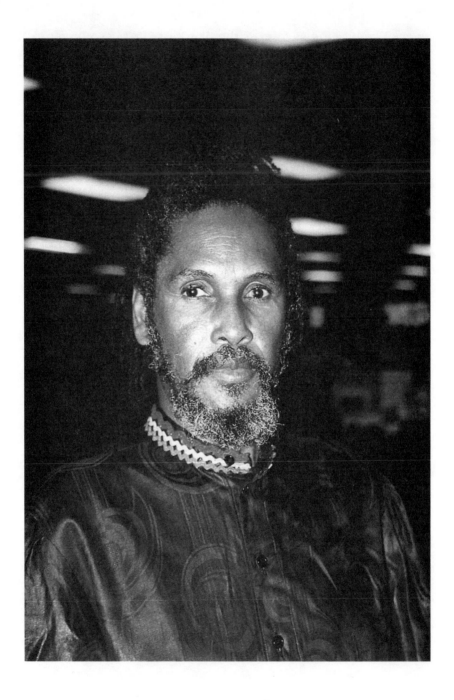

FOREWORD II
By the High Priest Kofi Kwatamani

This book, subtitled "Enhance the Powers of Your Mind, Body and Soul," is a guide to the path of the most supreme spirit of divinity. To follow this path, you must understand you are a sum total of all that you consume mentally, physically and spiritually. Any vibration or energy you call upon to carry you to a higher state of being, must be the energy of divinity if you expect to communicate with the most supreme spirit of divinity. Therefore, you must have divine fuel within your temple, or you will never get there.

If you do not consume the proper fuel, raw and living fruits, vegetables, seeds, nuts and grains, then you cannot expect to reach any level of divine consciousness. That is very difficult for people to understand because the death industry has perpetuated a fantasy, a false reality.

If you consume the energy of death and devitalization, your prayers are going out to the energies of death and devitalization. No matter how you call upon a holier than thou frame of reference, what you consume will determine who you are calling upon, because the fuel will take you into the energy of the force, spirit, mechanism, and thought waves of where you are going or where you end up.

The body is the ultimate physical machinery of the universe. It functions on the very same laws that have been created by the thoughts of minds. If you expect to reach a higher body of essence, mind, body and spirit, you must have a higher essence of the energy.

You must clean up the mind and the body; then, you can experience the amazing power of the supreme spirit. This book will help you free your mind, enhance your body, and release your soul from the misinformation, which has kept you trapped within a false reality. The information in this book gives you the keys to unlock your own potential and journey into a much higher level of consciousness.

—The High Priest Kofi Kwatamani

INTRODUCTION

There is proof that if one makes the transition correctly, today's age limit would be far exceeded. We would live beyond 70 or 80 years, and 100 years would not seem as amazing as it does today. It's very possible that if we follow all the laws of Nature, we can live 150 to 200 years at least. This is a very realistic goal as long as the laws of Nature are followed. However, it is not very realistic today because most people are so far from living by these laws. Given today's average lifestyle, there is no way man can live to these ages, but with a lifestyle change it is possible. I did not invent these ages; the proof exists. These ages have been reached and continue to be reached. There is much documentation of humans living to these great ages and beyond. If they can do it, we can too. Why haven't we up to now? Because the knowledge of how to do so was incomplete, even largely missing. I will explain how and give the knowledge to do so. That is why this book is entitled "Raw Knowledge." The rest is up to you.

Many believe that to reach these advanced ages, they just need to improve their diets and eat more raw foods. They think that is all they must change to reach great age and achieve excellent health. But there is more to it than just changing the diet to include more raw foods. A raw food diet plays a very important part in achieving that goal, but it is not the full answer. There are many variables to it all, many parts to the health puzzle. To reach optimal health, you must be at your optimum in all areas of your life. Spiritually, emotionally, and physically, you must be in harmony with yourself, your environment, and all the people with whom you interact in that environment. You must get a good balance of these things if you want to go far beyond what most people today call "good health."

When many of us think of health, all we talk about is diet. Certainly diet has much to do with good health, but as I've stated, diet alone is not the complete answer. Eating an all raw diet without considering the other aspects will not ensure good health. Of course, an all raw diet is the best way to go in terms of diet, but there is much more to it. There is a level of health much higher than simply eating a raw food diet. Eating healthfully is just part of the picture, not the total answer as so many people believe. Many eat a raw food diet, thinking they will suddenly obtain good health, while ignoring all the other important aspects. Many end up being sick. On the other hand, I know many people eating a cooked food diet, yet living a very happy life, who have outlived those on a raw food diet. These people understand that it's not what you put into your body that ensures good health. It's what you leave out that makes an impact. Leave out the booze, cigarettes, drugs, animal protein, and the processed foods, don't overeat and get enough water, rest and sunshine and you will do fine. The key is not to be 100% perfect, but to be 100% happy. The more raw organic food you have as your diet, the better you will do. However, as I stated, eating a raw food diet doesn't ensure good health. There are other important aspects. Even if eating an all raw diet, if you binge on fruits regularly and mis-combine foods and overeat, chances are you will run into trouble. Many long-term raw food eaters are getting cancer and other diseases and can't understand why. We need to do this intelligently, people!

I believe that Dr. Fred Bisci is the foremost expert on this topic; he is a living example of his own knowledge. It is through his teachings that I have learned much about health and how the human body truly works. I still have much to learn, but I can tell you that I have seen and experienced many of the answers, and I want to pass them along to everyone who cares to listen.

It's simple: just follow the laws of Nature! Don't put things in your body or your mind that don't belong there, and you won't experience disease or any other problems with your health. In my first book, I stuck to this simple and basic rule, and that is still what I recommend. The simpler we keep things, the better.

When I first learned about the raw food diet and health, I kept it very simple: I followed the laws of Nature. These laws declare to eat as you would in Nature. I did that and found it very easy to do. But as I met more and more long-term raw food eaters, I learned that it could sometimes be harmful. I am not questioning whether a natural diet of raw foods in their most natural state is best or not. There is no doubt in my mind that eating fresh, whole, ripe, organic fruits is best for our bodies. But here is the catch: they are the best foods for our bodies ONLY IF WE ARE LIVING IN NATURE!

Yes, fruit is the perfect food for man, but "today's man" is not ready for an all-fruit diet. Today's man is born toxic. It is not only what we do in our own lifetimes that matters. We must also take into consideration the lifestyle and habits we inherited from our ancestors. That is why today's man is born toxic, and why people are in nowhere near the condition they enjoyed many thousands of years ago when humans *were* capable of living on an all-fruit diet. The reason such a diet might be harmful to most of us today is that our bodies are not ready for it. If you eat a mostly-fruit diet (90-95% or 100% fruits), you might do very well for a couple of years, but eventually you will run into problems. I wrote this book to help you realize there are many variables to consider when learning about purification of the body and achieving optimum health.

If we were living in Nature, it would be best to eat a diet of mostly fruit. We wouldn't need to eat anything else, take any supplements, give ourselves enemas or take colonics. But we are not in Nature. We are very far from Nature. On our road

27

back to Nature, there are some "unnatural things" we can do to help put our bodies into the best state possible. I now feel it's okay to do some unnatural things while following this natural path. They can really help rid our bodies of the poisons we have put into them all these years.

I'm not perfect and I don't claim to know it all. I still don't even know how much I don't know. Yet, I'm always learning and applying new information that makes sense to me, and that is what I recommend you do also. No matter what you feel the best way to go is, in terms of diet right now, consider that one day those ideas might change. When you were a kid did you think candy was bad for you? Do you think candy is bad for you today? If you're a vegetarian now, when you used to eat meat, didn't you think it was good for you? Do you still think so today? The point is you keep learning, growing and your ideas change. No matter what you decide to do, it's important to have an understanding of what you're doing and to do it with a smile and to be happy. That is the only way to succeed. You don't want to be healthy for only one or two years; you want to be healthy for the rest of your life. So why not be happy at the same time? Enjoy what you're doing. Only do what makes sense to you, no matter who is telling you to do it. Follow the people who are in the shape you want to be in. Remember to enjoy and have fun with it. SMILE! ☺

In this, my second book, I'm holding to my same message while adding more information. Please don't get confused by this new information. Enjoy it and learn from it. If it doesn't make sense to you, don't try it. Only do what makes sense and take pleasure in it. I did not make up the information in this book. I've met many people all over the world who have been eating a raw food diet for many years. I like to focus on what they did to succeed, but I also looked at their setbacks and recognized some mistakes they might have made. This book contains information that can help you avoid these setbacks and pitfalls. Ranging from the thoughts we put into our minds to taking certain supplements, I discuss how and why these can help us avoid certain setbacks. I always say, "Why make things difficult for yourself if you don't have to? If you're sure two roads will get to the same place, why take the harder road?"

To all the purists out there, I am content in straying from Nature's laws sometimes. One of the most important things I've learned is we have to be willing and open to try new things in order to move forward. If you stay opinionated and headstrong, you can run into many problems. The more objective you are, the more answers will come to help you solve the health puzzle. I am not trying to argue against Nature. I am not suggesting that you can't live on a raw, vegan diet without any supplements; I know you can in the right time and place. But most of us are not yet in that time or place, and there are some things we can do to help get closer to that place. This is not about ego or being perfect, nor is it about being 100% raw. It *is* about being 100% happy. If you're new to a raw food diet, your goal should not be to eat 100% raw foods today, instead focus today on eating better than yesterday and eating even better tomorrow, if that means eating some cooked foods, that is fine. Keep moving forward at your own pace and be honest with yourself, and when you're ready you'll know it, and then you will get there.

To those who have been eating an all-raw diet for many years, open up and consider what I have to say. I'm not claiming you have to add anything to your diet or lifestyle; all I'm saying is, why make things harder? Why not take the easier road? There are far more happy people on that road. I meet many unhappy raw food eaters and vegetarians. You *can* change and become happy while eating a healthy diet. Appreciate and enjoy reading this book.

As you're reading, remember this: don't focus on experiencing health, but focus on experiencing freedom, the freedom to make your own choices, freedom from all diseases of society. With this freedom, you will be as healthy as you can be and you will be happy. In this book, I give you the knowledge to acquire this freedom.

It's not easy to gain this freedom today, because we live in a one-choice society. We're trained and brainwashed to accept a single choice, unaware there are other choices. That is how most people think. They are not leaders; they are followers. If you want to become a leader or just get control of your life, stop listening to "common" sense and start listening to your own "body" sense. Learn about ALL of your choices. With only one choice, you can only have one outcome. With two choices you will only have confusion, but with many choices, you can have many outcomes.

Successful, happy, free people look at the choices they have in life and put themselves in a win-win situation. A win-win choice is whenever both or all of your choices have positive outcomes. People who are unsuccessful, unhappy and trapped, look at their choices as bad or worse. They feel happy and satisfied in picking the bad choice instead of the worse choice. Positive changes and outcomes can only come from positive decisions. Setting yourself up with choices of "good" or "better" is a win-win situation.

How you do anything is how you do everything. If you try something and fail, no matter how many times you attempt to succeed in the same manner, you will fail again, unless you change your approach. If you reevaluate what you're doing and try other means then you'll accomplish your goal. Unsuccessful people look at failure as an end. Successful people look at failure as a beginning to manifest new ideas.

With one idea you can only have one outcome. With many ideas you can have many outcomes, and you can discover which is best for you. To accomplish a goal you have to start somewhere. It's like building a house: the stronger the foundation, the longer the building will stand. If you have a poor foundation, the building will fall apart. The body works the same way. There is a level of unsurpassed health we can all reach but we need a good foundation. It all starts with mind, then the body, and then the soul.

If you want to be healthy, you must purify and thrive. One leads to the other. Simply put: the only way you can thrive in life is if your body is clean on the inside. If you want to keep your body young, you must purify your body. Make it unadulterated and spotless. The dictionary, under the word "pure" reads: "free from what vitiates, weakens, or pollutes". There it is! That is the answer right there. You must free your body from weakening and polluting substances if you want to live a healthy life.

Today the average life span of people in the United States is 77, when it has been proven that we have the potential to live to 177, disease-free. Purifying the body is the difference between surviving and thriving, between sickness and health, comfort and discomfort, and between life and death. This book teaches you the best ways to purify your body and more importantly, your mind. It all works together. Keep the body clean, the blood clean and flowing, and the body will stay young and healthy for a very long time.

Go at your own pace and don't try to copy anyone else. The reason for this is: no two people are in the same place at the same time. In my first book, *The Raw Life*, I reported many interviews with long-time raw food eaters. It was interesting to find that some of them gave completely different answers to the same exact questions. Who is correct when it comes to these differences? They all are. They all did what they had to do to be successful at that particular time in their lives. Since no two people are in the same exact situation, there can't be just one answer. They all agreed the best quality food for the human body is raw, whole, fresh, ripe and organic plants. They also all agreed that diet alone would not heal completely.

The type of food we put into our bodies is very essential, but just as essential is the amount of food we put into our bodies. It's just as harmful to over-consume the highest quality foods as it is to eat very little of the worst foods. Why is this? Because the more food we put into our bodies that it cannot use, the harder it has to work to get rid of it. I am not saying a diet of little amounts of bad food is the best diet. It is not! I am suggesting it is best for people to eat small amounts of the best quality foods. That is the best diet. Eat relatively small amounts of raw organic foods in conjunction with the other important health factors discussed in this book and you will thrive.

The body is an amazing machine as long as you let it do its job. Assist it, but never interfere with its work. Nature made no mistakes when our bodies were designed. We have to understand everything happens for a reason. When something seems like a negative symptom, perhaps it's really a positive symptom of cleansing. Unfortunately, in today's world, instead of following nature's course to allow the body to heal on its own, we go against it, interfering with the process because we fear symptoms. That is where the problem starts. Once we understand how the body works and recognize what is actually taking place, we can cease to be afraid of symptoms.

"As time goes by and we put more stress on the body by putting things in it that don't belong there, the most import element of health, breathing, becomes more and more shallow. When this happens a lessened supply of oxygen is given to the lungs, and the result is that a gradually increasing supply of carbon dioxide gas finds its way into the circulation, deadening and poisoning the nerve cells throughout the body. This process is like an anesthetic. The body is over time like rocking itself to sleep. The final result is death without knowledge of the fact that we are really killing ourselves."
—From *Death Deferred* by Hereward Carrington

Don't focus on food. Continue to work toward the goal of doing better everyday. As long as you are moving in the right direction, you will get there. It might take you longer than other people, but as long as you're going at your own pace and not someone else's, you will be safe and you will succeed at your goal. Just keep moving forward and you will do better than you did the day before. As long as you continue to go at your own body's pace you can never run into danger. If you go too fast you can run into big danger. That should tell you the answer right there.

Dr. Bisci once told me something about the human body I will never forget, and it holds true for the mind as well: "The body either moves forward or backwards; it never stands still. If you stop, you are moving backwards." So the key is to keep moving forward, but move forward at your own pace. If you go too fast that is when you can run into problems. The human body has an amazing ability to adapt. When we are in a toxic environment, we can be very toxic and still seem to be fine. The body adapts, but when we are toxic we are slowly killing ourselves without even knowing it. This is why we must keep moving forward. The longer you move forward, the cleaner you get. However, as the body gets cleaner, if you don't continue moving forward, you can run into problems. As your body becomes cleaner and less acidic, it is adapting to a different environment, a less toxic one. Once you have rid yourself of toxins and begin to move backwards after having moved forward for so many years, it can become dangerous. This is why I stress again, move at your own pace. Also remember, if you're going to change your body from dirty to clean, it would be a very wise idea to change your environment from dirty to clean as well.

It is my wish that you accept and learn my message about how harmful it is to feed the body what doesn't belong in it, and how that will cause a negative reaction in the body. It is also vital to understand that what you feed the mind is just as important. It is even more important, because it all starts with the mind. That's why I subtitled this book, *Enhance the Powers of Your Mind, Body and Soul.* I didn't choose that order because I dreamed about it. That is the order in which the body works. If you want to have a clean body you must first clean the mind. What you feed the mind is so important. The body survives more on mind food than on body food. There's a saying I once read: "Life without learning is death." That is so true. Feed the mind with positive messages and create a complete and correct belief system and there is no limit to what you can accomplish in life. However, feeding the mind with anything less would be deadly. The body is whole: mind, body and soul. I wish people would understand this more thoroughly. If they did, they couldn't be brainwashed so easily. This world wouldn't consist of followers and dreamers, it would be filled to the max with leaders and doers.

Believe that you're not a body with a mind, but a mind with a body.

The most common negative food with which people feed their minds is so harmful to the human race. In my opinion, it is responsible for leading to as much disease as devitalized food, drugs or any other poison. I feel it is much worse, because most people don't realize what it is doing to them. This negative food for the mind is television programming. My wish is that after reading this book, you will realize it.

Watching television is one of the most harmful things in the world today. Once considered a luxury, so many people now consider it a necessity. In reality it is a poison box that relays deadly messages to people every single day in their own homes. Through television we are programmed by the media to do what they ask us to do. That is why they call it programming. Anyone who is watching television is addicted to it. Just as disease, you either have it, or you don't. You either watch television, or you don't. There are many educational shows on television that are good for the mind, but even with these shows we are controlled to watch them at certain times, instead of when we want to sit down and watch them. Another problem with these programs are the commercial breaks which are usually filled with some form of negative message.

The only answer is to either never watch television, or watch it on your own terms by VCR or DVD player. That is the only way you can be sure to watch what you want to watch, and when you want to watch it. That puts you in control of yourself. When you are programmed, someone else is in control over you.

In this book, I write much about the human mind and how we base our decisions on our belief systems. One of the most popular places our belief system comes from is television. It is my belief that people in society would be less brainwashed if they stopped watching television programming. This would lead people to think for themselves and listen to their body sense instead of what is sense to the common society, called "common sense." If you listen to common sense you will suffer from the same common unhappiness, sickness and disease of the common society. If you want to be a leader and not a follower, listen to your own body sense. It is there you will find the answers that will lead you to the free happy world, Nature's paradise: The Raw Life!

If you ask me, as many have, where I can start on the road to health, I'd tell you to start by not watching television. Start living life instead!

Move forward now to enhance the power of your mind, body and soul.

1 | THE JOURNEY BEGINS

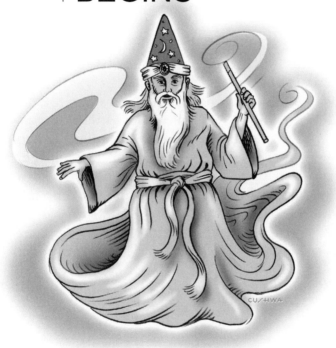

You wake up in a gigantic room filled with many strangers. You don't know how you arrived there or where you are. It's not a nice-looking room. You're cold and scared, as in a bad dream. You just want to be back in your warm, comfortable house. Suddenly, in front of the room, a very large person appears out of thin air looking like a floating wizard.

"Please be seated," the personage tells everyone. He goes on to explain, "This is not a dream; it is your life and you are in a castle: the Castle of Knowledge. This is a very old castle, haunted with many ghosts and goblins. There are many dark rooms and hallways filled with many old, yet still active, booby traps. For anyone walking through this castle, one false step can mean the difference between life and death."

You, as well as everyone else in the room, are very scared. The wizard asks, "Would anyone like to leave the castle now and be back home?"

Everyone immediately replies in unison, "Yes!"

"But this is the Castle of Knowledge. Don't you all want to spend some time here and learn?"

Everyone is frightened, and would rather be home. You, too, are scared by the unfamiliar surroundings. But just before saying you'd rather be home, you look around and notice that all the people there have something in common: they all look sick and unhappy. You realize that if you make the same choices they do, you might be sick and unhappy too; so it's a

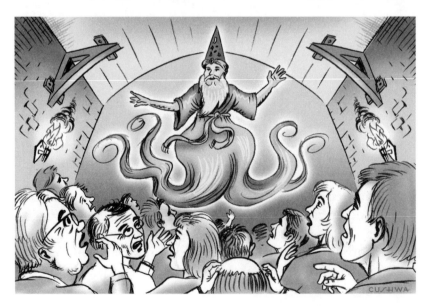

better idea not to make the same choices they do. They're all saying they want to leave, so you decide to stay. Before you can say another word, everyone around you is gone. Now, it's just you all alone.

You're not scared, just curious. You try to leave the room, but the door is locked and there are no windows. There is no heat in the room, and you're beginning to feel a deep chill. Then the light goes out and you start to get a little worried. The mystical wizard again appears out of thin air to hand you a key. You ask, "What's this?"

"This is the key to leave this room; you've earned it."

"How did I earn it?"

"You've earned it by being the only person in the whole bunch to stay, because you were open to seeking new information. You stepped out of your comfort zone to see what's out there. The key will open the lock on this door; this door is the first of many in this Castle of Knowledge."

Key #1

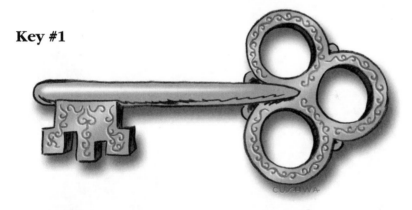

"Have an open mind!"

"Who are you?" you ask the strange, mystical man.

"I am the owner of this castle, and I share it with everyone who is willing to seek knowledge. Most people don't want the key you've just earned. They would rather be as far away from this castle as possible."

"Why don't they want to stay here and learn?"

"There are many reasons. Some people are scared, some lazy, and some just don't know any better."

You meekly ask, "What's your name?"

"Call me 'SCM' for now."

You timidly inquire, "What does SCM stand for?"

"I will explain that later; now, it's not important. What is important now is that you use the key you've earned to leave this room and roam around the castle as if it were your own."

"How long can I stay?"

"That's up to you. You're welcome to stay as long as you like. I must go now. Have fun and enjoy a good journey."

After using the key to unlock the door, you put it in your pocket. Upon opening the door, you perceive a long hallway with many doors.

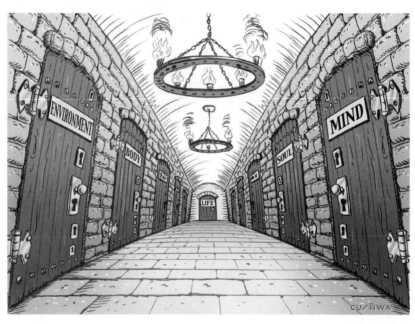

As you're walking down the great length of the hallway, all you can see are doors around you with words written on each one. Finally, you come up to a door with a sign that reads "LIFE." This is on the very last of many doors, all the way at the hallway's end. There are many locks on this door. You take out your key and try it in each one. The key works in one of the locks, but it doesn't work in the others. You can't get through that door, so you try to unlock some of the other doors along the hall. All of them have many locks and the key isn't capable of unlocking any of them. After spending hours and hours trying to get these doors open, you give up in despair. You implore, "SCM, I want to go home!"

SCM appears and asks, "What seems to be the problem?"

"I can't open any of the doors along the hallway and I'm getting bored just walking back and forth."

SCM offers, "If you go inside the rooms, maybe there will be something to keep you busy, so you won't be bored."

"I would love to, but I can't get in because all the doors are locked and I don't have the keys to open them. I can't get into the rooms to see what's inside."

SCM calmly replies, "That is correct. You must find the keys."

"Where should I look for them?"

SCM declares, "Just as you've earned the first key, you must earn all the others. All the keys are here, but you must not look for them on the *outside*, you must look for them *within*; within yourself, that is. That's where you will find these keys."

SCM then further reveals, "The castle is not as big as it appears. It is small and simple. But the Castle of Knowledge has an extraordinary effect. After you've looked into all its rooms, upon leaving you'll be a different person."

"How so?" you ask.

SCM replies, "You will understand the 'how' after having visited all the rooms. Just enjoy the Castle and open as many doors as possible." SCM vanishes. Now, you are left alone to find the keys and explore...

41

Environment

Even though you haven't gotten any new keys, you keep trying to open some more doors anyway, thinking one might just be unlocked. BINGO! After trying eleven doors, the twelfth, bearing a sign reading "ENVIRONMENT", opens.

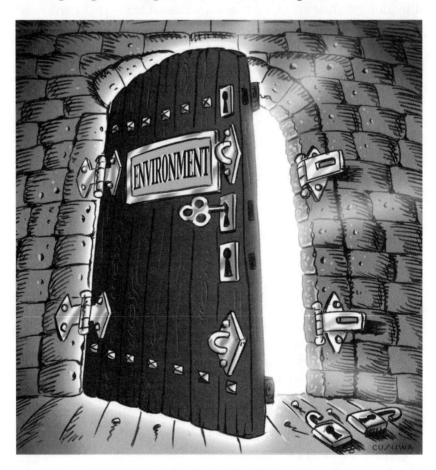

You go inside. On the floor, there is a key with a note. It reads, "Before going into any of the other rooms, in order to make your journey easier, you'd do well to put yourself into the best environment, the most helpful environment possible." That makes you start thinking. You begin to realize that SCM wants to create a positive environment for you. Right away, you say to yourself, "It's much easier to get through this castle with SCM guiding me, than it would be had I to do it alone."

You can't see SCM, but you can hear him say, "Why is that? Why do you think it's easier with me around?"

"Because you give me help and support."

You think, "How awful it would be, were he here without helping me. Even worse, how difficult it would be, had I wanted to stay in the castle, but he kept trying to talk me into leaving. That would create a negative environment, making it all the more of a challenge for me to succeed."

SCM concludes, "Thank you for enjoying my company. Because you've learned another lesson, you've earned another key. The lesson you've learned is that an unsupportive environment makes things harder. It's never a good idea to make something harder than it has to be. It's always best to be in a supportive environment. Life is so much better when surrounded with support."

Key #2

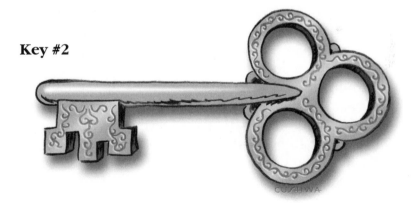

"Surround yourself with positive people and put yourself in positive environments."

"Does that mean I should surround myself with people who agree with me all the time?"

SCM reflects, "No, not necessarily; the people with whom you choose to surround yourself in life don't have to agree with you, but if they're open-minded they will support you. Negative people make everything so much harder, adding too much stress. If you weren't in a positive environment before taking this journey through the Castle of Knowledge, you'd do best to get into one. Either find the most positive environment or exchange your negative environment for a positive one. It all begins with your environment. Be happy that you've found an unlocked door. Knowing that some of the doors in the castle are unlocked helps create a positive environment. That is why this door was unlocked. It's a sign that my castle offers a positive environment. You needn't focus on the challenge of getting all the keys and opening all the locks. You'd be well advised to focus on welcoming and giving thanks for the little surprises, such as the unlocked doors. That is what will keep you happy. If you want to be successful in effecting serious changes in your life, it is helpful, and of fundamental importance, to put yourself in the best environment possible. In fact, if you try to make changes, without being in the best environment to do so, it can add extra stress to your life; so it might do more harm than good. Do you understand?" SCM asks.

"I do understand, and right now I understand that I'm in a good environment with you, SCM, as my friend helping me find the keys to open the doors."

"Good," says SCM. "Now, that you have earned this new key, you are ready to open some more doors. If you want to find all the keys, you have to stay focused on happy thoughts and keep moving forward."

2 | The MIND

Key Number One to the Mind:
Have an open mind and be open to
all information.

As you're walking down the hall, you come to a door that says 'LIFE'. You're looking at the door to 'LIFE' thinking to yourself, "How am I going to get in there?" Looking more closely at the sign, you observe a note. Because it's dark in the hall, you light a match to read: 'THE KEYS TO THIS ROOM CAN BE FOUND IN THE MIND ROOM.'

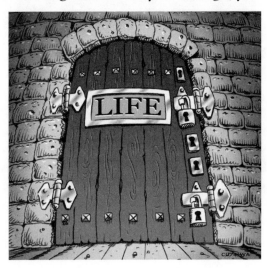

You get excited and run down the hall looking for a door that says 'The MIND.' At first you don't see it, but you keep running, and finally you do see it all the way at the end of the hall. When you get to the door, you see the word: 'MIND.'

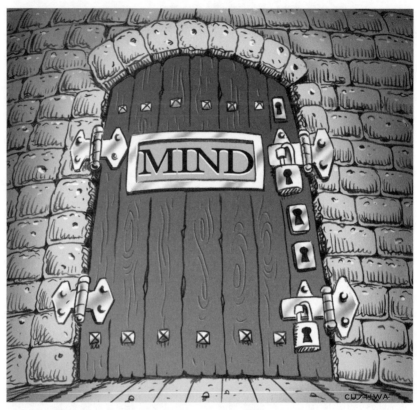

You realize that it has got to be the first door. You passed many other doors as you ran down the hall, but this one is all the way at the end. The door called 'LIFE' is all the way at the other end of the hall, and you conclude that if 'The MIND' is the first door, then 'LIFE' must be the last. Now you're looking at all the doors and realize that they're in a basic order, all starting with 'The MIND.'

SCM, popping up out of nowhere, says, "You've just figured out something very important and helpful. The key to each door is in the previous room; you've got to go from one room to the next. You've earned the key to the 'MIND' room by being open to new information and stepping out of your comfort zone to see what's out there. That is called having an 'open mind.' When you use the key to unlock the 'MIND' room, you have an 'open mind.' "But," as SCM explains, "The key you have now only works for the first big lock on the 'MIND' room door. There are other, smaller locks that must be opened before you can get into the mind. The first key is to have an open mind, and the next step is to use that open mind to find other keys."

Key Number One:
Have an open mind.

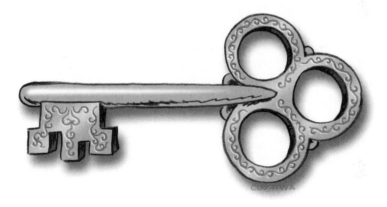

You are given a key and you unlock the big lock to the MIND room.

Key Number Two to the Mind:
Belief.

After the initial excitement of opening that first lock wears off, you're calmer. You can't seem to find any more keys. Starting to worry, you think the rest of the doors might never be opened. But then you look within, realizing that perhaps if you believe, anything is possible. SCM said you would find the keys within. You realize that you must believe before you can do so.

SCM, now popping up out of thin air, says, "Wonderful, you have found the next key. This is a very big key: your belief system. It all starts here. Do what makes sense to you. Listen to your body, not someone else. If you do what you believe, you will succeed. You must believe. That is where the power behind all ideas comes from. Listen to this great saying from my friend James Allen's classic book, *As a Man Thinketh*: *As the plant springs from, and could not be without, the seed, so every act of a man springs from the hidden seeds of thought, and could not have appeared without them."*

SCM nodding, tells you, "The thoughts you think are the result of the seeds you plant. If you've planted a healthy seed, your thoughts will be healthy. But, if the seed that has been planted in your mind contains false information, you will live with false beliefs. You must change those beliefs, if you want to be healthy."

You agree with SCM, "As long as people believe false information, they will never come up with the correct solution to the problem. We must have beliefs based on facts, not on popular choice."

SCM continues, "That's correct. When it comes to belief, it's all about having many choices. In today's society, we are brought up with only one choice, the most common choice. One choice leads to only one outcome. It is obvious that the choice that is most common today does not lead to the best outcome. In any and every aspect of life, the common choice leads to sickness, death, corruption, greed, jealousy and many other negative outcomes. You must break away from this one-choice society."

You tell SCM, "I know that the common choice is not always the correct choice; in fact, it's rarely the best choice. But how do you know when it is or isn't?"

SCM answers, "The best way to tell is, instead of listening to 'common sense,' you should best listen to your 'own sense'. If you listen to your own sense, you will have more choices to make in your belief system. One choice will lead to one outcome, two choices will lead to confusion, but many choices will lead to many possibilities. You can choose to live in this one-choice belief system or you can choose to break free. There is nothing greater in life and more important than FREEDOM. To experience freedom, you must live your own choices."

SCM continues, "In the old days there were many bright people who believed this. They went against popular society's opinion about many so-called facts. Their body sense told them something different. There was a time when most people thought the world was flat. If you said the world was round, they looked at you as if you were crazy. Since most people thought the world was flat, it was accepted as 'fact.' But that did not make it correct. The people who visited the castle knew the truth. They knew the world was round."

Today the same thing is going on. Most people believe what they are brought up to believe, because if most people believe it, then it must be 'true.' This creates our belief system. This is the premise of our opinions and thoughts. Great people question this system if it doesn't make sense to them. They are the people who are successful at what they do. Mark Twain knew this many years ago. As he put it, *Whenever you find that you are on the side of majority, it's time to pause and reflect*. He knew that just because you are of a differing opinion, it doesn't mean you're wrong. Truly, if you are open-minded enough to question popular beliefs, you might have knowledge others don't have.

Unfortunately, most people do not know this. They don't

think that way. This is the first thing you must overcome if you want to be healthy or successful at anything in life. SCM explains, "You must unlearn the misinformation you've been given, before you can learn the new information. Here is a revealing story about a student of karate. He and his master worked together for many years. One day the master told the student that he had nothing left to teach him; he had taught him everything he knew. If the student wanted to continue learning, he'd better move on to another master. The student, who thought he knew it all, agreed. When the student met his new master, the student said, 'I know it all'. The new master asked him if he wanted a drink and proceeded to take out a cup. He started pouring the drink into the cup and kept pouring until it started to overflow. The student said, 'What are you doing? The cup is overflowing.' The new master looked at the student and said, 'This cup is like your brain, and the drink is like information. You have a lot to learn, but you must first empty the cup of what you already know, if you want to learn anything new.' Most people are like that student. They think they know it all. Their brains have no room to learn anything new. In order to get the correct answers, which are not necessarily the most popular answers, you must first empty your mind of the information you have been conditioned to believe, and learn other viewpoints."

SCM adds, "It seems as if you already had this big key of belief; you just needed to bring it out. In today's world, people tend to accept what they hear on the nightly news or what they read in the daily newspaper, without ever questioning it. People are brainwashed about health; they are taught lies and myths. Finding out the truth is the first step to becoming healthy. No matter how hard you work, if you don't have an open mind and if you don't keep learning, you will not get the results you desire."

"You're right SCM, this key is big, but as you said, I already have it. I know it already, so can we move on?"

SCM shouts, "Don't be a fool."

"What do you mean?"

"The three most dangerous words in every human language are 'I know that.' A very wise man was once wonderfully quoted: 'If you ever meet anyone who tells you he knows everything, he knows nothing.' If you ever meet someone who thinks he knows it all, he, in fact, knows very little. You can't know what you don't know! That's the big problem with most medical schools. They think they know all there is they need to know about health. As the quote would reveal, they know very little about health. They know a lot about drugs (which they call 'medicine') and controlling disease (which is what medicine does), but that has nothing at all to do with health. True health is about preventing and purifying. If anyone tells you otherwise, they simply do not understand. The reason they don't understand is that they're not open to new information. They think they know it all. They have been conditioned."

You ask SCM, "Why don't they get it? What is the problem?"

"The problem is that they're basing their information on fiction and not the truth. Do you know the difference?"

"Yes", you say.

"To get the facts, people must first change the belief system they were conditioned with as they were growing up. They must be open to getting more information, not just settling for what other people say is true. When people stop listening to doctors and start listening to their body sense, they will be healthy and happy."

"SCM, what should I tell people when they ask me about their belief system?"

"You can tell them that when it comes to their belief system, they should listen to people, read books and access all available knowledge. They would do best to believe what truly makes sense to them, no matter where it comes from and regardless of how many people believe it. Don't just take someone's word as truth because he or she is a doctor or professional. Apply what makes sense to you. Don't worry yourself with what other people think. If something makes sense to you, then embrace it as being the truth. That is how you can recondition your belief system to make sure it's based on your own true feelings and thoughts and not just everyone else's. If you can do that, you can acquire a belief system that will allow you be successful at gaining health."

"Remember, as you go through this castle, to be open to all the information. That is the only way you'll get the keys you need. It all starts with building a solid belief system based on correct information. Too many people have strong belief systems that are based on incorrect information. You must have a true base. Believe in what works, not what fails."

"You didn't follow the crowd out of the castle. You listened to your own beliefs instead of listening to everyone else. You believed you could survive and you did, and now you are entitled to the next key. It's a big one. Keep up the great work!" SCM glows in praise of your accomplishment.

Key Number Two:
Have a correct belief system and listen to your beliefs, not anyone else's.

"They themselves are makers of themselves."
—*James Allen*

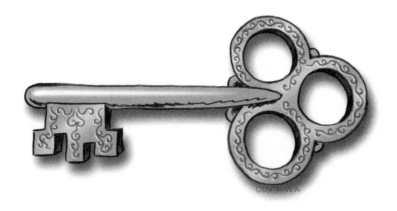

You are given a second key and unlock another, but smaller, lock to the MIND room.

Key Number Three to the MIND Door: Knowledge.

As you're walking down the hall, SCM asks, "How are you going to support your belief system? With what information?"

"I thought I already had the answer based on my old belief system, but I guess my belief system was incorrect. How can you help me get more truthful information to support a more effective belief system?"

SCM winks at you, saying, "Seek knowledge! You need knowledge to support your belief system. To have a valid belief system, you must let go of fear. The way to do that is to understand that knowledge and fear are opposites. You cannot have both at the same time. If you have any fear in life about anything at all, you just don't have the correct knowledge. Once you get the correct knowledge, all fear will just melt away."

Self knowledge is the beginning of wisdom and the end of fear.

People fear the unknown. Once something is known, your good sense might tell you not to do it, but that is no longer fear. You would be afraid to do anything to which you don't know the answer. When you know something, there will be no fear; once you know the answer, you might still think it's fear, but it's not; it can't be. Because once you know the answer, you can make a decision if you'll still go through with it, based on the outcome. You cannot make a sensible decision if you don't know the outcome. So the answer to all of this is to get knowledge about what you want to do.

The body is the servant of the mind. It obeys the operations of the mind, whether they are deliberately chosen or automatically expressed.
—James Allen

Fear can be a good thing. It is a great sign. It can let you know that you don't have the knowledge you need and can motivate you to get it. It can push you to strive. Is there a simple way to find out if what you know is fear or sense?

SCM confides, "Many people who come to this castle are frightened by myths about changing their diets. Where will I get my protein? Where will I get my calcium? What about weight loss? Those are common questions. But once they understand what is happening to their bodies and how the body works, once they get the knowledge, all the fear melts away. This is how you'll know if you have the best knowledge on which to base your belief system. If there is any fear in your belief, then you can be certain you don't have the knowledge you need. It doesn't necessarily mean the information you have is wrong. It could mean that, but in reality it means that it's incomplete.

Nothing in life is to be feared. It is only to be understood.
—Marie Curie

People fear illness because they don't understand what disease really is, or how the body works. In this castle, you will gain that information. If you let go of the old common belief system with which most people were brought up, and listen to your body sense instead of common sense, you will not fear things the common person fears. People are trapped because of fear, and that leads to disease.

It all starts with getting the correct information, and creating a belief system based on that correct information; then you can move forward from there. Remember, if you have any fear about anything, then you just don't have the correct information or the right amount. Having knowledge is the only way to eliminate fear. Many people are afraid to go against society because they don't have knowledge of the outcome. The reason so many people struggle to make the change to a healthy lifestyle is that they don't have the knowledge of why certain things are happening to their bodies. They fear detoxifying, fear losing too much weight, fear discomfort. Once a person gets the knowledge of what is really going on, all that fear disappears. The person then realizes it's a good thing, that the body is working to get rid of waste, and might feel worse before feeling better and might look worse before looking better. These things might happen, but once you have the knowledge of why they're happening, dealing with them will be easier.

You tell SCM, "There is a lock that this key you just gave me will open. If you're going to give me the keys to the other locks, then why don't you just give them all to me now, so I can get in?"

SCM replies, "You're right; I gave you that key. But don't expect that to happen too often. I just gave you that one because so many people take so much time to get it, and it's getting late. I wanted you to get into the room sooner."

"Am I going too slow, SCM?"

"No, you're doing fine, but I just wanted to help."

"Thank you, SCM."

You are never too young nor too old to learn. The more you increase your understanding, the more doors of association and opportunity will open up.
—Morris Krok

Key Number Three:
Let go of fear. Replace it with knowledge.

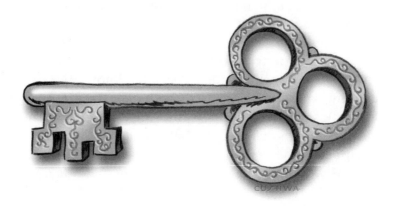

You've found the key and opened the lock.

Key Number Four: Exercise.

SCM says, "Here is one more little key I will give to help you. It is about doing? You can try or you can do. You must do. Create action with what you know. Having the correct knowledge is very important, but it's not enough. The knowledge you have gained must be exercised. No matter how much knowledge you have, if you don't use it, and if you don't exercise it, it doesn't mean a thing. If you have knowledge and don't use it, depression sets in. You must constantly exercise everything you have learned. Some call it exercise, others call it practice. The bottom line is, use it, or it will go to waste. If the good knowledge you have goes to waste, in time, you too will go to waste. Make sure you exercise everything you've learned."

If you want to make this easier, replace the word exercise with another word that means the same thing, but causes less stress. 'Movement' is a good replacement. That's exactly what exercise is. It is movement. You must move every day, your body as well as your mind. Take action! Make action!

Key Number Four:
Exercise or practice your knowledge and put your belief system into action. Use it or lose it.

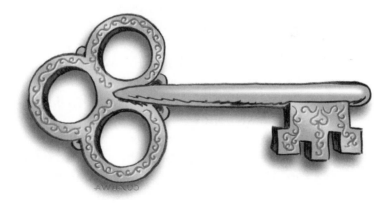

You've found the key and opened the lock.

Key Number Five: CONTROL.

"How do you feel?" SCM asks.

"I feel okay, but I wonder how many people got into this MIND room before me."

"Why do you care about them?"

"Because if I knew how they did it, maybe it would help me. Also, I'm worried whether or not they were successful. What if they weren't able to unlock these doors? What if these doors won't open? What if I can't find all the keys?"

SCM reassures, "Remember about knowledge and fear? If you don't have the answers to the unknown, fear will be there. Just get the knowledge and…"

"And what?"

"Well, that's the next key. It's about control."

"What about control?"

"Well, I don't want to give you the answer, but you must know what you can control and what you can't. You can only determine the outcome of ideas or plans over which you have control. To find the answers to getting this key, stop trying to do things you can't do. Focus on whatever is within your control. You must learn to distinguish between what you can and can't control. To understand this, you must not look outside yourself at what others do, but you must look within at what you can or can't do. Do you understand?"

"Yes. I must only use my energy for things and in situations over which I have control."

"Right. You have control over many things, events and ideas. What you choose to do in many situations is under your control; but too many people waste time and energy focusing on things over which they have no control, not today, not ever. They waste so much time focusing on these things, that they don't have any time to focus on what *is* under their control."

So now you think you have the key to open the lock. You

try it, but it's not opening.

SCM hints, "Ask yourself what is under your control."

You can't seem to come up with an answer.

SCM clues you in, "The things under your control are your own opinions, aspirations, desires, and whatever repels you. These are very important to you, and they should be. You always have a choice about them, because they reflect the inner you, and that's where your next key is. Don't focus on things that don't or shouldn't mean much to you, such as how others regard you. Those things are external and should not be your concern. If you try to control what you can't, you'll only hurt yourself. Focus all your attention and energy on whatever you can control, and then you'll find the right key to open this lock."

"Okay, SCM, I understand. From now on I will only focus on the things over which I have full control."

"Very well. You have just earned the next key."

Key Number Five: Control what you can, not what you cannot.

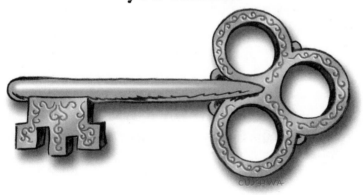

You've found the key and opened the lock.

"Wow, so far I've opened five locks on this door and still there are more. When will it end?"

SCM tells you, "The mind is an amazing thing. Most people use only 10% of their thinking power. There are many locks to the MIND room, but once you get inside, everything will be much easier to open. And once you're inside, you will acquire the key to the biggest lock on the next door.

Key Number Six:
YOU.

SCM informs you, "For the next key, you must mind your own business."

You ask, "What? What do you mean by that? Mind my own business?" Then you finally get it, "I must focus entirely on what is truly my own concern and not use any of my time and energy on anything or anyone else. What belongs to others is their business and none of mine."

You ask SCM, "Did I get it right?"

"That's correct. As long as you can do this, you'll be free and effective. Your energy won't be used on trying to find faults in others. With this lesson, you've just earned the next key."

Key Number Six:
Mind your own business,
not someone else's.

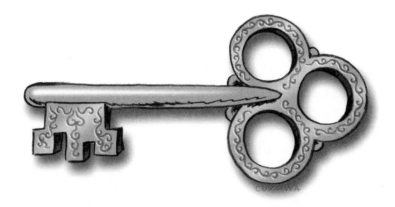

You've found the key and opened the lock.

Key Number Seven: Perception.

SCM says, "The door is almost open. The next key pertains to how you perceive things. Many people have different reactions when they experience the same situation. What makes them have different reactions to the same situation is how they perceive it. Two people can be in exactly the same situation and see it in a completely different way. You can choose to perceive things with a positive attitude, and that is your best choice."

"Of course, SCM, everyone knows that."

"That is not true. Many people look at failure as the end and give up. Others look at failure as the beginning, pushing them to keep going until they find the answers. This is the biggest difference between people who are successful at achieving their goals and those who are not."

You ask SCM, "What about how we perceive pain?"

SCM replies, "When it comes to getting hurt, you can't blame anyone but yourself, if it's mental and not physical. Anyone can hurt you physically, but you are the only one who can hurt yourself mentally with how you perceive what is being said to you. You also have total control over how you feel about things. If you ever feel hurt or upset, don't blame anyone but yourself. Better yet, don't let yourself feel hurt and don't get upset."

"Okay, SCM, I understand. How we perceive things will determine the outcome."

"That's correct. You have just earned another key."

Key Number Seven:
Events don't hurt us; it's how we view them that does. We cannot always choose our external circumstances, but we can always choose how we respond to them.

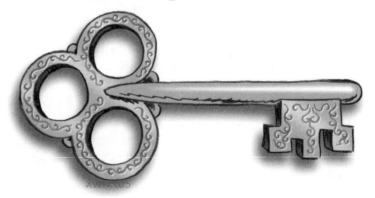

You've found the key and opened the lock.

All the locks are open now and it's time to open the door to the mind and see what's in the room. Are you ready?

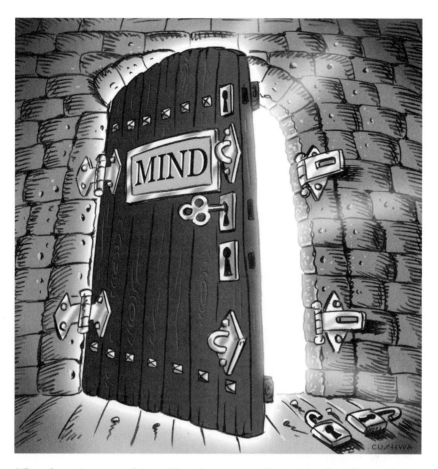

The door is squeaking. Slowly, you walk inside. Holding all the keys you have gained so far, you are now inside your mind. Right in front of you is the ANSWER to controlling your mind and being able to deal with everything, everyone and any situation. There it is, the thing that will make you a success in anything you decide to do. Once you understand what you are about to get in touch with, you will have successfully fulfilled the learning challenge provided by the first door in this castle. This is where it all starts.

Emotions

As you enter the room, you see a big book on the floor. A certain page is earmarked. You're not sure if you should read it or not. SCM asks, "What are you waiting for? Aren't you going to read it?"

"I would like to, but I remember you told me there are many traps in the castle."

SCM assures you, "This is not a trap. You've worked so hard to get into this room, so now you should read the book. That is how you will get the key to the next room."

Opening the book, you start reading: *No matter how much knowledge you acquire and how much you use it, how you deal with your emotions is what will determine how effective you will be. This is the MOST important key when it comes to the mind. Very few people even know what emotions really are. Finding out and getting in touch with them separates the healthy people from the unhealthy, the happy from the unhappy, and the satisfied from the unsatisfied. Once you learn how to get in touch with your emotions, you will become successful at everything you put your mind to. Understand that:*

Emotion = Energy in motion.
Learn to use your emotions to think, not to think with your emotions.

SCM, interrupting your reading urges, "If you want to be successful in life, you need to learn the reasons why you do things. Doing things that are well planned and make sense will keep you safe and in control. Doing things because of emotions is very dangerous and will take you out of control. That is one of the biggest problems today. People don't think; they just act on their emotions. Getting control over your emotions is getting control of your life."

When a man dwells on the pleasures of sense, attraction for them arises in him. From attraction arises desire, the lust of possession, and this leads to passion, to anger.

From passion comes confusion of mind, then loss of remembrance, then forgetting of duty. From this loss comes the ruin of reason, and the ruin of reason leads man to destruction.

But the soul that moves in the world of the senses and yet keeps the senses in harmony, free from attraction and aversion, finds rest in quietness.

In this quietness falls down the burden of all her sorrows, for when the heart has found quietness, wisdom has also found peace.
—The Bhagavad Gita

Continuing to read the book: *Being in control of your emotional state is a very important aspect of the growth of consciousness. The less developed you are in your consciousness, the more you tend to get caught up in unpleasant emotional states. As your awareness expands, your emotional life will become more integrated and channeled toward the experience of more positive effects. Conflicting and unhappy emotions such as anger, jealousy, fear, depression and guilt are left behind. Instead, the energy which gave rise to these states is experienced in a more refined and purified form as joy, peace, love and compassion.*

Emotions are simply urges people have. If they act on those emotions they are acting on their urges. Common urges many people have today deal with sex, food, sleep, and self-preservation. There are many urges and emotions we deal with everyday, but those four seem to be the most common. Emotions spring from desires, which are human creations. Animals do not have the same urges. Instead, ani-

*mals have control because they are not products of adver-
tisements, and they are not brought up brainwashed as
most children are today. They are given the freedom to make
choices based on their own sense. They are "taught" at a very
young age to be leaders. Children, on the other hand, are
"trained" to be followers. In humankind, the basic urges have
grown to an almost unlimited number of desires for specific
experiences. We spend a great deal of our time trying to satisfy the many desires that have grown out of these few basic
urges. It is in seeking to obtain and keep objects of our desire
that we become emotional in one way or another. Thus it is
said that desire is the mother of all emotions.*

*When we obtain the satisfaction of a desire through a par-
ticular object or situation, we experience pleasure. When
this becomes a habit, we become dependent on, or addicted
to that experience. Usually we use the word addiction to
refer to dependencies on particular intoxicants such as alcohol or narcotics. However, if we analyze our desires for
other objects, we will see that we relate to them with much
the same kind of dependency. We become intoxicated with
many experiences, people, and objects in the world. Our addictions are much more numerous than most realize. We are
all aware of the intense or even violent emotions that may
be experienced by an addict who cannot obtain what he
craves. This situation is merely an exaggerated version of
experiences that bring about unpleasant emotions in all of
us. Also, we are not only addicted to pleasant things. The desire to avoid unpleasant experiences can also lead to unpleasant emotions. The intensity of our emotions is related
to how massive our addiction is to a particular object. Who-
ever has not yet found the key to controlling his emotions
experiences negative and positive emotions, without control over either. Some of the most common negative emotions include anger, jealousy, fear, greed and depression.*

"Wow, I can't believe what I'm reading. It is so powerful. I'm grateful for this information."

SCM explains, "Emotion is stronger than thought power. When a violent emotion arises, it disturbs the entire thinking process. You must attain emotional maturity. Once you do, your thoughts can be guided properly. All control is emotional maturity. Emotion is a great power if properly handled, but very dangerous if not understood."

SCM adds, "You have all the information you need to handle and transform your emotions into a positive force right here in the MIND room. All the keys you have received so far will help you achieve the very realistic goal of all successful people today: to get control of their emotions. We all experience emotions; that is only natural. However, it's common, but not natural, to lose control of our emotions. Once you break out of the one-choice society of followers, you will have regained control of your emotions. Once in control of your emotions, you'll be able to change negative emotions to positive ones, such as love, peace and joy. If you do things to satisfy your positive emotions, you will experience positive results. Don't get me wrong. I'm not suggesting eating cake because you 'love it.' I am suggesting that avoiding emotions doesn't work. You must deal with and get control of your emotions, as long as you're living in today's society. If you can get control of your emotions, you can transform them from unpleasant to pleasant. This way you'll stop acting out of fear and start acting out of sense. Doing things to satisfy your unpleasant emotions will make you an unpleasant person. Doing things to satisfy your pleasant emotions will keep you a happy and loving person. You won't eat because you need love, instead you will become filled with love and give it to all around you."

"Is there a way to tell when I've earned this key of controlling my emotions?"

SCM illuminates, "There is one clear sign: forgiveness. Forgiveness is an essential virtue for developing love. When you get control over your emotions, step out of your comfort zone and start thinking about the purpose of life and its various aspects; then you will experience the value of forgiveness. Then, and only then, will you have this key."

SCM reflects, "Money is not the key to being rich. Many people with little or no money are among the richest in the world. Wealth comes not with money, but with love and forgiveness. Without love and forgiveness, one cannot attain divinity. It cannot be bought. Love means giving selflessly; forgiveness means going forward and not dwelling on the past."

SCM adds, "Earlier, I mentioned that the three most harmful words in any human language are 'I know that.' Well, the three most powerful words in any human language are: 'I forgive you.' You can't just say it; you have to mean it. Once you say it and mean it, your whole demeanor will change. Your attitude and personality will change dramatically. Instead of being tormented by the hate and vengeful feelings that are carried inside, in seeking justice, you'll experience a warm expansiveness. You would do best not only to forgive others, but also to forgive yourself for mistakes and errors that you've made in the past that have kept you so angry inside. Once you do that, the sense of rigidity and being shut off within yourself is replaced by a feeling of comfort. All of this is achieved by simply saying, 'It's no big thing. I don't have to get even. I'll just let go.'"

SCM further urges, "When practicing forgiveness and love, you'll find that others begin to treat you differently. Instead of reacting to your vengeful attitude with their own closed-off distrust, people begin to open up and share their warmth with you. As they become aware of your forgiving attitude, they realize they no longer have to fear your judgment and wrath. They can be themselves and be comfortable with you. Some people will appreciate this to such a degree that they will open themselves to you, and give whatever they can.

The more you use this key, the more you will be in control of your emotions and the happier you will be."

"That is some serious information."

"Never forget it," SCM admonishes. "It will help you in life more than anything else. That is why this room was first. It all starts here in the mind."

"Am I ready to go to the next room?"

"Yes, but before you leave, there are a few other keys in this room you might want to look into."

Other Keys in the MIND Room:

The Language Key.

As you turn to the next page in the book, it reads 'Words'. Looking at SCM you ask, "Should I read this?"

SCM nods affirmatively, "By all means; be my guest."

Words

Think before you speak. Sometimes, the greatest means of expression is silence. Before we even discuss sickness and poor health, let's take a look at language and how it affects our decisions in regard to health. People don't realize it, but words affect their decision-making process so much. Every day, people make decisions based on the words that are used in the problem, to come up with an answer. Depending on choice of words is the answer and the outcome of the situation. If negative words are used, you will have a negative outcome. Positive words will produce a positive outcome. How words are perceived in today's society is what makes a word negative or positive. There are also words that are negative or positive no matter how they are perceived. 'Can't,' 'No,' 'Never,' 'Impossi-

ble,' etc. are negative words and hold you back when you use them. 'Yes,' 'Okay,' 'Sure,' 'Can,' 'Will,' etc. are positive words that will push you forward if you use them.

"That is so true," you confide in SCM. "When I tell people about my diet, and how I eat and live, the first thing I hear many people say is, 'I can't do that.'"

SCM replies, "If they say that, then they won't be able to do it. Instead of saying, 'I can't do that,' they would serve themselves better by saying, 'How can I do it?' or even better, 'I can do it!'

When they say, 'How can I do it?' it opens their minds toward examining the possible ways to achieve their goal. When they say, 'I can't do that,' it closes their minds to any possibility of attaining their goals."

SCM counsels, "Say, 'I can and will do that!,' over and over again. Then you will achieve your goals. The way you speak about your goal and the way you perceive it will affect its outcome. Speak positively and that is what your outcome will be."

Language is not just important in terms of speaking positively and negatively; the very words you choose are also important. Take some common words that are used today and change them. It will produce a different decision and a different outcome. Many people don't realize how words mess with their minds. Once they realize the importance of what they say and how they say it, they can start moving forward and stop moving backwards.

The Word 'Disease'

Take the word 'disease' for example. Many people get so worried when they hear this word. They think about death and all the other things that doctors have them believe about it. Change the word 'disease' to 'discomfort,' because that's all it is. These two words mean the same thing. 'Disease' is just a word. 'Disease' is used by medical doctors and people in general every day in such a negative way. It is one of the most negative words in the English language, not because of what it means, but because of how the word is used. Disease itself is actually a good thing (which we will discuss later), but because of the way the word 'disease' is used, people think disease is a very bad thing. Most people think it's a death sentence. When people hear the word 'disease,' right away they think they're going to die. They think, 'I caught something and my life is over.' Not only is it a negative word, but also, it is almost always used in a serious tone. How can we change this to make it positive? Well, what is 'disease'? Let's look closer: dis-ease, meaning 'disease of the body,' 'uncomfortable,' or how about 'discomfort.' Now here is a word we don't hear used often but let's use it. How weird it would be to walk into a doctor's office and hear the doctor say, 'You have a discomfort.' This word is so much better to use than disease, even though it means exactly the same thing. A dis-ease of the body is a discomfort of the body.

Everything you say, you also hear. Speak negatively and you will have negative reactions that will produce negative results. Speak positively and you will have positive reactions that will produce positive results.

You can't see SCM, but you can hear his voice, "It's time to go to the next page in the book."   •

The Will Power Key

SCM says, "Everyone 'can' be here in the castle with you, but how many people 'will' be here? There are say-ers and there are do-ers." The book advises: *Everyone has will power, but many people do not use it. Your will is what will get you through the hard times. Your will equals your drive. Your drive is what will keep you moving forward. Consider your will power key to be a key that will help get you out of a jam when you have no other option. You will always have this*

71

key with you, just as everyone has will power inside. It won't mean a thing unless you put it to good use. With good use of your will power, nothing can stop you from accomplishing your goals.

Ready to Leave the MIND Room?

You have spent much time in the MIND room. You've seen much, but there is still much more to see. But you are too excited, and you want to move to the next room to see what is there.

SCM, popping up out of thin air, spouts wisdom, "Slow down! One of the biggest problems people have, even those who have gained these keys, is they want to rush everything. They have no patience. You should take your time and enjoy the room. The other rooms aren't going anywhere. But if you must go ahead, the room in your mind is very open and big. People make such little use of the room in their minds. It's okay to store things in your mind that you don't yet understand at this time. Pick up as much information as you can and store it in your mind. One day when you need it, it will come to you and you will understand it. Don't pass up anything."

Take everything that you see, hear, and touch in life as a lesson, a lesson of life. Put it in your mind for future use. One day you might need it, and it will be there. Everything happens for a reason. Don't use all your energy trying to understand the reason; just accept it and move forward.

3 | THE BODY

While you're walking along the hall toward the next room, you spot a door with a big sign on it: 'BODY.'

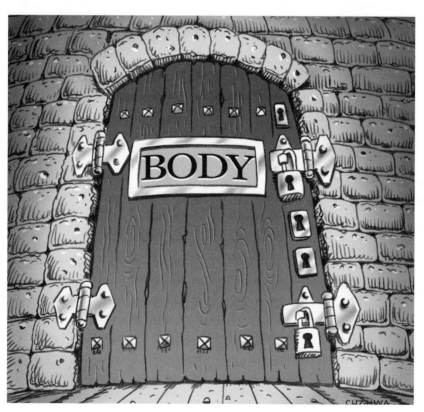

Thinking that the set of keys you got from the last room will open this door too, you try all the keys in all the locks; but none of them seems to work. The keys don't even fit. The locks on this door seem different from those on all the other doors. You call for SCM who appears 'poof' right in front of you. Thinking to yourself, "That is so cool how he can just show up out of thin air whenever he wants to."

You confide in him, "I would like to be able to do that someday."

He chuckles, "No problem; I can show you how later. But, do you have a question?"

"Yes, why can't any of the keys I have unlock the BODY room?"

"The body is a very complex system, but at the same time it's all very simple. At one time, the locks on this door would open easily, but time has taken its toll and they don't work as well as they used to. Some locks might not work even if you were to use the correct key."

"How am I supposed to get in to learn how to cure disease inside the body?"

"You do have much to learn. Before you can learn how to heal people from disease, you must first learn what causes it, and before learning that, you must learn what disease is."

"How can I learn if I can't get in?"

SCM instructs, "These pieces of information are the special keys you'll need to learn before you can open the old locks and get inside. I must go now, but before I do, here is some advice: Let nature take its course. Don't interfere, and you will experience good health. If you assist nature without interfering, then all the answers you need will come to you. If you interfere, as so many people do today, then and only then will you run into problems and experience disease. That is the real answer on how to avoid disease. But most people reading this already have one disease or another, so they must learn what it really is, and then try to get rid of it. Understand that you've created these problems for yourself, and only you can get rid of them. You will have to find many keys to unlock this door to find the cure to the problems you've created. Look and you'll find the information you'll need for healing. Once you have that information, you'll have many special keys to use to unlock the door to the BODY, also known as the door to health.

You'll also need to use the keys you've found in the MIND room; so don't ever get rid of them, if you want to achieve your goals."

Finally, you blurt out, "If you already know all the answers, SCM, why do I have to keep looking for them? Why can't you just tell me everything?"

"It wouldn't do any good if the answers were given to you. You have to figure them out for yourself before gaining understanding. These rooms contain the information that will help you figure it all out and understand all there is that you need to know to heal your body."

"Can you give me any helpful hints?"

"Okay." SCM agrees, and explains, "There are two main places to look in each room. One place keeps the information very simple, while the other goes deeply into scientific answers."

"Which is better, the scientific one or the simple one?"

SCM imparts a pearl of wisdom, "Why take the harder road if you don't have to? The simpler road is much easier and provides the same answer. If you want to make this easier for yourself, you'd do best to leave out all the confusing scientific information that most people don't understand anyway, and use the answer that is presented to you in the simplest form."

You are ready to get some keys to health, but before you start looking, you begin to have doubts. You think, "Maybe I'm not doing the best thing. If I had the keys to health, I would be different from most people. People might not listen to me because I'm not a doctor. I would be considered abnormal.

I wonder if I'm doing the right thing by being here, and if I'll be able to fit into society when I come out of the castle."

SCM offers choices, "Ultimately, you'll have to make a choice between the quality of your own health and your feelings of social acceptability. If you choose a path of natural health, which so many people today avoid, it's true you might become a social outcast. However, if you do choose this path of natural health, it will reward you with a long, happy, pain-free, comfortable life. Choosing the popular path, will give you a short, unhappy, painful life. Which way would you prefer to live? Which one would you choose? Why would you choose it? Which one are you actually living? Why are you living that way? No one is exempt from the consequences of his or her actions, no matter what is involved. Every decision a person makes, or fails to make, is a decision to move closer to life or closer to death. All decisions must be made in the context of a lifetime. You can give up now, or you can keep moving ahead, gaining knowledge."

SCM challenges you, "What will it be?"

"I'm going to do it! I'm going to find the keys I need to open this door and all the doors!"

In an instant, SCM is gone, and you are ready to move on. Looking down at your feet, you see a note that wasn't there before. You pick it up to read: "Good choice!"

Key Number One:
Know What to Look for (What is Disease?)

You are walking through the hall reflecting upon the things SCM has told you. You remember what he said about disease, "In the castle, were you to see a big sign on a door that reads: 'POISON - KEEP OUT' or 'IF YOU ENTER THIS ROOM, YOU WILL DIE,' you'd avoid that room at all costs. You would never even think of going into that room. But what if you saw the same door with no sign? There would be no warning, and you would have no reason to stay out of that room. Even worse, what if the sign on the door read, 'WELCOME'? Then you might really want to see what was in there, right? Well, that's the way life is when it comes to disease of the body. The door leading to disease is there, but until you recognize it or know which one it is, it's like a door without a sign. Once you know what disease is and how the body really works, you'll see big signs on the doors you won't want to enter.

What it comes down to is this: how can you get rid of disease or discomfort, if you don't know what it is? Before you can cure yourself of disease or avoid it, you must first understand what it is. Once you do, then you'll know what to avoid."

"Where do I get this information?"

SCM says, "You'll find the answer if you go back to the room you've already opened, the MIND room. There you will find the information about what disease is and how to identify it."

Upon going back to the MIND room, you spot a big book on the floor entitled: 'The Book of Knowledge.' It's really big. You'll have to read extensively to get the answers you're looking for. But now, you're only looking for the key to identifying disease or discomfort, so you turn to that chapter and read:

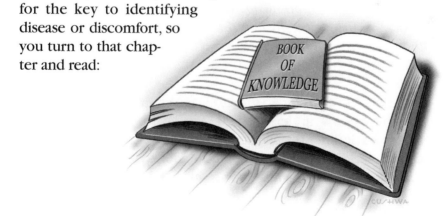

Discomfort is something that happens to the body when it is trying to tell you that you have done something wrong. It is a good thing. There are two kinds of physical discomfort. First, there is an immediate reaction if you do something hurtful to yourself on the outside. For example, if you drop a hammer on your foot, you will feel discomfort. If you did not have this feeling of discomfort after dropping a hammer on your foot, something would be wrong. Your body would not be working correctly. Your body would not give you a warning sign, so you would think that it is all right to drop a hammer on your foot. But it is not all right, and it is not a good thing not to feel pain or discomfort. It is harmful not to feel these warning signs that something is wrong. Luckily, if most people today drop a hammer on their foot, slam a car door on their hand, or do anything else that is hurtful to the exterior of their bodies, they will feel it. Their bodies are still able to react appropriately.

The other discomfort is a reaction to when people do something hurtful to themselves on the inside. Unfortunately, their bodies are not working well enough to feel this pain right away. The warning signs are not there, so there is no way for them to know that what they are doing is wrong. This is happening to so many people today. Their bodies are not able to feel the signs of discomfort. Without these warning signs, there is no way for people to know they are doing something harmful until it all builds up and they experience a huge discomfort that the body cannot overcome on its own power, the way nature intended.

You've now understood, according to the book, disease means something is hurting. It's your body telling you, 'You're causing me distress.' This is an important and very helpful signal.

"Wow!" you exclaim, "This book is filled with the knowledge I need. What it says about pain is so true."

You tell SCM, "It reminds me of a story I once read about a

boy who couldn't feel any physical pain. Something was wrong with his brain; the part of it that senses pain just didn't work. Because he was a little kid, I thought that sounded just fine. Everyone you knew hated pain and tried to avoid it, including me. I thought: 'Wow, that boy was lucky not ever to feel any pain.' But as I grew older, I realized that not feeling any pain was not as good as it once had seemed. Just because the boy couldn't feel any pain didn't mean he never got hurt. When the poor boy got hurt, he couldn't feel it because he was not able to feel any physical pain. If he were to drop a hammer on his foot there would be no pain. But he could have broken his foot and not even have known it. Had he bruised his foot without knowing it was damaged, he would have just kept walking on it as if nothing were wrong, making it worse and worse. If he could feel pain, he would have known right away that something was wrong, and he could have given special care to the area where he felt the pain or discomfort. Pain is actually a good thing."

SCM approving, "That's a fine story. There are many people today who are in the same situation as the boy in your story. They can't feel pain, and they don't know when they're being hurt. Keep reading."

Pain happens when you put things into your body that don't belong there. Most people today are so internally dirty, their bodies clogged with mucus and slime, that they've lost the ability to feel pain. Thus, they don't realize they're injured. Since they don't feel pain, they continue to injure themselves day after day. Putting things into your body that don't belong there should cause pain. Some people think they are unlucky when they have an allergic reaction to something, but actually it's a good thing. They are the people whose bodies can still feel pain and react. If you try to eat glass, you should want to feel pain. Pain is your body telling you that glass doesn't belong in it. Many people have allergic reactions to certain foods. That is good, because those foods don't belong in the human body. But there are many more people who eat these same foods and do not get a reaction. This means their bodies have become so over-filled with excess mucus and slime that they have lost their ability to react. Once they stop eating those foods and start to clean out their bodies, they will no longer be able to eat those foods without a reaction, without having some sort of pain. Then their bodies will become clean and they will be healthy. So, pain or discomfort or disease is a good thing, a very good thing. It is your body talking to you.

You think, "Yes, it's all so simple, but not as simplistic as it appears. The cleaner my body becomes, the more sensitive I'll become to things that are not good for me. When that happens, I'll experience discomfort. When people don't have knowledge of the human body and how it works, they take this discomfort for a sign that something is not working, but in fact, it is working, and working very well. Detoxification is part of the process."

"Do you understand what this means?" SCM asks.

"I think so, but it's starting to get dark and cold, and I hope I don't get sick."

"I guess you don't get it yet!" SCM exclaims. "You can't catch a disease from someone else, because disease is a problem with your own body. You can never 'catch' a discomfort that someone else is experiencing due to his or her detoxification or healing."

"Okay, sorry, I was just kidding. I do understand. It's just as if a friend were to hurt himself with a disease or an injury. It's the same thing. You might feel sorry for that person or it might bring your spirits down, but if your friend breaks his leg, you can't feel pain in your own leg, and you can't catch that pain unless you break your own leg."

By now, you have some idea why disease is good, but you

want to know more. You want to know how the body works and what the stages of disease are. You continue reading the book. As you turn the page, you see the answer right there in front of you. Before you read it, you realize that all the answers to life are easy to find, as long as you ask questions and don't settle for a common or popular answer that doesn't make any sense. Now you go on to read:.

The Stages and Signs of Disease

1. ENERVATION or NERVOUS EXHAUSTION: the condition of imbalance in the ratio of available body energy to necessary task performance energy. This happens when nerve energy is reduced to the point that you feel exhausted and very tired all the time or lazy and you feel like not doing anything. The energy that your eliminative organs need to operate efficiently is being slowly depleted. It is like a clogged pipe. Nerve energy can no longer get through to the rest of the body. When this happens, it creates a gradual physical and mental weakening. Result: It creates an overload of poisons in certain part of the body. If not corrected, it continues to worsen and further debilitate the body. It is caused by overeating, lack of water, and lack of sleep. Get rest!

2. TOXEMIA or TOXICOSIS: when the body does not have the energy to eliminate toxic substances, an excess amount of toxins accumulates in the blood, tissues, lymph system, interstitial fluids, and the cells of the body. This is caused by putting too much food and too many negative thoughts into the body. Result: the functioning of your tissues and organs is impaired. Clean up your diet and clear up your mind! Stop putting these things into your body. Take control!

3. IRRITATION: the result of the nervous system detecting an overabundance of toxic material. The area in the body where the toxins are stored the most is greatest where the cells and tissues become irritated. This may create an itch, sneeze, queasy feeling, jumpy, antsy, intense body urges, arousal, or general annoyance. You may feel queasy, nauseous, irritable, and "on edge." This is your body telling you that something is wrong with your lifestyle. Result: if the ingestion of toxic materials is not discontinued, the body will then introduce the next stage of disease. Cause: continuing to overindulge and ignoring your body's message. Cure: listen to your body! Be frugal in your diet and lifestyle.

4. INFLAMMATION: a local response to toxemia and injury on a cellular level. The body often amasses this saturation within the weakest tissue or organ, which then becomes inflamed with the intoxicants. Pain and noticeable discomfort are experienced. Because of the pain and discomfort at this stage, the sufferer usually contacts a physician. Drugs are often administered for relief which only add to the toxic build-up. Cause: not listening to the signs of your body and lack of knowledge. Result: pain and discomfort. Cure: listen to your body, and if you feel pain, rest. Rest is the only true cure. Rest your mind and body by relaxing, sleeping, fasting and meditating.

5. ULCERATION: characterized by a break in the skin or mucus membrane with a loss of surface tissue, often accompanied by an accumulation of pus. Canker sores, open sores, and stomach ulcers are common examples. This is often painful and aggravating since the nerves may be exposed. The body creates this condition in order to relieve itself of an over-abundance of toxic material. Excessive or extreme build-up of toxins necessitates extreme measures to cleanse. Medical doctors will perscribe potent drugs, which may lead to surgery. If the body is left to rest, the body at this point can heal itself, repairing the wound. Cause:

avoiding the signals of the body or suppressing them if they are too strong (painful). The outcome is a serious stage of disease. If cleansing measures are taken, the body will heal itself, but if none are taken, the body will continue to get worse and finally get to a stage where it will no longer be able to heal itself. Cure: LISTEN TO YOUR BODY! Get knowledge and understand how and why this is happening. Your body created it, and your body can heal it.

6. INDURATION or SCAR TISSUE FORMATION: long-term inflammation and ulceration continues unless over-saturation from toxins is stopped. If not ceased, a hardening and filling in of empty space will occur. Under these conditions, normal localized cellular regeneration ceases, and the tissues harden to a hardened fibrous sac. This is a defensive move by the body in order to isolate toxins from the rest of the body. These sacs are commonly referred to as tumors, cysts, polyps and warts. At this point physical pain and emotional distress intensify. This is the last intelligent thing the body will do before the last and final stage of disease. Cause: continuing to go against your body's own intelligence and suppressing your symptoms with drugs. Result: if not taken care of, the result will be an irreversible form of disease that not even your body can overcome no matter what natural methods you use. If you don't wake up now, your body will never be able to wake up again. Cure: WAKE UP! Clean your mind and your body.

7. FUNGATION or CANCER: mutation or proliferation of cells. The cells and tissues go awry and become disorganized due to disruption of their genetic encoding by poisonous substances. These mutated cells obtain their nourishment from lymph fluid but do not serve the body. As long as the nourishment is available, the cancer cells continue to thrive and divide. This stage is chronic and irreversible. The body degenerates past the point of no return. It is usually fatal, but no one can ever tell you when you have reached this stage. Caused by continued long-term saturation with poisons that compromise cellular integrity. The result: fatal disease that the body can no longer overcome. Cure: never stop trying to heal and eliminate, and give the body the rest it needs. There is no way to tell if the body is at this of point of no return or if it isn't. Wake up now or never! Don't ever give up no matter what anyone says. At this stage, some medical doctors might tell a patent that there is nothing that can be done and it is just a matter of time before death. That is the worst thing they can tell anyone, since there is no way for them to be sure if the patient is at that stage or not. There is absolutely no way for them to be sure. The present moment would be your only and last chance to help the body and stop going against it. Give it what it needs. REST! At this point you have nothing to lose if you try.

You put the book down and say, "WOW! That was a lot of information," but it makes perfect sense to you. So now you understand that DISEASE IS NOT THE PROBLEM, BUT THE CURE! It is not the problem, but the result of cleansing, also known as a detoxification. Listen to that word, 'detoxification.' It is the opposite of 'intoxication.' As opposed to putting toxins into the body, detoxification is the body releasing its stored toxins.

You look up, and SCM, right in front of you, suggests, "Imagine that you had to wash a dish with food stuck to it. If you took a course steel wool pad, such as Brillo, and scrubbed the dish very hard to get the dirt off, it wouldn't feel very good to the dish. Well, the same thing happens to the body. The scrubbing might hurt or cause a discomfort, but it gets the body clean. That is what you want, a clean body with no more dirt. That is why during healing, you sometimes feel worse before you feel better. Once you understand this, everything will heal much faster."

However, just because disease is the cure and a good thing, doesn't mean we have to live with pain, nor should we want it in our lives. Not having any pain or discomfort is best, and you should want to strive to have no pain. But you want to avoid pain by not having it at all, not by not feeling it when you do have it.

Key Number One to the Body: You must first learn what disease is, before you can cure or avoid it.

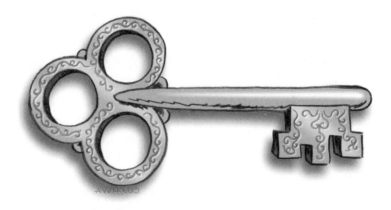

You've found the key and opened the lock.

Key Number Two:
The Causes of Disease

So now you understand what disease is, but you are wondering what is its cause, or the causes of discomfort in the body. SCM comes out of nowhere with the answer: "Disease can be a result of one thing that you are doing wrong or a combination of many things. There are many causes of disease. I could name many, but to keep it simple, let's focus on the major causes that many people overlook."

SCM explains: "The major cause of disease is stress to the body. Stress makes the body work harder than it should have to. When you have too much going on inside your body or mind and not enough energy to deal with it, stress is created. Therefore, stress is the cause of all disease. You will never see a healthy, happy person with stress in his or her life."

You ask, "What causes all this stress?"

SCM explains: "The major causes of stress leading to disease are:

PUTTING THINGS INTO YOUR BODY THAT DO NOT BE-LONG THERE.
They can be mental or physical: The body was made to thrive on certain material, just like a car is made to thrive on gasoline. If you put anything into the gas tank other than gas, you will cause harm to your car. The body works the same way. If you put anything into your body that it doesn't need, it will treat it as a foreign substance, causing the body great harm. Your body will do all it can to rid itself of these foreign substances. The process the body goes through causes it to use too much energy, overburdening it. This energy overburden is known as stress. All this stress is not healthy. It becomes very harmful. The human body is allergic to anything that doesn't belong in it, and the result is stress, disease, illness and pain. If you do not respond to it, death can result. The most common

86

things we don't need are, negative thoughts, cooked food (which just turns to ashes inside the body), poor combinations of food, polluted air, polluted water, etc. They all stress the human body, causing poor health.

CONSUMING TOO MUCH OF THE THINGS THAT DO BELONG IN THE BODY: OVEREATING AND OVERDRINKING. YES, YOU CAN HAVE TOO MUCH OF A GOOD THING: Too much of any food, good or bad, will create stress in your body, leading in poor health. One of the most common causes of disease is overeating. Even eating too much good food can cause many problems. Look at it this way," explains SCM, "If you have an empty room and you keep filling it up with stuff, once it runs out of space, there will no longer be room for any more stuff. If you keep trying to put more stuff into it, ignoring the fact that there just isn't any more room, eventually the stuff in the room will overflow and come out any way it can, through windows, doors, or any opening it can find. If the openings are blocked, the walls might even break and crumble. The body works the same way. The more you eat, the more room you take up in your body. The bad food you eat clogs the body's openings, and this excess waste has nowhere to go. That is when the body will start to crumble just like the walls of the room. No matter how good or bad the food you eat is, if you eat too much, it will be harmful to the body. It will cause your body to work harder than it can, leading to loss of energy. That will lead to many other health problems.

IMPROPER DIGESTION AND IMPROPER ELIMINATION: What you put into your body is not the only problem. What comes out is an even bigger issue. Or I should say, what does not come out is the bigger problem. If you put too much of something into your body and it stays there, chances are it will rot, ferment and putrefy. That is when the real problems happen.

87

NOT DRINKING ENOUGH WATER ALSO STRESSES THE BODY IN A MAJOR WAY:

Not drinking enough water can dehydrate your body. Many people think that the only way to become dehydrated is to do something like running a marathon on a hot day, but that is not the only way. You can become dehydrated just by sitting inside your house watching television or reading a book. Eating any food that does not have water in it will dehydrate you no matter where you are. When you eat food that has no liquid in it, as soon as you swallow it, that food will absorb water from your body, just as if you swallowed a dry sponge. You are either dehydrating or rehydrating your body. When you're not putting liquid into your body, you're allowing it to dehydrate. Your health is declining. Having a good amount of water is important. It cleans the body. It is nature's soap. When you don't use this soap, you become very dirty. If you're not drinking enough water, you're building up mucus and slime, letting it sit there to harden.

LIVING IN UNNATURAL ENVIRONMENTS CAUSES A LOT OF STRESS TO THE BODY:

Living where people were not meant to live is not in nature's plan, and is highly unnatural. An extremely cold or excessively hot climate can be harmful to your body, adding much stress. It is not natural for humans to live in extreme climates. It has been proven over and over again that living in these climates adds stress to people's lives.

LIVING IN A NEGATIVE ENVIRONMENT, SURROUNDED BY NEGATIVE PEOPLE:

You become like the people around you. If you associate with negative people, their negativity will influence you, and you might become negative as well. Being around negative people all the time will add much stress to your life.

NOT SMILING:

If you are a negative person, then you probably don't smile often. Smiling releases stress. There are many studies proving that being unhappy adds stress to your life. The best way to tell if you're healthy or not is the sign of smiling. No matter how well you eat, if you're not smiling, something is wrong.

NOT JUST WHAT YOU EAT, BUT WHERE YOU EAT:

If you're not comfortable where you're eating and continue to eat in uncomfortable environments, you'll have much stress in your life. Eating, surrounded by people you dislike, or eating in very noisy or dirty places will affect your digestion, adding to your stress level.

NOT JUST WHAT YOU EAT, BUT WHEN YOU EAT:

Eating when you are angry, anxious, upset, or while experiencing other moods will add stress. Eating late in the day or when it's dark outside is also very harmful. The human body slows down when it's dark outside. That is the time to sleep and rest. If you eat at this time, you're going against nature and your body will catch up with it, creating much discomfort.

NOT JUST WHAT YOU EAT, BUT HOW YOU EAT:

Not chewing your food can hinder digestion, introducing a huge amount of extra stress into your body, as will eating your food too fast. Drinking with your meals will also hinder digestion.

NOT GETTING ENOUGH SLEEP AND REST:

Most people do not get enough sleep. This is very harmful to the body, because healing takes place during rest and sleep. If you cut your sleep short, you cut healing short as well. Under-sleeping is the biggest cause of not being able to heal.

CLEANING OUT TOO FAST:

Do not try to speed the healing process. Go at your body's

own pace, not someone else's. You can clean out too fast, which will cause more stress than your body will be able to deal with.

POOR BREATHING:
Nothing will kill a person faster than not breathing. We can live for months without food and days without water, but only a few seconds without air. Most people do not breathe full breaths. When the breathing becomes more and more shallow, a lessened supply of oxygen is given to the lungs. That causes much stress to the body. The opposite of breathing is suffocation. Most people do not breathe to their fullest capacity. Oxygen is the most important element of life. Without it you cannot exist. With small amounts, you can only have so-so health.

POOR AIR QUALITY:
Breathing poor quality air causes more stress to people's bodies than they realize. Breathing poor air is living a slow death. Your health decreases with every breath you take."

The book on the MIND room floor reads:

Most people eat for the wrong reasons. They eat for taste or emotional and social factors. If you eat for the same reasons as most people, then you will get the same diseases most people get. If you are eating unhealthful food because you don't want to be different from others or you want to avoid difficulty in your relationships, you are eating according to reasons that have no relevance to the objective nutrient requirement of your biological nature. Neither listen to 'common' sense nor do what the common person is doing. People today are brought up in a one-choice society, conditioned to do this. Be different! Be healthy!

Key Number Two to the Body:
You've learned that disease is a good thing; a sign that should always be responded to.

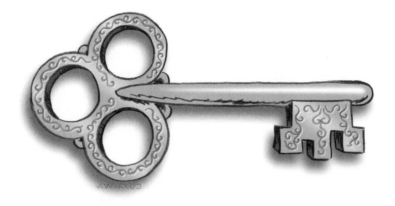

You've found the key and opened the lock.

Key Number Three:
The Results of the Causes of Disease

Now you have the information about disease and its cause. But you wonder, "What are the results of the causes? What will happen if I ignore my body sense and continue to indulge in practices that will lead to a diseased body? What will happen when I finally experience disease?"

SCM elucidates, "Once you start to experience disease, your body will get so filled and clogged with excess mucus and slime that it can no longer feel pain. But, just because your

91

body doesn't feel pain doesn't mean it's not there. Poisons will keep building up. Years and years of filling your body with excess mucus and slime will make it so dirty that you will not be able to feel the body's signals, i.e. pain. If your body can't hear the wake-up call, you won't get the message and be able to react. The longer you don't react, the dirtier your body will become. If you continue to ignore signs of disease, your body will not be able to work the way it was meant to. Your body will not have enough energy to deal with the stress in your life. If you continue on this path, the result will be sickness; and not changing your poor habits will lead to a very painful death."

The results of the causes:

PUTTING THINGS IN YOUR BODY THAT DO NOT BELONG THERE:
When you do this, you feed harmful bacteria into your bowel. The bacteria, fed with more junk food, continue to grow. Your body will then have to work even harder to deal with this growth, resulting in overworking the body and not giving it the rest needed to heal. This creates a waste of energy, nutrients and enzymes. Even worse, it creates a number of other harmful by-products in the body.

OVEREATING:
Overeating creates havoc in the body. When you eat more calories than your body needs, the excess calories get burned off in a process called 'futile cycles' which literally burn up the excess. Burning up this excess material produces a large quantity of 'free radicals,' some of the substances in your body that cause aging, deterioration of bodily functions, and the build-up of residues in the cells themselves. These futile cycles also use up the cells' energy, reducing the efficiency of their functions. But the most harmful thing that this excess material produces is fermentation which can lead to an imbalance in blood gases,

which could lead to problems. Overeating also clogs the body. As you continue to stuff your body with junk, slime and waste, not only do you clog the body, you also clog its exits. The food builds up inside with nowhere to go. This food then finds a place to stay in the body, resulting in poor digestion and energy loss. This leads to fermentation and putrefaction in your system, eventually leading to sickness and death. One of the factors in poor health is overeating.

IMPROPER DIGESTION AND IMPROPER ELIMINATION-
When the large intestine retains food longer than it should, harmful bacterial action occurs in the bowel. The result is that gases and toxins are formed. They are absorbed by the tiny vessels on the walls of the bowel and poison the entire blood stream. This is known as auto-intoxication.

Dr. Carrington explains in *Fasting for Health and Long Life:*

"When food is not properly digested, it causes trouble! An excess of protein results in putrefaction; an excess of carbohydrates, in fermentation. Both are bad; both result in unpleasant and ultimately serious symptoms. Gases and poisons are formed within the body, which pass into the blood-stream and affect the tissues and organs, and even the delicate nerve-cells of the brain. The mental and emotional life are affected, no less than the grosser physical elements. Waste material accumulates, toxins are formed, which poison and block the tiny blood vessels. The body becomes choked with the excess. Desperately, nature tries to get rid of this load by driving the eliminating organs to greater and greater efforts, until they break down under the strain. When this occurs, the patient is already in the throes of illness. He is now a really sick man."

NOT DRINKING ENOUGH WATER ALSO STRESSES THE BODY IN A MAJOR WAY:
Water is the liquid of life. Life could not exist without it. Depriving your body of water will dehydrate it. When you dehydrate your body, you deprive your life of an essential material it needs to live. The result is sickness and death.

LIVING IN UNNATURAL ENVIRONMENTS CAUSES A GREAT DEAL OF STRESS TO THE BODY:
When you live in an environment you were not meant to, your body does not perform optimally. Your body can adapt to unnatural environments, but that doesn't mean it's healthy. It gets stressed without the signals that something is wrong. Living in excess cold or heat hurts your health, slowly creating much stress in the body.

LIVING IN A NEGATIVE ENVIRONMENT, SURROUNDED BY NEGATIVE PEOPLE:
Always being around negative people can lead to depression. Depression is not the state in which humans were meant to live. Depression is a mental disease. Relieve it or suffer the consequences.

NOT SMILING:
If you live a grumpy life, chances are you will get some form of disease. The key to consistency is to enjoy what you're doing; if you are doing anything you don't enjoy, you will get sickness that you won't enjoy.

NOT JUST WHAT YOU EAT, BUT WHERE YOU EAT:
If you are eating in an uncomfortable environment, your digestion will be poor, thus leading to many problems. Poor health is the result of poor digestion.

NOT JUST WHAT YOU EAT, BUT WHEN YOU EAT:
You body works best during the middle of the day. At night-time, it slows down and tries to rest. If you eat at that time, your body will have to work when it should be resting. This can lead to loss of energy, stress and poor digestion.

NOT JUST WHAT YOU EAT, BUT HOW YOU EAT:
Rushing eating and not chewing well will make the body work much harder than it has to. Your body will have to use extra energy to digest the food, and then will require more rest. The more stress you add, the greater the chance that your body will not have enough time to get the rest it needs to heal. Also, drinking liquids with your meals interferes with the process of digestion. Digestion starts in the mouth with saliva. When you mix liquid with saliva, you are diluting it, thereby compromising digestion, leading to many harmful problems.

NOT GETTING ENOUGH SLEEP AND REST:
Having excess waste in your system, along with all the added stress your body has to deal with, is too much for the body to endure. The only way to heal from this excess stress is to sleep. But due to your busy schedule, there is a good chance that you're not getting the amount of sleep you need for heal-ing. When that happens, you curtail the healing process. If your body does not heal, it will continue to get worse. When you prevent your body from getting the rest it needs, you're creating stress. Each cell of the body requires a specific amount of energy supplying/rebuilding nutrients. Give them to your body or suffer the consequences.

CLEANING OUT TOO FAST:
If waste comes out of your body too fast, or if you detoxify too fast, too many toxins will enter the blood at one time. The stress can make you worse than you were before you started

cleaning in the first place. Some people are so toxic to begin with, cleaning out too fast can kill them.

BREATHING: HOW•YOU BREATHE:
The result of poor or shallow breathing is a gradually increasing supply of carbon dioxide gas. The more full breaths you take, the more oxygen there will be to neutralize and clean this gas. When too much carbon dioxide gas finds its way into the circulatory system, it poisons and deadens nerve cells throughout the body. The opposite of breathing is suffocation. Breathing is life. Suffocation is death.

BREATHING: WHAT YOU BREATHE:
Breathing the best quality air will keep you nourished. Breathing poor air will cause disease. When you breathe poor quality air, positive ions in that air will enter your lungs. They then go on to enter your bloodstream, suffocating the cells of your body. Breathing poor quality air can also trigger various harmful responses in your body such as the release of excess serotonin and histamine. Most people today are breathing poor quality air. What deceives people is the body's amazing power of adaptation. After a time, the body will adjust and adapt itself to a very dirty atmosphere, and people will be able to breathe without noticeable discomfort. If you were to put a healthy person in the same poor air, it would seem intolerable to him. This adaptation is termed "immunity." According to this theory, man becomes immune to a condition or poison if it does not kill him on the spot. Such adaptation can occur only at the expense of general depression of all the vital functions, which necessarily becomes injurious if long continued or often repeated. It is in this condition that people die by inches while being treated for some "mysterious disease." Every sneeze, every cough, every cold, and every headache are the first warnings that you are breathing polluted air. Most people do not understand what health is and what the body needs, so

they take poisonous remedies further depressing the vital functions and stifling the symptoms, while they continue to breathe the same vitiated air. Man was never made to live in an atmosphere so foul that each breath puts more poisons in his body. Breathing should be a process of purification rather than of a process of poisoning. The body is so perfectly equipped with the power of adaptation that it will adjust itself in time to tolerate an atmosphere so poisonous that it would kill a vital, healthy man in a few moments if he were to suddenly walk into it. Due to the body's power of adaptation, people can live constantly in polluted air and, on the surface, suffer nothing more than coughs, colds, hay fever, sore throat, and other mild ailments of the air organs. Yet they are dying by inches from the effects of that air and don't know it.

ONE CAUSE OF DISEASE IS OVEREATING, which leads to fermentation and putrefaction of food, which leads to a rise in toxic gases in the blood, which lead to toxemia of the blood.

Key Number Three to the Body: You've learned what happens as result of disease.

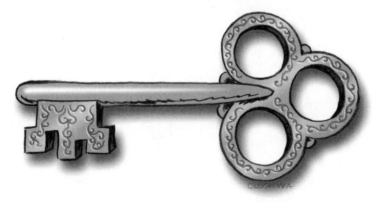

You've found the key and opened the lock.

Key Number Four:
How to Recognize the Signs of Disease

SCM tells you, "By now, you should understand that disease is a warning sign and should not be suppressed, but released. Before you can cure disease or release it from you body, you must know how to recognize it.

In a clean body, you will have no physical discomfort and you will feel good ALL THE TIME! Many people today believe they are supposed to experience some form of discomfort when they reach a certain age. That is not true. The fact is, as long as your body is clean, you will never feel any physical discomfort. If you have any discomfort in your body, then you are not yet clean; you are diseased. That is a clear way to tell. Feeling discomfort is the best way to tell if you are not clean, but sometimes a person can be so toxic that his body is not be able to feel. When you cannot feel discomfort due to your illness, you have to pay really close attention to your body and its functions. Learn what is supposed to be happening. If it is not happening, then take it as a good sign that something is wrong, whether you feel it or not. Monitor your digestion, energy, sleep and feelings.

A great way to tell if your body is working as it should is by paying close attention to your digestion. If you are eating three meals a day, you should be going to the bathroom three times a day. Anything less would be constipation, which is a good sign your body is not in perfect working order and something has to change.

Another good way to tell is by your energy. Your energy should be at a high level all the time. If it is not, then you should be resting or sleeping. If you can't fall asleep, but have little energy, take that as a sign that something might not be right.

If you don't feel at your best emotionally, you can also take that as a sign that you are doing something wrong. In nature's plan you will always feel great physically and emotionally. Your body is the best messenger to tell you otherwise."

SCM asks, "Turn to the page in the book with the heading: *THE BODY AND ITS SIGNALS*. Below that it reads: *If you put things into your body that shouldn't be there, the result is disease and illness. Any discomfort is a sign that you're not giving your body the resources it needs to thrive. If you eat anything besides fresh, organic ripe fruit and vegetables, you will clog your body. Lack of oxygen will be the immediate result, and the final result is death.*"

SCM says, "If you put things into your body that do not belong there, or if you put too many things into your body, even good things, your body will tell you. It will try really hard to tell you, and it won't stop trying to eliminate. Most people think it's a bad sign when the body keeps pushing toxic substances out, but it is a good sign. It shows that you are either putting in things that don't belong there or simply putting in too much. Do not suppress what is coming out, the way most people do. Do not interrupt nature; just assist nature and take this as a sign that you are over-indulging.

If food doesn't come out of the body quickly enough, your body will tell you by eliminating foul odors from the body, breath, skin, etc. This is a good sign that food is staying inside your body longer than it should. Other signs are constipation, laziness, pain and disease.

If you're not drinking enough water, there are good ways to tell. When you drink water and do not have to go to the bathroom within a few hours, that is a possible sign that you don't have enough water in your body. Another way to tell is if your urine is very yellow and has a strong odor to it. These are clear signs of dehydration."

You ask SCM, "Is being thirsty is a good sign?"

"Yes, but that is the last sign of dehydration, not the first. Dehydration is also a result of overeating."

As for the climate you live in, SCM says, "If you have to wear heavy clothing all the time, you can take it as a good sign that you belong in a more natural, warmer environment. As for the people around you, if everyone around you is negative, or no one supports you, or no one has an open mind, that's a sign that you're in a negative environment. You become like the people around you, so look for signs they show. How do they act?

One of the greatest signs that the body is healthy or diseased appears on the face: your smile. You can tell by your smile or the lack of one whether you are ahead of the game or behind. No matter how sick you are, if you can smile, you still have the will power and reserve to heal. If you can't smile, take it as a sign that you are in poor health and fix the problem.

As for where you eat, if you have any distractions, that is a sign that you are eating in the wrong place. As for how and when you eat, if you are always eating late at night or when it seems to be dark outside, that is a good sign that you are not eating at a good time. If you are not able to concentrate on your food because you are driving or talking or doing something that takes your mind off the food you're eating, that is another good sign that something is wrong. You should be able to relax when you eat. Make sure you eat your food slowly and chew it well. If you are not able to do this, that is a very good sign you are not eating in a healthy way.

How do you feel? If you can't feel how you feel, how do you appear to others? You should not seem lazy and you should not be yawning all the time. You should want to be up and high on life all the time. If you don't feel this way, then take it as a sign you need more sleep.

If you are following all the guidelines for a healthy lifestyle and still do not feel your best, that is a good sign you are detoxing at a faster than optimal rate.

If your body is not working perfectly, whether you feel pain or not, that is a major sign of disease. If you don't feel great most of the time, you can take it as a sign that you have some form of disease.

Fever is a sign that putrefaction and fermentation might be taking place inside the body. Fever can be generated by fermentation. Fermentation and putrefaction could lead to an increase in temperature.

One of the first places people feel the effects of fermentation and toxemia is in the upper parts of the body. They get a headache or a toothache. The fermentation produces warmth, and we soon become conscious of the rise in the temperature of the body. That is what fever is. Fever can therefore only occur when foreign matter is present and the natural exits are closed (where there is no regular motion of the bowels, urination is deficient, pores are obstructed, and the respiration is weak). So fever would be a clear sign that fermentation and toxemia is taking place in the system and something is wrong. Chills are another sign that something is wrong. When all the exits of the body are open for toxins to be released, blood will be able to reach all parts of the body, but when these tiny blood vessels are obstructed, especially in their minutest branches, the blood can no longer reach the exterior skin. One of the causes can be cold feet and hands and a chilly feeling all over. Chilliness is thus a precursor of fever, and it would be a mistake to ignore it.

Starvation is another big sign, but so many people misunderstand starvation. It is not something we necessarily feel or see. It just happens if we don't give the body what it needs. Most people today who eat a lot of junk food and breathe poor air and don't exercise are starving. We spoke before about the toxic gases of the body. Well, all starvation is the gas destroying the cells. If a person doesn't do the right things, that person can't be healthy. So only undernourished people can starve. A healthy person in a healthy environment

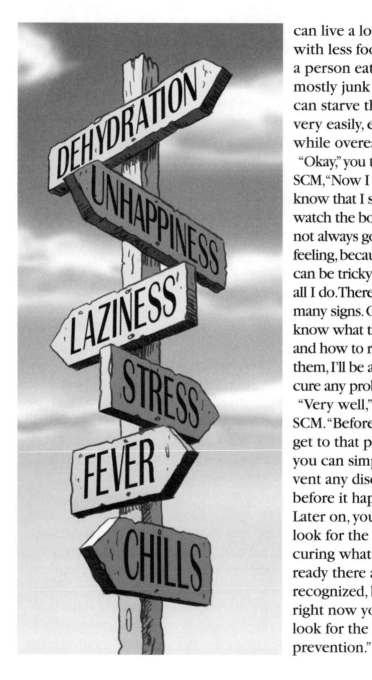

can live a long life with less food, but a person eating mostly junk food can starve the body very easily, even while overeating."

"Okay," you tell SCM, "Now I get it. I know that I should watch the body but not always go by feeling, because it can be tricky if that's all I do. There are many signs. Once I know what they are and how to read them, I'll be able to cure any problem."

"Very well," says SCM. "Before you get to that point, you can simply prevent any disease before it happens. Later on, you will look for the key to curing what is already there and recognized, but right now you will look for the key to prevention."

Key Number Four to the Body: You must know what to look for, so you can avoid it.

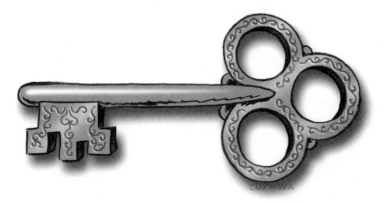

You've found the key and opened the lock.

Key Number Five: Prevention (How to Avoid Problems)

SCM instructs you, "The key to prevention is in the book." You read:

To prevent disease, you must understand what maintains, sustains, and keeps your body clean. Once you understand that, then all you have to do is avoid things that will interfere with the system. Health doesn't start with what you add to the diet; it all starts with what you eliminate and avoid. Take out the bad and only leave the good stuff, the stuff that maintains, sustains, and keeps your body clean. What will be left? What will keep you bodily system running at its best? The answer is raw organic food, sunshine, water and the air you breathe.

You must give clean oxygen to your body for all its cells to support life. If you stop breathing, you will stop living. If you breathe dirty air, you will have dirty blood. Blood is the stream of life. It carries oxygen to the cells of the body. The cleaner the blood, the more efficiently this system will work. But if the blood is mixed with mucus and slime, getting oxygen to the cells will not be easy. The function of respiration is the key to living a healthy life. This has been proven, but it is overlooked by most health professionals. In his writings, Hilton Hotema states that to maintain and sustain the living organism, three things are required:

Constant breathing.
Constant absorption by the blood of gases in the lungs.
Constant elimination of the toxic substances produced in the body.

The way to prevent any unnatural disease is to follow the laws of nature. If the laws of nature were always followed, there would be no need for any unnatural potions, ills, or supplements. The best and most natural things for your body are small quantities of whole, organic, ripe, fresh fruit. The most important things are clean water, sunshine, rest and clean air.

Because most people do not follow the laws of nature when they are growing up, the human body today is not what it once was. Through generation after generation, it has gotten weaker and weaker, and it is no longer able to work the way it once did.

There is no question that if food stays inside you longer than it should, it will become waste. The more waste inside your body, the more you waste your life away.

The condition of the body depends on the condition of the blood, and the condition of the blood depends on the air you breathe, the fluids you drink, and the food you eat. You must keep your blood clean and keep it flowing smoothly without disrupting or blocking its flow. Clean blood will keep you healthy and supply your body with everything it needs. If you eat just enough of the right foods without overeating and you exercise, rest, smile, drink clean water and breathe clean air, you will avoid most, if not all diseases. Don't get stressed over the things you cannot do right now. Do the best you can!

You ask SCM, "From what I just read it seems that all the body needs is air and water. Besides air and water, what does the body need to thrive?"

SCM answers, "It needs the best quality foods; raw, organic, whole, fresh foods, as well as sunshine and love. If you give it all those things, you will be fine. The cleaner the body is, the less food it needs. Eat a wide rage of fruits and vegetables to make sure the body gets a good balance of all these foods. These high quality foods have the highest concentrations of nutrients. Avoid foods that have little essential nutrition relative to their calorie content."

"SCM, if we get clean air and water what is the role of food?"

"The food you eat determines the quality of your blood and that will determine the quality of your body. The better the quality of the food you eat, the better the quality of your blood."

It is important to have clean blood. The blood is an important transport system. The main reason you eat and drink is to give your blood the nutrients it needs to keep it clean and flowing. The less you eat, the cleaner you keep this transport system and the better it will work. Most people overeat. Overeating causes this system to become faulty.

"What about water?" you ask, "How does that help?"

SCM says, "Prevention and good health don't start only with what you eat, but also with what you drink. Drinking a good amount of water can help keep you from overeating. Not overeating will help you avoid all the problems that come along with overeating. Eating the highest quality food in small amounts is best for most people. More people get sick from overeating than from under-eating. Many people think they must eat a lot of food to keep up their strength and be healthy. That is not necessarily true. The body can last for days, weeks, and even months without food. Missing one meal a day will not harm you. Man's strength and vitality depend on the the quality of the air he breathes and the quality of the food he eats, not necessarily the amount eaten, just as you've read in the book."

"But what about the nutrition we get from food? Would more food give us more nutrition?"

SCM replies, "Quality food creates quality blood. The quality of your blood creates healthy cells and tissues. The cleaner the blood, the more oxygen it can carry. Cell by cell, the body divides and builds. The body is the product of electrons, atoms, and molecules, which build the cells, which build the body. These 'building blocks' are not only the product of food. They are also the product of the air you breathe. Overeating, even good quality food can lead to lack of oxygen in the blood, which can lead to suffocation and disease. One of the keys to prevention is to avoid overeating.

SCM turns to a page in the book and asks you to read it:
When the body is given the exact amount of food that is needed and no more, the metabolic efficiency will continue to increase up to the 50 percent level. You end up with more vitality, physical energy, and robust health. By restricting your diet to only the amount of food your body needs, you produce fewer substances in your body that cause aging

106

symptoms and you preserve energy.

If you follow the laws of nature: eating the most natural food and not overeating, your body will work optimally. The chart below shows the length of time that each type of food would spend in the stomach if eaten by itself with no other food (called a mono meal) and if your body were working properly and provided that the most natural food were eaten: raw, organic, whole, ripe, and fresh fruits and vegetables. The faster out of the system, the better.

Food	Time in Stomach
Water	*10 minutes*
Melon	*20 minutes*
Fruits	*1 hour*
Vegetables	*2 hours*
Starches	*3 hours*
Protein	*4 hours*
Slop, mis-combined foods	*up to 12 hours*

SCM clarifies, "That is how it would be had you been eating healthfully since birth.

You can see from this chart what eating healthfully is by looking at the best and worst foods for you. Because of all the junk people put in their bodies while growing up and because of the poor environment they live in, the chart for the average person today is not the same. For today's average person, change the word 'hour' on the chart to the word 'days,' YES, DAYS! That is how long food stays in the stomach of the average person today. Just because someone goes to the bathroom once a day doesn't mean he or she is not constipated. If people eat five times a day, they should go to the bathroom five times a day. If a person eats two pounds of food, a lot should come out, not a little.

Constipation is one of the first steps in the dirty body

disease process. This is how a chart would look today for most people:

Food	Time in stomach
Water	*10 minutes*
Melon	*20 hours*
Fruits	*1 day*
Vegetables	*2 days*
Starches	*3 days*
Protein	*4 days*
Slop, miscombined food	*up to 12 days*

You want to get food in and out as fast as you can. Otherwise, you are in trouble.

You must keep your body clean, eating only the foods that will leave it rapidly."

SCM has already told you, "A great deal of stress is caused by living in an unnatural environment. To prevent this, you should move to where it is most natural for your body: places where you can be in nature freely and enjoy your life. Tropical climates are the best and most natural places for you. Also, make sure the people you surround yourself with in your environment are open-minded and supportive. This will keep you happy and healthy. When you are happy and healthy, you are able to smile. The healthiest people are the happiest people. If you're in control of your life, you will smile. When it comes to prevention and eating, make sure you eat in a controlled environment; that is, under your control and no one else's. The more in control you are, the better your meal will be digested. Also, eat when you are relaxed and in control of your emotions. If you are in control, you will eat slowly and be relaxed. That, too, will keep you healthy and happy."

Now you seem to understand. You think the reason most people get sick is that they don't get enough rest and sleep, where true healing takes place. Rest is essential in avoiding disease and sickness. Fasting is another important form of rest. Sleep, rest, and fasting will keep you healthy. I can sum up this whole book right now: the major causes of sickness and disease are overeating and under-sleeping. If most people were to change those two things, they would get better much more quickly and stay healthy. When it comes to sleeping, many people get a lot of sleep, but still not enough. There is a big difference between a lot and enough.

SCM says, "That is correct, good job. Another problem is that people go to sleep too late at night. The best hours for the body to heal and for you to be sleeping are the hours before midnight. They are the most important. Every hour you sleep before midnight is like two hours. After midnight, every hour you sleep in like half an hour.

For example if you sleep from 10:00 p.m. to midnight, that is like getting 4 hours of rest, but if you sleep from midnight to 2:00 a.m. that is like getting only one hour of rest. Even though you slept the two hours both ways, there is a big difference between when the two hour periods took place. More harmful than any drug or any polluted environment is something most people sleep next to every night: an alarm clock. It deprives the body of the important healing rest it needs. No matter how much you stress the body, if you give it enough rest, the body will heal. The problem is that people are adding stress to the body and cutting their rest short. Sleep is the best healer of any and all discomfort. It is important to get enough. There is no such thing as oversleeping. It is impossible to oversleep, but very common to under-sleep. The more energy you use, the more rest and sleep you need."

Now, a little confused, you ask SCM, "You mean energy comes from rest and not from food?"

"There are two types of energy: one is caloric energy from food, which gives your body fuel through calories; the other, and more important type, is the energy you get from oxygen. This energy, also known as prana, does not come from food; it comes from breathing clean fresh air. The best way to maintain energy is to rest. The less energy you use the more you will have. Eating less rests your body inside and out. That's the best way to save energy. Sleeping and resting your body, inside and out, is the best way to conserve energy. Eating food consumes much energy, especially eating junk foods. To rid itself of them, the body has to work extra hard. It is a fact that digestion uses more of the body's energy than anything else. Digesting food takes energy away and doesn't give energy as so many believe. The more complex something is, the more work it will require to break down. The more you eat, the more you need to sleep. To avoid stress, get to bed early, if you can, and get enough sleep. The length of time for enough sleep is different for everyone depending on his or her lifestyle, and it is always changing. Don't just take one answer for it all. Listen to your body, and you will be fine.

To avoid disease, you must go at your own pace. Make changes when you feel you are ready, physically and mentally. Otherwise, you will run into some problems. No two people are in the same place at the same time. You must move at your pace, not someone else's. If you go at your own pace, you will not be able to go too fast and run into problems."

You say, "Wow! Now I have all this information about avoiding disease. I wish I had known these things years ago."

SCM advises, "Don't focus on the past. You have the information now, so use it."

"SCM, of all the great things I've learned, which is the most important for avoiding disease?"

"They are all important, but it all starts with the air you breathe and how you breathe it. When you breathe fully, you are releasing toxic gases. As long as the body can consistently release these gases, you will feel well, but once you start to get tired and not take full breaths, then the trouble begins."

"SCM, I've heard that exercising purifies the blood. So isn't that just as important?"

"They are both important. Breathing purifies the blood by oxygenating it, and exercise helps it to circulate. You should do both. But you only have to do one of them to live: you must breathe. Both are very beneficial."

SCM directs you, "Look at the book on the floor near your feet. It's open to a page that's worthwhile reading: *Getting oxygen is of fundamental importance. The air in your lungs is composed of oxygen. The blood is the medium through which oxygen is carried from the lungs to the body's trillions of cells. The blood also carries off poisonous substances produced by disintegration and disposes of them through the channels of elimination.*

"There's so much information and talk about toxic gases in the blood, I wonder how to avoid getting toxic gasses in the blood?"

SCM explains, "To avoid getting toxic gasses in the blood, avoid fermentation and toxemia. In a properly working body, decomposed matter will be disposed of before fermentation can occur. Toxic gases in the body are developed by fermentation, which is not at all instrumental in building up the body. If you avoid fermentation in the first place, you won't have to worry about toxic gasses in your blood. The way to assure yourself of this is when eating, make sure the food you select will go through your body quickly and easily. The safest way for that to happen is to have a good digestive system. If you overburden you system, you can't have a good digestive system. So don't overeat, and breathe to you fullest capacity!"

"But the air pollution where I live is so bad. Where I live, it's so dirty and...."

"Whoa, slow down," SCM begs you. "You're talking, but do you even understand what poor air quality means, and how it can help you avoid disease and maintain health? Many people hear about clean air and dirty air; and breathing polluted air will create poor health. That is spoken of all the time, but do you know why it's true? Do you really understand why polluted air is so bad? And do you realize that polluted air *will* cause poor health? But, what is more important, and what you should be thinking of, is that certain quality of clean air which can nourish your body, to help avoid disease. This magic air can even help the body to cure itself from poor health."

"Wow! Really? How so, SCM?"

"There is no doubt that the healthiest people in this world live in more natural environments. Throughout history, people living in forests, near waterfalls and near oceans were much healthier than people living in big cities. The reason is the air in these natural environments is so powerful. There is much that can be seen and is already known about the human body and how it works. There is also much that cannot be seen. Some people know about these unseen things. Many people believe if you can't see them, then they don't exist. But, just because you can't see some things doesn't mean they aren't there. They are there and in the air; magic in the air."

"What are they?" you rush to ask SCM.

"Ions; air in all environments contains ions. They are molecules that carry a charge of electricity. Ions are produced by the action of natural phenomena such as cosmic rays, lightning and radon from the earth's crust on atoms in the air. At such times, some atoms lose or gain electrons and become either negatively or positively charged. So, all air is electric air. Some of it is just good and some is bad. A negative air ion is an oxygen atom or molecule that has gained an electron and a positive air ion is usually a carbon-dioxide molecule that has lost an electron. Just as batteries wear out, your body wears out. But if you are able to breathe this good electric air, you'll get reenergized.

Even though these molecules are everywhere, they are so small they can't be seen by the human eye. But trust that they are there. As soon as you start breathing them, you will feel the electricity in your body.

The reason these ions are so beneficial in natural environments is that the natural environment around them recharges their energy. In big cities and unnatural environments, they have their energy sucked right out of them. The ions that have lost their electricity or their electrons are called positive ions. Ions with their electricity or electrons are called negative ions. When it comes to ions in the air, you want the negative recharged ions in your body.

It is not just the type of ion that's important, but also the size of the ion. Not all ions are the same size. Negative ions come in small, medium and large sizes. Small (ingestible) negative ions are highly mobile and biologically active. Medium to large negative ions are sluggish, slow moving and serve just to clean the air. You want negative ions in your body, but you want them to be as small as possible. Only small (ingestible) negative ions can be inhaled. When they are inhaled, they can have positive biological effects. If they can't be inhaled, as is the case of larger clusters of negative ions, they are simply air cleaners and have no biological effect on your body. Inhaling this air, highly charged with small ingestible oxygen ions, is the key to the 'recharged' feeling you have in natural environments. The smaller the negative ion, the better.

The smallest negative ions are found in the most natural environments such as near waterfalls, in pine forests, and at the seashore where waves are breaking on the rocks. They are naturally produced by the action of cosmic rays, lightning and radon from the earth's crust. The best generator is lightning, followed by ocean surf and waterfalls. Negative ions are also abundant in mountains and forests (all plants give off some ions).

Positive ions are found indoors and in most other unnatural environments. In healthy people, there is a perfect balance of negative and positive ions, favoring the negative. What happens in today's unnatural environments, where most people live, is a balance in favor of positive ions. This leaves these people with a lowered electrical charge, leading to loss of energy and poor health.

Negative ions have been called the 'vitamins of the air.' It is most important to keep the balance of negative and positive ions indoors as close to the balance outdoors, where they are almost equal. Indoor and poor unnatural environments containing many positive ions will cause an imbalance of positive over negative ions. Some common equipment people use everyday to cause this imbalance are air conditioners and heating devices which actually strip the air of negative ions. Static electricity is created by non conductive synthetic building materials, wall coverings, fabrics, carpets and furniture. Electro-magnetic fields are created by radiation from electrical supplies such as high voltage cables, big transformers, etc. and in offices by electrical appliances such as computers, telephones, etc. Negative ions are also carried by small airborne particles. They attach themselves to these particles found in dust, tobacco smoke and pollen, and then lose their charge. They also attach themselves to particles of moisture in very humid rooms.

Negative ions only exist for a short time. They are destroyed by air pollution, whereas hot electrical discharges such as sparking, electric motors, furnaces, etc., generate an excess of positive ions. Furthermore, air moving through metal ducts, as in air conditioning, is stripped of any negative ions it may contain.

The problem arises when staying indoors. An airplane, for example, is filled with positive ions. There are oppressive concentrations of dead air indoors, causing germs to flourish. Get out in nature as much as possible to offset staying indoors. If you must stay indoors, it can help to use a negative ion generator or an ionizer. Good negative ion generators, or ionizers, produce a large volume of negative ions, restoring the ion ratio.

Negative ions are so important to human health. They not only recharge our batteries, they raise the percentage of ionizing "organism ion" minerals in the system, purify the blood to slight alkalinity, and allow for much easier absorption of nutritive substances. Simple waste material is readily eliminated from cells, and the increased circulation and exertion improves metabolism, helps the power of resistance, naturally strengthens the body's defenses against viruses and diseases, reduces tiredness, improves emotional calm, and reduces allergies of the respiratory system."

The Raw Matrix:
Our universe is electrical and so is the air we breathe.

In ancient textbooks on yoga, that venerable mystic discipline of the East, it's suggested that a student wishing to perfect his body and mind through breathing exercises should practice near a waterfall, in a cave or (best of all) in a cave under a waterfall. While it's obvious that pure air is better than polluted air, the proposition that there's more energy in one kind of pure air than in another would, to many people, seem specious, if not superstitious. But science over the past 20 years has proved that some air does give us more energy than other air.

Two of the most important things for our health are air and water. They are so powerful; you can't grab either one in your hand, yet they can keep us alive forever or kill us in minutes. **—Paul Nison**

115

**Key Number Five to the Body:
Breathe clean air with full breaths,
drink clean water, eat small amounts of
the highest quality foods and get enough
rest, and you will avoid most diseases.**

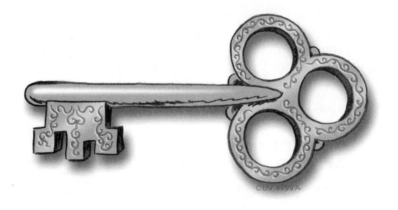

You've found the key and opened the lock.

Key Number Six:
The Cure (If You Already Have Disease)

"SCM, I wish I had known all this information about avoiding illness when I was younger, but what do I do now if I have disease? How do I cure it?"

He explains, "To cure disease, you still have to follow all the rules of nature. You need to do the same things you would do to avoid disease, but your body might need some extra help. This is where some unnatural things may need to be done to help you get better.

Remember that during the curing of the disease, you might experience detoxification symptoms. As long as you go at your own pace, they will not become dangerous. You can monitor your progress through these detoxification symptoms. If you go at someone else's pace or go too fast, they can become very harmful, so go slowly, but keep moving forward.

There is no special food or magic pill that will get rid of disease. To clean your body, you must use nature's soap: water. Consider it the soap that will cleanse the dirt from your body. The key is to have the cleanest blood possible. The cleaner the blood, the more oxygen it will carry and the more vitality you will have. You will have to regain the vitality you lost. Staying alive and thriving depends on how clean your blood is, because the blood is the oxygen carrier. Were a person with clean blood to stop breathing, he would survive up to a few minutes, but if his blood were dirty, he would die in seconds after stopping breathing because his blood contained very little oxygen. You must clean your blood if you want to get rid of your disease!

Cleaning your body internally requires it to go through a detoxification. You might look worse before you look better, and you'll feel worse before you feel better while your body is undergoing detoxification. This scares many people only because they don't understand detoxification. Many worry about detoxification, thinking it's a bad sign. But it's a good sign. You will understand detoxification if you remember this: 'Energy is always noted in its expenditure, never in its accumulation. Whenever one feels stronger, he is often getting weaker, because he is expending his strength more rapidly. On the contrary, when feeling weakest, strength is often accumulating most rapidly. It is accumulating and hence unnoticed.' That piece of information can help so many people understand why eating healthfully and cleaning out will sometimes make them feel worse before feeling better. Healing requires consuming the foods that are best for your body. The best way to avoid bodily dehydration is to eat the foods that will keep your body clean and free of excess mucus and slime. The more water you have in your body, the cleaner you will be. If water is your soap, then you want to drink a lot of it to stay clean and free of debris. The best foods for the human body are those that contain the most water (liquid). Water will help you stay clean and remove the dirt that has been there for so long, causing disease/discomfort."

"How can I tell which foods contain the most liquid?" you ask SCM.

"Picture a juicer. As you put different foods through the juicer, which foods contain the most liquid? Melons, juicy fruits and green leafy vegetables. If you put any cooked food through the juicer, you won't get any liquid. If you put dehydrated foods through the juicer, you won't get any liquid. If you put dense fruit and veggies through the juicer, you won't get as much liquid. For example, if you try to put a piece of bread through the juicer, the juicer will work very hard but nothing will come out. The juicer will work very hard until it breaks under the pressure. Well, your body is like a juicer. If you put food into it that has no liquid, it will break and you'll experience disease. You'll experience discomfort. Your body is the best juicer on the planet. If you feed it foods that will go through it the easiest, it won't break; it will work perfectly for a very long time. Keep it simple."

SCM reminds you, "You're in the MIND room, still looking for keys. Once again, it goes back to one of the keys you've already found: words. Look at the word 'carbohydrate'. Many people hear the word 'carbohydrate' but don't even look at it. Usually, it is preceded by another word, either 'simple' or 'complex.' Simple carbohydrates have the most liquid, so putting them in your body is like putting them through a juicer. They are easy on the body. That is why they are simple. Now look at the word 'complex.' 'Complex' means hard, difficult. Complex carbohydrates make your body work hard. Just as bread would make a juicer work very hard because it has no liquid, complex carbohydrates make your body work very hard, until it finally breaks down. 'Simple' is a good word. You want simple. 'Complex' is a very dangerous word. It will kill you. You must avoid it at all costs if you want to live life to its fullest. Cooked foods are complex; that's what is wrong. Just keep it simple. Go for the liquid, go for the raw, simple carbohydrates".

You have learned so much. Realizing you might have the answer that has eluded the medical community for so long, you ask SCM, "If I wanted to heal someone who is sick, I would start by telling him not to overeat. But how do I find out how much food is considered overeating?"

"Do you overeat?" SCM asks.

"I don't think so."

"Most people in this country overeat. If no one in this country overate, the words 'I don't like that' would not be in the English language. Anything and everything would taste wonderful to you, if you were really eating with true hunger. People in this country and throughout most of the world don't eat out of hunger; they eat for pleasure. Don't focus on not overeating; there is nothing wrong with a little pleasure. A little pleasure has never hurt anyone. However, a lot of pleasure has killed many. Learn to control your pleasure. You must gain control. It's okay to experience the pleasure of food, but overdoing it is overeating. Learn to ensure that all your nutrient needs are met while reducing your caloric intake of food to the amount needed. The right number of calories is different for everyone, but you can be sure that the higher the quality of the food, fewer are the calories needed.

When you eat less than you are used to, you might get a headache or feel weak. This is not caused by a lack of food, but rather by toxins being loosened into your bloodstream. Eating stops your body from cleansing and thus stops the toxins from being released. It might feel good to stop discomfort this way, but over time it is very harmful, because all the toxins continue to build up in the body. When you eat something, it might seem that the food is energizing, but this can be due to the food's stimulating properties and not to the food's strengthening power. Overeating makes your body use much energy; it does not give your body higher amounts of energy, despite the stimulating effect. The way to conserve healing energy and build strength is either to eat very little or to fast, depending on what level of health you're in. This will give your system a chance to clean itself, to dislodge and get rid of poisons in the body, to get rid of disease and to heal."

It's not the amount of food that will keep you alive. It is the amount of food your body can use. The excess will just cause trouble. You can eat a lot of food and still starve to death if the body's cells cannot use anything in the food. It's not how much you eat, but how much of what you eat the body can use.

"There was a man who visited the castle a very long time ago and got this key," SCM reveals. "He tested and proved the recuperative powers of the body. His name was Luigi Cornaro, a Venetian nobleman born in 1467. When he came to the castle, I asked him about his health. He said that he became a chronic drunkard at the age of twenty-five. By age forty, he was a physical and mental wreck. The physicians told him repeatedly that he would not live. Then he quit drinking and turned to Mother Nature. Within one year, he had recovered health. He regained health to such extent that he lived to be one hundred and two. His wife adopted the same course, and bore children very late in life, also living beyond the century mark. Cornaro became the greatest of modern experts. He found that a simple diet of 12 ounces of solid food and 16 ounces of unfermented wine daily was best for him. Except for a twelve day period, he lived on this ration for over sixty-three years.

On his seventy-eighth birthday, Cornaro's friends urged him to increase his ration. Reluctantly, he agreed to a 14-ounce allowance of solid food. In twelve days, he was stricken with fever and had pain in his right side. He immediately returned to the 12 ounce ration, but he suffered for thirty-five days. That was his only illness in 63 years. He wrote several books, the last when he was over the age of 95. In his book entitled *Birth and Death of Man*, he said of himself: 'I am now as healthy as a person of 25. I write daily six or seven hours, and the rest of the time I occupy in walking, conversing, and occasionally attending concerts. I am happy. My imagination is lively, my memory tenacious, my judgment good, and what is most remarkable in a person of my advanced age, my voice is strong and harmonious. We can all be like this man. He didn't even care about the kinds of food he ate, just the amount, and he got better. Can you imagine how long he would have lived if he had eaten the best quality foods?"

So you ask SCM, "What do you recommend to start with?"

He says, "Keep it as simple as possible.

Here is a simple rule. I call it the 5-5-5-5 rule. Use this to start and have as a final goal a 1-1-1-1 rule. Now remember, you may never get to a 1-1-1-1 rule, but this is not about perfection. It's about being positive, and moving in the right direction at your own pace. Here is the 5-5-5-5 rule:

- Never take more than 5 minutes to make a meal.
- Use no more then 5 ingredients in the meal.
- If the meal is in liquid form, make sure it doesn't exceed 5 cups. (You can eat a whole meal, but think of how many cups it would be if it were in liquid form. Try it in liquid form the first time if you have to, so that you know the amount.)
- Consume no more than 5 small meals a day.

Follow this rule. When you are ready, go to a smaller number. If you go at your own pace, you will eat less and less, and eventually be able to cure yourself of many of your discomforts.

"What if that doesn't help me?" you ask SCM.

He explains, "If your digestion is poor and you feel you are not getting food out of your body fast enough, there are certain herbal formulas that can be helpful in getting the job done. High Colonic Irrigations and enemas can also be very helpful. The most important thing is to drink a lot of water and make sure you are not overeating.

By putting water or liquid into your body, you are cleaning away all the excess mucus and slime that is causing problems to your health. Not getting enough water into your body, also known as dehydration, is a major cause of stress in the body that causes disease. Dehydration is the problem. The cure is to hydrate your body. So, the cure is to find a way to hydrate your way to health! The best way to do this is with water. You remember when I told you that to cure yourself you must keep things simple. Water is the simplest liquid there is. The next is juice, and last is food. Yes, even food with a lot of liquid is not as good as water, because the more there is to something, the more complex it is, and the more it has to be broken down, thus requiring more work and energy. Simple things require very little work and very little energy. Water is simple. It's the best.

Water, the simplest liquid available, is the only liquid that cleans the body and at the same time doesn't require any energy to digest. But you must make sure the water you are putting into your body is the cleanest you can get. Putting dirty water into your body will also cause problems. You wouldn't try to clean the outside of your body with soap that had oil on it, so why try to clean your insides with dirty water? Drink plenty of clean water, and you will be clean, happy and feel great."

"About three-quarters of the human body is composed of water, and the circulation of water throughout the body is

immense. Every day, more than six tons of blood is pumped by the heart throughout all the ramifications of the numerous blood vessels along tubes, large and small, which circulate throughout the body. One of the great contributory causes of old age is lack of sufficient water in the system. Lack of water is also one of the greatest causes of constipation, which is the beginning of most diseases. Drinking enough water throughout the day will help wash your body out. It will give your body an inner bath."
—Hereward Carington from Death Deferred

Now you are confused. You tell SCM, "I see so many people who are healthy eating a raw diet, and they drink very little water."

SCM says, "Yes, but they are eating a great deal to get their water from their food. That can lead to another problem: overeating. However, if you have clean water, your body can thrive on less food."

"Why can't I just eat a little food with liquid in it, such as fruit and nothing else? Isn't that best for the body?"

"At a time in the past that might have been true, but because of our poor heath habits over the years and the damage we've done to our foods and our environment, we need to include more vegetables in our diet as well as fruits. The reason we eat it is different from the reason most people think. People need food so they don't kill themselves. They don't only need food for nutrition, but also to hold back all the toxins in their systems. Without food, these toxins would be eliminated too quickly. Were people in the perfect environment, they would still need to eat to control and hold back the toxins already accumulated in their bodies, not only from what they consumed when they were growing up, but also from what their parents ate and what their grandparents ate and so on. But you can eventually get to a level where your body is clean enough for you not to have to rely on food to hold back these toxins, once all those poisons are out. That is the only time it is safe to do so.

Most people will not reach that point in this lifetime because it took them a long time to get all those toxins into their bodies, and it will take even longer to get them to come out. The toxins go back a long time. But when it comes to food and the body and not eating, anything is possible, if done intelligently and not rushed. Remember, one of the greatest things is freedom, and freedom from food is a great feeling. Overeating on food does not keep you alive, oxygen does. Water helps to move the oxygen around in your body along with breathing and exercise. The cleaner the body, the less one needs to eat."

"How can the body thrive on so little, SCM?"

"It was made to do so, that's how."

"How can we know when we get too much of a good thing?"

"If you overdo something such as eating, it will cause ill health, and that's how you know you're overdoing it. There are some things you can never overdo or get too much of. The proof is that it doesn't cause a problem and you only benefit from it. Sleep and rest are perfect examples. You can never get too much rest or sleep. If your body is lazy or tired, it is that way for a reason. Maybe you are doing too much of something else. But giving your body the rest it requires is the answer, not the problem. If you eat too much, your body has to work harder, so it requires more rest and sleep. If you eat less, your sleep needs will diminish and you will have time to enjoy life."

You ask SCM, "What if I get enough sleep and don't overeat? Will that cure any diseases I might have?"

SCM explains, "It's not just what we do, but where we do it. If you're living in an unnatural environment, it will put a lot of stress in your body. If that is the case, you would have a better chance to heal if you moved to a less stressful environment. Follow the sun, and be where there is a tropical climate. That will help cure any disease you might have. You must also surround yourself with open and supportive people. Once you can do all that, you should enjoy a big smile all the time, and then you'll know you have found the cure. The other thing you can do to help cure yourself is to live as close to nature as possible. Eat outdoors when you can, and try not to eat during darkness or during the late hours of the day."

SCM says, "There are many cures, but only one main cure: rest."

"I know that already. You've told it to me many times."
"I'm going to tell it to you again, because it's so important to deeply understand. No matter how healthy or sick you are, you must always get enough sleep and rest if you want to be healthy. If you want your body to heal, you must give it the rest it needs to do so. That is the only way to heal a tired, stressed system. In order to give the body the rest it needs, you have to sleep, sleep, sleep. There is no such thing as oversleeping. It's impossible to sleep too much, but very easy to sleep too little. Your body will require many hours of rest to heal, and that is the only way it will. Got it?"

"Got it, but why?"

"Many important functions are performed during sleep. Your body is not only able to rest, but the food you've eaten during the day is broken down, and after you awake you are able to eliminate. If you keep eating without ever giving you body a chance to do this, you will be constipated. During sleep, the body also performs natural dialysis. Along with a good diet, rest and quality sleep is important."

"Good sleep? What's the difference between good sleep and bad sleep?"

125

"There is a big difference. The best healing of the body takes place during phase 4 (deep) sleep, and it's very important to get enough. There is a big difference between a lot and enough sleep. True healing takes place during this phase 4 deep sleep, when your body recharges its nerve energy. Alarm clocks, a big problem today, interrupt the body, preventing it from getting this important rest. It's very hurtful to the body to be awakened out of any resting or sleeping phase, but it's most harmful to be awakened out of phase 4 sleep. The best way to wake up is gradually, so your body can safely and easily awake. Most people today are literally 'shocked' out of phase 4 sleep. This curtails the body's healing process and causes damage to the nervous system."

"How can people know if they're awakened from this deep sleep stage?"

SCM imparts another pearl, "You know you've been awakened from phase 4 sleep if you don't know where you are or can't even speak or remember your name for a few moments after awakening."

"But, SCM, so many people feel they must use an alarm clock. If that's the case, what should they do?"

"If you must use an alarm clock, you'd be better off using a more natural approach such as the *Sunrise Natural Clock.** It's nowhere near as harmful as the common alarm clock. The *Sunrise Clock* gently awakes you to a soft glow of light rather than with a jarring noise in a dark room. This innovative wake-up system is based on medical research on morning light and human behavior. Scientists have demonstrated that in the early morning, even while you're still asleep, the biological clock is sensitive to low intensity light. Dim light, gradually getting brighter simulating the natural process of a sunrise, can result in a smoother transition to wakefulness. This natural approach is akin to waking up with the sun on a beautiful summer morning. You wake up in a better mood and feel

*(Sunrise natural clock available from **www.rawlife.com**)

126

more refreshed as you begin your day. The Natural Clock's light slowly begins to shine half an hour before the wake-up time setting, gradually illuminating the room and becoming brighter until it's time for you to get out of bed. The clock also has a back-up beeper alarm (but most people won't need it). The adjustable light in the *Sunrise Clock* doubles as a fine bedside lamp. This lamp/alarm clock will help bring you to a lighter phase of sleep just before the alarm rings. It will let you know if you didn't get enough sleep... you'll be awakened by a beep."

"Is that all, SCM. Do I have all the keys I need to open the door to the body?"

SCM says, "No. Before you start to heal, you have to know where to go. No two people are at the same place at the same time, so there is never one cure for everyone. It will be different for everyone. What might help one person might kill another and vice versa. If you start from the wrong place, you can harm yourself no matter how good the food might be. Don't go too fast. Determine where you are right now and start moving forward slowly but surely. Be cautious, but make sure you're having fun and enjoying life. Remember, you want to be consistent, and the way to do that is to have fun. Exercise is also a very important part of the cure, as are breathing exercises. Learn breathing exercises and practice them everyday. You must also focus on your outer environment. A clean and natural environment will help you very much. Make sure you use natural materials as much as possible, such as wood, cork, clay, brick, coconut fiber, hemp, organically grown cotton, etc. Wear natural fabrics as much as possible, such as hemp, organic cotton, linen, wool, or silk so that your largest organ, the skin, can breathe. Avoid static electricity from the movement of synthetic fibers. Ensure that fresh air gets into a building without causing a draft and low temperatures. The humidity should ideally be between 40 - 50% to prevent the loss of too many negative ions. If there is a problem with humidity, install a humidifier with automatic humidity control. Install an electronic filtering unit in each room to filter out airborne particles, smoke, bacteria, and viruses in the atmosphere to reduce respiratory and other infections. Surround yourself with growing green plants. Thriving plants provide two important benefits. First, they show they are living well in an ion-enhanced atmosphere, especially if they have a marked increase in size and growth rate. Furthermore, they tend to gather negative ions around themselves. This is particularly true of evergreens and ferns, which focus negative electrical charges on the pointed tips of their leaves. The body absorbs light energy as a form of nourishment, but normal fluorescent lighting does not possess the combination of wavelengths of color found in natural sunlight and should be changed to full spectrum fluorescent lighting tubes."

"Whoa, slow down. That is so much to remember."

SCM says, "That's because there is a lot to it. Remember when I said it's simple but not that simple? Well, the things you have to do are simple, but there are so many to do. Most people can't do them all."

"What is the most important thing?"

"That depends on who and where the person is. That's why there is no one answer for everyone. One must do what works best for him and makes the most sense at that time in his life. Also, not everyone can do it all, so do the best you can."

You have gained many keys and opened many locks. There are only a few more left. You ask SCM, "Can you help me?"

"Okay, here are some other keys that will help.

Going without food will give the body a good amount of rest and is very helpful when it comes to healing. Fasting is another way to rest your body so you can overcome disease."

"How do I know if I'm ready to fast. Isn't it dangerous if I'm not ready?"

"Yes, it can be, but most people can fast for one or two days without harm. Answering this question is a good way to find out: Can you go the whole day without eating anything, without having any cravings at nighttime? If you can do that, then you might be ready, but if you have cravings at nighttime, then you're not ready and you should eat during the day. But, don't eat too much.

Another excellent key is to skin brush. The biggest elimination system of the body is the skin. You must keep it clean so it can do its job. It only takes a few minutes a day to skin brush the body, and it aids so much in the healing process."

"Okay, SCM, now I have so many little keys, I can't carry any more. I want to open this door already." Pointing to a lock on which 'SUNSHINE' is written, you ask SCM, "What about that one?"

"That's another very important key that most people in this society tend to think they should avoid. Contrary to popular belief, sunrays are good for you. As long as you don't abuse them, they will never cause harm. The rays of the sun are actually the source of all life on this planet. Animals, plants and humans would not exist without them. You should get exposure to the sun everyday. When the sun is up and out, you should be up and out. The sun going down is nature's way of telling you, it's time to rest. Your body slows down and gets ready to sleep. It is unnatural and unhealthy to be awake after the sun goes down. The longer you wait after sundown, the more unhealthy it becomes. Because of society's demands, many people find it unrealistic to go to sleep at sundown.

Health and happiness require exposing your skin and eyes to the sun on a regular basis. The cleaner your body becomes, the more you'll realize this. You'll burn less and tan faster. Even being in the sun for many hours will not bother you. The sunlight will actually keep your skin soft and beautiful. However, no matter what state of health you're in, burning of the skin is never healthful. It's just another sign that the body is telling you the true answers of life. If you ever experience sunburn, it's time to get out of the sun; you've had more than enough for that day, whether it's five minutes or five hours. It's different for everyone. Do not stay out long enough to get burned. Anything short of that should be fine.

"Thanks so much for all your advice SCM. I'm going to open this door.

But, before I do, can you tell me about enzymes?"

"That won't be necessary because you can read about them in the books in the MIND room."

Back in the MIND room, you open the simple book first. In the chapter on enzymes, it is written: *The big problem with cooking is that it destroys and eliminates all the enzymes in the food. Enzymes are energy. They are life. If you remove them, you are taking all the energy and life out of the food. Then you are left with food that has no energy and is dead. If you eat that food, you will have no energy, and you will move closer to illness, discomfort and death.*

In the big detailed book, it is written: *Enzymes are the primary motivators of all the biochemical processes in the body. They are present in all living plants and animal cells. Foods in their natural uncooked state contain all the enzymes necessary for their digestion. When a food is cooked at a temperature over 110 to 115 degrees, all of its enzymes are destroyed. This is why, if cooked food is part of your diet, there is a great need for enzyme supplementation. Vitamins, minerals, carbohydrates and protein are all nutrients that support our cells' growth, life and energy. Without enzymes, these nutrients are not available to our cells. Enzymes are needed for every chemical reaction in the body. All living organisms are made of chemicals, proteins, carbohydrates and lipids. Enzymes generate the spark of life. They are composed of groups of amino acids that act as catalysts to gov-*

ern the spleen for most of the chemical reactions involved in the metabolism of living systems. Enzymes are broken down into several different groups according to their activity. The three broad classifications of enzymes are: Metabolic, Digestive, and Food Enzymes.

Metabolic Enzymes are produced in every cell of the body to perform specific biochemical reactions in tissues and organs.

Digestive Enzymes are produced by the body, and are specifically used to break down or digest food.

Food Enzymes are not produced by the body. They are found in raw food, and are liberated during digestion.

As we age, the vital functions of our bodies become less efficient. In order to help slow down the aging process, we need to replenish our supply of biological materials and nutrients. We can help replenish our enzyme supply by eating fresh fruits and vegetables, which are rich in enzymes, and by taking enzyme supplements. When cooked food is eaten, vital enzymes that can be used for healing the body are diverted and sent to the digestive system to digest the food. Raw foods already contain enzymes that aid in their digestion. Since cooked food does not have these vital enzymes, the body takes enzymes from its vital storehouse. After digestion, these enzymes are eliminated with the body's waste. When enzymes are removed from the body after having been used in the process of digestion, the organ systems begin competing for the enzymes that are left. If the enzyme supply is not replenished, we will become enzyme deficient and our healing and restorative capacity may be diminished. If we are enzyme deficient, just going on a raw diet may restore all of our enzymes. Most fruits and vegetables only have enough enzymes to digest themselves, and do not contain extra enzymes for helping to replenish the body's supplies that were depleted by eating cooked food. In this case, an enzyme supplement is recommended. Make sure to use the best quality available. There are many brands on the market. Ask around, do research, try a few, and then use what you feel is best.

"Wow! Okay, SCM, is there anything else you would recommend I learn before I open the locks on the door to the BODY, with all the keys to health I've earned?"

"If you really want to heal yourself, once again rest is the key. However, sometimes the damage is so extensive, other, even unnatural, means may be needed to help. The main key to healing is to have an open mind and to try whatever makes sense. If you have an open mind and keep trying, you are sure to find the cure. Most people stop after trying a few things and never find the cure. Their minds are too closed. The door to health and the body will always stay closed to them."

Now you're ready to open the door. Using all the needed keys you've earned, you open it. Upon entering the room, you say, "Wow!" You realize that all the questions in the room are those SCM has already answered. SCM looks at you and says, "You had all this information even before you entered this room. To get the key to the next room, you need to sum it all up. That will be the key. How would you sum up health and the human body?"

"The cure is in the cause."

"Well done! Now you may take this key and move on to the next room."

Key Number Six to the Body:
The cure is in the cause.

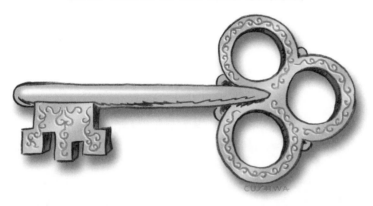

You've found the key and opened the lock.

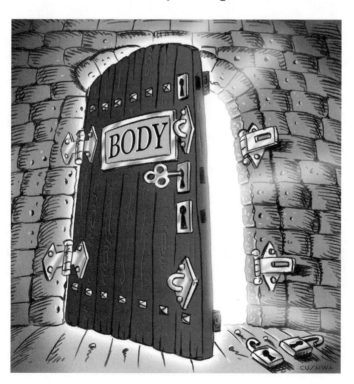

We are eating ourselves to death.
The following passage is from an extraordinary book called *Death Deferred* by Dr. Hereward Carrington. Right here is the answer to the cause, cure, and prevention of all disease.

"Of all the factors which go to making health, the food factor is doubtless the most important.

The food is the greatest producer of disease, and that its proper regulation, as to quality and quantity, is the greatest preventative measure, as well as curative measure, which we know. Why does the athlete always have to go into training for so long a period of time, and take so much exercise in his preparation for any contest requiring endurance? It is simply because his body is in such a condition that this is required, in order to get rid of a lot of useless material which should never have been introduced in the first place. We constantly overeat, and then have to take enforced exercise in order to burn up, and get rid of, this excess of food-material! If we did not eat so much in the first place, all this would not be necessary. We should prevent the accumulation of this excess of mal-assimilated food material, and then the toxic or poisonous products which result because of its presence would be avoided."

Have a good balance and you will be okay.
Hereward Carrington says:

"Every muscular effort we make, every thought we think, wastes the bodily tissues; they are broken down or destroyed by the effort. This loss is made good by the food we eat, so that, to maintain the best possible heath, the equivalence between the "income" and the "outgo" should be maintained.

We should eat just enough, not more and not less than is required to keep the body in this state of physiological equilibrium, "that just balance we call health." Less than this amount causes weakness, depletion, exhaustion, loss of weight, and all the symptoms of starvation. More than the required amount has the effect of clogging the body with an excess of effete material and choking and blocking it, and ultimately causing no end of mischief."

Paul Nison says:

The key to assure good health is not what we add to our diet but what we leave out. If we take care of our bodies and avoid putting things in them that don't belong, we will be clean and healthy. The surest way to know whether something belongs in the body or not is to listen to our bodies when they are still in the clean stages. At that point, the body is still able to react to this dirt, and begins to show signs of pain. For most of us, this happened when we were kids growing up. It is unfortunate that when we are sick or don't feel well, we are given drugs and antibiotics that actually make us dirtier rather than cleaner. We must do our best when we are young to learn what pain is and why we experience discomfort. If we eat pizza and soda or a hot dog and our stomachs gets upset, we must rest until we are better, and not put anything else into our systems. Just as we try to keep the outside of our bodies from getting dirty, we have to keep the inside of our bodies from getting dirty. It's all done in the same way: by not playing in dirt or with dirt. By avoiding dirt, we cannot get dirty. Since most of us didn't learn this lesson until now, we are already dirty inside. This dirt is what causes excess mucus and slime and other problems with our health. We will continue getting dirtier until we stop ingesting this dirt, and we'll continue to get cleaner as we rid our bodies of the excess mucus and slime.

4 | THE SOUL

You're feeling fine, walking along the main hall of the castle. You've found many keys that have let you inside to explore both the mind and the body even further. Excited, you can't wait to get into the next room to see what you'll find inside.

Upon seeing a door to your right, you stop. Turning toward the door, you spot the word: 'SOUL.'

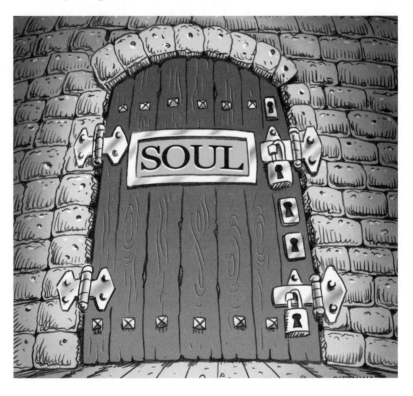

You stare at them for a second, but then you start walking away. As you continue down the hall, SCM, popping up out of nowhere, asks, "Where are you going?"

"I'm going to the next room."

"Why didn't you want to go into the SOUL room?"

"It never really interested me. My main goal is to find out about health, not about the soul."

"It would be a very smart thing to find the keys to the SOUL room before going to any of the others. Many people ignore this important room, but finding the keys to the soul is one of the pieces to the puzzle of life. Without these keys, your life will always be incomplete. Do you want to live an incomplete life?"

"Okay, okay," you stop, turn around, and start walking back to the SOUL door. But the hall is dark and you can't find it. As nighttime is approaching, the light from outside is dimming. The hall is getting dark and you're getting nervous. You ask SCM, "How can I find keys in the dark?"

"There's a lot of light inside the SOUL room, once you get inside, so hurry up and find those keys to the SOUL room, if you don't want to be left in the dark."

"Okay, I'll hurry, but where should I start?"

"You can start with the keys you already have to the mind and the body. Remember, if the soul is one part of the puzzle, that means you already have other parts. These parts will help you find the keys to the SOUL room."

Key Number One to the Soul: Don't Give Up!

Looking at the door, you see only a few locks, but they're big. You stare at the keys you already have and think about where you might find the keys to the SOUL room. You can't seem to come up with answers. It's getting darker, but you can see light under the door. SCM tells you, "The castle halls gets very cold and dark at night, but the rooms have light and heat. Keep thinking and you'll get it."

You spend hours thinking, but nothing happens. It's now very cold and very dark and you are about to give up when SCM tells you, "That's the problem with so many people. They can't take a little challenge. Once it gets dark, they run. If you want to be different, stay and figure it out. I know you can do it. So many people today commonly don't do anything but run around in the dark looking for light. Well, you know where the light is. All you have to do is find the keys to these few locks and you will be inside."

Deciding to stick it out, "You're right, I don't want to be like the rest of them. I won't run from the dark, I'll run toward the light."

"That's it." says SCM. "You have earned the first key to the SOUL room."

Key Number One to the Soul: Don't run from the dark, run towards the light.

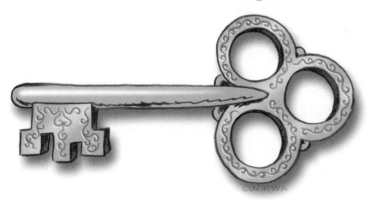

You've found the first key to the Soul.

Key Number Two to the Soul: Why We Need to Eat.

SCM congratulates you, "I'm glad you stayed and got that first important key. Now you must get the other keys. I must go now, but before I do, here is a hint. The physical body is like a car: the mind is the driver; the spirit is the gas. If you have the fastest car and the best driver, it won't get anywhere without the fuel to make it run."

SCM then vanishes into thin air. You continue to wonder how he pops up and disappears like that. In any case, you write down what he said and try to figure it out. Now you have two clues:

1. One of the keys you already have will help you find new keys.

2. The spirit is the body's fuel.

As you think about those things, you remember something else SCM told you earlier: "There are two roads to every destination, an easier road and a harder road. The key to having fun and being consistent in life is to choose the easier road. As long as they lead to the same place, why not? The easier road is not necessarily easy, but easier than the harder road. If you want to get into the SOUL room, the harder road would be to do it without cleaning your mind and body first. Yes, it can be reached without cleaning your body or mind, but why take the harder road if you don't have to? Take the easier road; in this case, to clean your mind and body first. That's the third clue."

As you think about those things, you come up with an answer: "The cleaner the car, the better the driver, the easier it will be to get to the fuel. Hmm," you think to yourself, "the soul is the fuel? I thought food was the fuel. That would mean that food only maintains the body (the car), but it is the soul that keeps it running. So if we don't need much food, all the overeating peo-

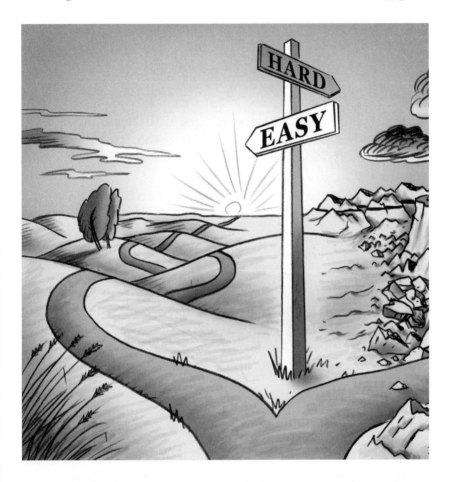

ple do just makes it harder for the body to get to the fuel (the soul). Earlier, in the other room, I learned that overeating is like taking the harder road. Overeating makes us unable to recognize the signs and clues that are already there. It would be unwise to drive a car and not see the signs. So to get to the soul, I must see the signs; and to see the signs, I must eat less food; and the food I eat must be very simple. Eating complicated food or even too much good food will put me on the harder road. When I eat that way, I feel grounded. That's what all that food does to people. The less people eat, the better off they are."

Now you're starting to sound like SCM. You feel you're getting close to the answer. It's still getting colder and it has grown very dark, but you're not letting that stop you.

"Many people are not used to being at a level of lightness. All the time, I hear people say that when they try to stop eating heavy foods, or cut back on fats in their diet, they feel lightheaded or not grounded and they can't handle it. Then, they eat heavy foods again and feel better. Maybe they just aren't ready to be at that place."

You can't see SCM anywhere, but you can hear him saying, "That's one of the keys. You've just found it."

"I did?"

"Yes, the real reason people eat is one of the keys."

"Okay," you say to yourself, "on one level, wanting to feel grounded, or just not being ready to be in a state of lightness, is the reason people eat. On another level, they eat to control their emotions. On still another level, people eat for taste. So when I think about the mind, body and soul, the key is to realize why people really eat: *

Mind - to control their emotions;

Body - for taste;

Soul - to feel grounded.

So overeating and eating bad food will keep the car from running at its best. Eating to control emotions is a way to avoid dealing with the mind. You need a good mind to be a good driver. Eating for taste is like damaging your car by putting things in it that don't belong. Overeating keeps us grounded, making it more difficult for the car to move."

*Food nourishes the body, but most people don't eat for this reason. They eat because of these reasons stated herein.

**SCM says, "Great, you've found the second
key to the Soul:
To reach the soul, you can't be
weighed down with food."**

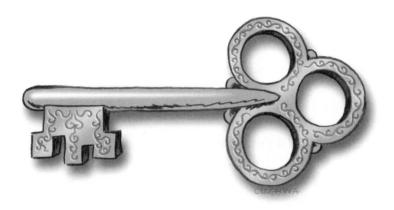

You've found the key, now open the lock.

SCM has appeared from thin air again. You can see him and hear him saying, "As you can see, the reasons people eat are not really what they think. Most people will tell you they eat to satisfy hunger. They think they must eat every day or they'll die. That is wrong. They don't eat every meal for nutrition or because they must eat. They eat for all of the reasons we've just discussed.

Eating every day is an acquired habit. People eat every day because they're accustomed to using food as a way to avoid other things. People do not eat for hunger. Were people to eat for true hunger, everything and anything would taste great. But, when people are selective with food, they're eating for other reasons besides nutrition. They're eating to satisfy appetite, not hunger. They're eating to control the three main areas I spoke of before: mind, body and soul. If they were truly hungry, they would not be selective with their food. They would eat anything, anywhere, no matter what it was. They wouldn't turn down something just because they weren't in the mood for it, or because they didn't like the taste. With true hunger, there would be no such thing. Everything would taste wonderful."

SCM goes on to say, "You did a great job. Not too many people have a key like the one you've just earned. Those who do, choose to use their God-given birthright: their minds. The reason many people do not get this key is because most people just listen to the network news. They're brainwashed, robots of society. One of my close friends, Stan Glaser, says it best about food when it comes to spirituality or the soul:

"I think a reason many people don't have much success on raw food diets is because they are not used to living on that level of lightness or that level of energy. People really don't get energy from food. They get energy from the cosmos. It is your God-given gift. This is why if you fast a little bit you have more energy than you know what to do with. You can't even sleep. So what we are doing most of our lives is using most of our energy to digest food. Not necessarily getting energy from the food. As you eat lighter and lighter, your body can process more easily without using all of its resources. When this happens, you will start to experience lots of energy. This newfound energy does not feel grounded to the normal person. This is when it is very important to have a spiritual context. I think spirituality at its best is teaching your body and mind how to deal with this infinite energy. If not, you won't feel good, or as I say, grounded, and you are going to wind up eating heavier foods to use the energy again. I think it is very important to have success with the raw diet." **—Stan Glaser**

SCM concludes, "Once we clean our minds and bodies, and are ready to live with the lightness that less eating and a clean body will produce, we will be ready to really get in touch with a much higher power."

"Thank you, SCM, for all your help."

"Don't thank me; you did it yourself. You figured out the answers. Now go and find the next key so you can get into that room. It's cold out here."

Once again, SCM disappears into thin air.

Key Number Three to the Soul: What Does SOUL Mean?

SCM says, "The next key has something to do with what you found in the MIND room."

You think about it, but you can't come up with an answer.

SCM tells you, "Words, or just one word: the *SOUL* room. Do you know what the word 'soul' really means?

"Not really."

"It could mean many different things. Some people call it spirituality; some call it religion. Although there are many different words for it, they all mean the same thing: to believe there is more out there than the physical form we're in, to believe there is a higher power."

From what SCM tells you, you deduce that there's a much higher level out there that we can all reach. There are different names for it, all meaning the same thing. Some people call it spirituality, some call it religion, and there are many other names for this level. The name doesn't really matter. Many people are searching to get to this higher level. Some will reach it, many will not. However, many will reach it, yet not realize they have, because their bodies are so toxic from a poor diet and incorrect thinking. Their toxic conditions will block them from noticing signs showing they've already reached a spiritual level. No matter what people call it, once they've cleaned their minds and bodies, they will recognize soul more easily and understand how this cleansing will lead to getting in touch with its powers.

"That's right," says SCM. "You see, this is the biggest change people go through when they cleanse their minds and bodies. Many people aren't even looking for it; it just happens. Even though they weren't looking for it, some of them sure are happy they've found it. Some people know how to handle it, some don't. Others are simply not ready.

So now you get it. Once you reach this level, you'll realize there is much more out there than just this physical life. You'll see everything in a different light. You'll see things that you didn't think existed, but were there all along.

The signs are always there, but people are not able to see them because they've put unnatural things in their minds and bodies. Once you clean the mind and body, these signs become so clear and evident."

Now you have another key.

Key Number Three to the Soul: Its name doesn't matter; it's a higher power we all can reach.

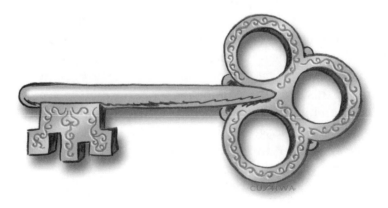

You've found the key. Now open the lock.

Key Number Four to the Soul: Spirituality Is Contagious.

SCM tells you, "The next key can be found in the same place as all the other keys. The hints are in all the rooms you've already visited. You've already found keys to open many locks on the SOUL door. Here's the next one:"

Remember when SCM told you in the MIND room, "The company you surround yourself with will influence you, so choose it wisely? Well, it's the same in this room as well. Being around people who are already at this level is a great help. Your body is electric and not just chemical. If you've ever seen pictures taken by an aura camera, you'd be able to see what I mean. The people already at this level of lightness have a special energy you can feel when you're around them, no matter what level you're on. The people you surround yourself with will not only make your life easier, but also feed you the energy of this higher power. This is an important key. But even more important, when you are clean in mind and body, you will recognize the signs. If a person is not yet there physically and mentally, he or she will still feel the energy, but not recognize it.

SCM says, "Now you've got it." Here is a quote from my friend Benito De Donno, from his book, ***Glimpses of Reality:***

"Spirituality is contagious; you can catch it from someone else. Spiritual energy is like heat or radioactivity; it emanates from a source and radiates in all directions. Everyone subjected to its influence is affected by it. That is why spiritually advanced persons cannot hide their secret for long. Sooner or later, someone will feel the elevating and uplifting influence of their presence and will tell others."

Key Number Four to the Soul: Surround yourself with special people.

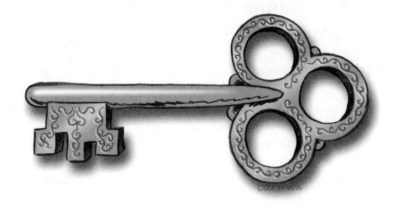

You've found the key, now open the lock.

Key Number Five: Nourishment of Soul and Body.

By now, all the locks on the door to the SOUL room are open, except for one. If you get this key, you can open the door. Then, you may enter this room. You start to think about it. By now, you've been in this cold, dark hallway all night. You can still see light under the door, but it's almost dawn outside. As the sky is turning from black to orange to blue, you realize that the sun will be up soon. You reflect on the information you've already received. You understand that this final key has to do once again with the nourishment of the body. You ask yourself, "What nourishes the body and how much of it do I need? I understand from what I've learned in the castle of knowledge that much food is really not needed in order to be healthy or to reach the special place of lightness to experience the soul. Taking all this into consideration, the answer to how much food the body really needs is: as little as possible.

In the right environment, if the body is ready, a person can thrive on very little food. This has been proven. As you noticed in other rooms of the castle, there is proof that man needs very little food. We do not get our major nutrition or energy from food. As the sun starts to come up, SCM, who you can hear but not see, asks, "So, where do we get most of our nourishment?"

You reply, "From spiritual energy."

SCM beams, "That's right. Spiritual energy is what gives the body energy. Do you know why?"

"Yes, because when you receive spiritual energy, your soul is energized. People who are not there yet are stimulating their bodies with food and they call that 'energy.' But the truth is: that is not energy, it's only stimulation. Stimulation works like a battery. It keeps us moving, but stimulation, just as in that battery, will run out. But spiritual energy will never run out."

"That's correct," says SCM. "If food were needed to keep you energized, then why is it that some people don't run out of energy if they stop eating?"*

You agree with him, adding, "As long as people keep eating, how come they lose energy anyway? That just proves that food doesn't give the body energy."

SCM agrees with you 100% and asks, "What material substances are needed from outside the body to produce energy?"

"Only clean air and clean water, if we are in the proper environment. They will keep us clean, and enable us to receive the pranic energy into our bodies to produce energy and sustain life.

SCM is impressed, "Wow, I didn't even think you knew about pranic energy, you are 100% correct. Can you tell me more about it? Now he is asking you questions, and you feel great.

*The cleaner a person's blood, the better he or she will feel on less food. However, the dirtier the blood, the worse he or she will feel on less food. This is because the ingestion of food holds back the toxins from getting in the bloodstream.

"Sure, there are many definitions of pranic energy. The term is used in yoga all the time. When our bodies are dirty it's hard for them to use this energy, but when we are clean and ready for it, then you will notice the tremendous feeling of this life energy."

SCM tells you, "To experience pranic energy, you must understand what prana is. Remember in the room of the body you learned one of the most important functions of life."

"Yes, it is breathing," you reply.

"Well," SCM tells you, "to a degree, that is what prana is. Actually it means controlling the breath, and thus calming the nerves. Once you can do that you can use it to control the mind and the body. Once you're in control over them, you will be able to feel pranic energy."

PRANIC ENERGY:
"As soon as the stream of creative energy enters the human body, it is split into two currents; one goes into the throat center, the other into the nervous system. The first combines with the oxygen in the lungs, and subsequently with the hemoglobin and red cells. The blood system will see to it that such life-giving energy is transported to all the body's cells. This will be the primal and only energy used to build all the tissues of the body, without exception."
—**From *Glimpses of Reality* by Benito De Donno.**

"When can you experience the highest amount of pranic energy?" asks SCM.

"When my body is clean and free of toxins, you reply. That is when I will feel it, and also see the signs I've missed all these years. If I have a dirty body, I will not be able to feel it, or recognize the signs."

"Is there a way to recognize all of this?" SCM asks. "When one is ready, is there a sign to tell that this level has been reached?"

"There is a space between our eyes that some people call the third eye," you tell him, "the eye of knowledge. I call it the first eye. When people eat cooked foods and put things in their bodies that don't belong there, their toxic build up keeps that eye shut. As people start to eat cleaner more healthful foods, that eye starts to open. In time, they will be able to see all the signs that passed them by when their first eye was closed. All of us have this eye, and we just have to open it to see the unseen.

There are signs everywhere once this eye is open."

"Very well," SCM jubilantly exclaims, "you have found the last key!"

Key Number Five to the Soul:
The body derives its nourishment not from food, but from pranic energy. That is what nourishes the body; most food merely stimulates it."

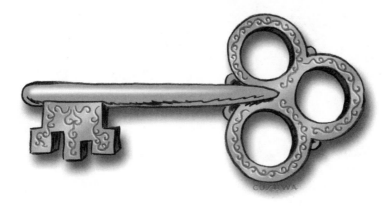

You've found the key; now open the lock and the door.

Upon opening the SOUL door, you whisper to yourself, "Wow, this is such a beautiful room." Just as you open the door to the soul, the sun comes up, bathing your face in brightness

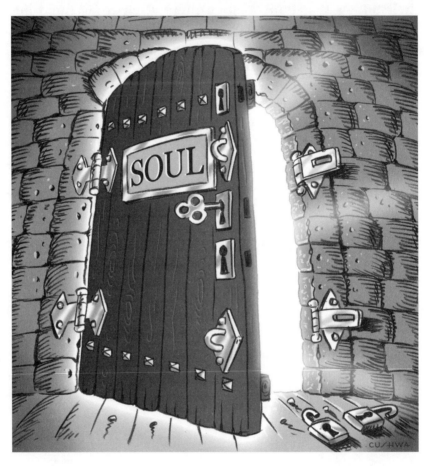

and warmth. It was perfect timing to create the most beautiful moment.

Once inside, you experience many amazing visions. Then you spot a sign that reads: 'You have said enough. Say no more about what is in this room. Each seeker must find out for himself. The keys you have earned to arrive here will also help many others get here and recognize the same signs you did; a job well done. Spend as much time as you need in this room and enjoy all it holds. Earn some more keys, and move on to the next room. Keep moving forward. Never stop.'

5 | THE ANSWER: ALWAYS LOOK WITHIN

After you've spent a long time in the castle, SCM hands you one last key, a big one.

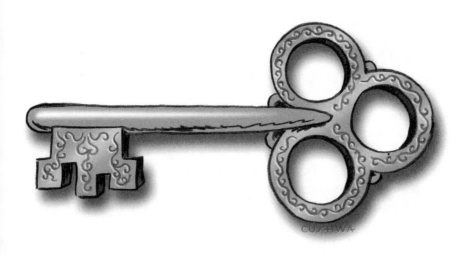

You ask him, "What's it for?"

SCM says, "You've spent so much time here learning, you haven't realized one of the main keys."

You ask him, "Which one is that?"

"Having fun," he replies. "Although your work is important, seeking knowledge is also important, and you can find fun in doing both. But, most important of all is having fun and enjoying yourself, no matter what you decide to do in life."

"That sounds great, but SCM, what's the key for?"

"It's the key to the castle, and it's for you. You've spent so much time here working to get the keys, it would be a good idea for you to leave the castle. Take a vacation and enjoy yourself. Have some fun! This big key is to the front door of the castle. You can come back and visit as much as you like, but for now you'd do best to go out and enjoy yourself."

"Thanks, SCM, but I still have two questions. What does SCM stand for? And how does SCM always pop up out of thin air?"

SCM reveals, "Here is the answer to your first question: I am you. SCM stands for Sub Conscious Mind. When you were talking to SCM, you were talking to yourself, simply asking yourself questions. Every time you thought you were looking to SCM for an answer, you were actually asking yourself. Your subconscious mind was giving you the answer your conscious mind could not.

The answer to your second question: Since SCM is, and has always been, part of you, SCM would always pop up whenever you needed help. SCM will always be with you. As you learned from the beginning, whenever you have a question, before looking outside for the answer, always look within, deep within. Do that, and chances are you will find what you are looking for."

"Now that I have the knowledge of the mind, body and soul, I own the castle of knowledge. I can visit it whenever I please. We all own a castle of knowledge and have that choice;

we just have to get past fear. The way to do that is to visit our castles and get the knowledge...

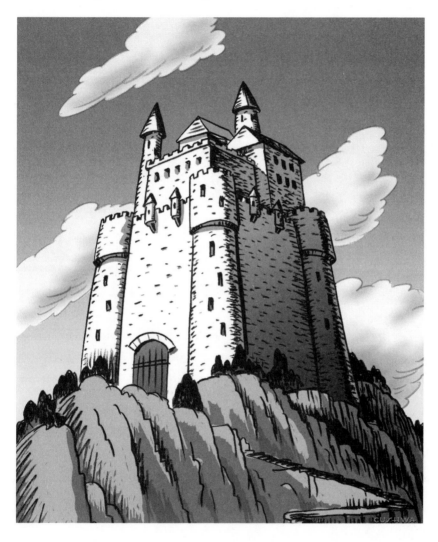

I've just found a very special room in the castle: the Museum of Knowledge. In this room interviews are found with some of the most knowledgeable people in the world. They own the biggest castles of knowledge, and here in the museum they will share their knowledge with you. They'll share information with you that you can harness to make *your* castle as big as they've made *theirs*. Go to the next chapter and find out their keys to success."

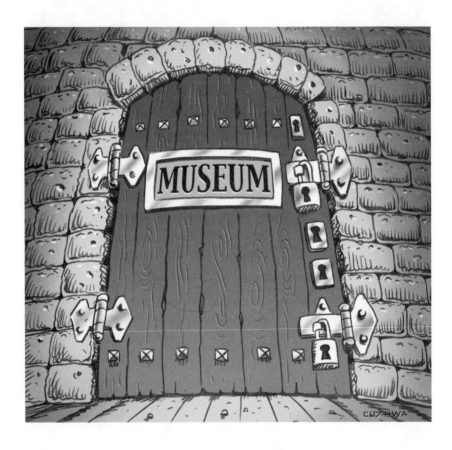

6 | THE INTERVIEWS

Many readers of my first book have asked, "Why not more interviews?" They were pleased with the interviews they had read and told me what a great learning experience they had provided, not only to hear about my background, but also to hear how many people had discovered the great message of how to achieve health and happiness. Since then, I've been working hard to meet and interview as many people as possible who have been successful in this endeavor. To say the least, the response has been overwhelming. Not only has it personally brought me great insight, but also I've made many new friends who have shared information that has proved very important to my growth progress. The interviews I held with these far-reaching pioneers will give you great insight as well.

First, I would like to clear up some confusion. After having read the interviews in my first book, many people also expressed some confusion, asking why the pioneers I interviewed answered the same questions very differently.

In this book, I have tried my best to get the point across that there is never one answer to it all. No two people are in the same place at the same time, so the answer will always be different. The people I interviewed did what made the most sense to them at that time in *their* lives. Read what they did

159

and if it makes sense and gives you ideas to try something, that's great. But, if what they did doesn't make any sense, don't try it. If you understand what they are suggesting, chances are it will make sense to you. But, just because you don't agree with something they said or did doesn't mean they are incorrect. At the same time, their word is not set in stone as being correct. Read the information and process it. After thinking about it, if the information makes sense and you think it can help you, then, do it. There is information in these interviews for everyone. Read them all and you will find what you are looking for.

Many of my readers ask me who is right and who is wrong, or whose way is best. They are all correct because they did what worked for them at that time in their lives. I have my personal favorites and I'm sure we all do. I have met and interviewed many more successful people than those included in my books, but these are my favorites. I do not agree with all of them 100%, but what I value in all of them is the same great accomplishment they have in common: they are successful in achieving their goals. They did what they had to do to get it done and continue to do so.

When writing **Raw Knowledge**, I set a goal to include some more great interviews to share with you. I planned to have at least the same number of interviews that were in my book, **The Raw Life**, which was nine. I have more than doubled that number this time. After seeking and finding the world leaders in this movement, gathering all the interviews and putting this book together, I came to the realization that there is simply too much material. Another of my goals is to keep the size of the book as small as possible in order to keep the price as low as possible, yet, at the same time, to get all the information out to you. First, I decided that I would select only the best interviews. But, after reading all of them again and again, I couldn't come up with a best list because they all contained important information that I didn't want to keep all to myself. What was I to do? I could have put all the interviews in this book and had a very big book. But, instead I decided to have two books: Part I and Part II. Thus, I could place a few interviews in this book, *Raw Knowledge, Part I*, and the rest in *Raw Knowledge, Part II: Interviews with Health Achievers*. And that is what I did. In no special order, I included half of the interviews in this book and the remainder in *Raw Knowledge, Part II*. All these interviews contain a message for everyone, and I recommend you get both parts and read them all.

At the end of this section is a list of the experts whose interviews appear in Part II, along with a brief bio about them. But first, here are the interviews I included in this book. If you would like to order *Raw Knowledge, Part II*, you may do so from:

Paul Nison   Or you may call:
PO Box 443   **866-RAW-DIET**
Brooklyn, NY 11209   (866-729-3438)

Or you may order it from my website:
www.rawlife.com

Now, here are interviews to give you the raw knowledge to be successful and happy in life, whether through eating a healthy diet or achieving the goals you might have.

A final note about the interviews: Many of the people I interviewed are 100% raw. They eat only raw fruits, vegetables, nuts and seeds. However, some still eat small amounts of cooked food. I included their interviews to help get an important message out. That salient message is: It's not about being 100% perfect, it's about doing the best you can and being 100% happy!

Now, here are the interviews. Enjoy!

*Many of the people I interviewed have donated some of their delicious raw recipes. You can view them all in the recipe section at the back of this book.

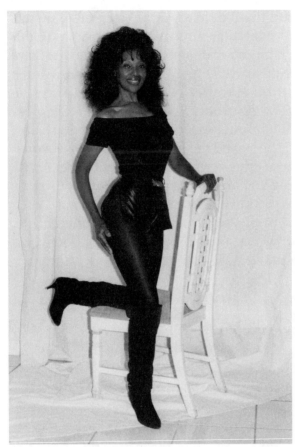

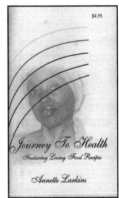

Annette is the author of a great little booklet titled *Journey To Health*, featuring Living Food recipes. To speak to Annette, contact her at the information below.

Web Site: www.annettelarkins.com
Email: Annette@annettelarkins.com

PO Box 770097
Miami, FL 33277
305-238-1169

Annette Larkins

At sixty and still beautiful, Annette's secret has been a raw food diet for many years. When I learned this about her, I knew that an interview with her would enhance my book.

I almost met Annette a few years ago when I was in Florida giving lectures. One of my lectures was canceled and so we did not have the chance to meet at that time. After interviewing Annette on the telephone about a year later, I was so moved by her message, "Enlighten and enhance your existence through living foods," that I decided to go to South Florida and give her a visit. I now have another friend who understands the benefits of the raw food diet.

How many years have you been on the raw diet, and what got you into it?
I became a vegetarian thirty-nine years ago; I have been a living foodist (eating live and raw foods) for seventeen years. I view the transition from vegetarian to living foodist as a natural evolution. The more I learned and the better I felt, the more I wanted to learn and the better I wanted to feel. It makes sense that foods in their natural raw state offer optimal nutrition.

How was your health before you started the diet?
I was not ill when I became a vegetarian, but after becoming one, I noticed that my immune system became stronger, my energy level increased, and I was not sleepy after a big meal as I had been when I ate animal flesh.

Who are some people who have inspired you to do this?
Ann Wigmore and Norman Walker were great sources of inspiration to me.

Is there any one person who has inspired you the most?
Most of the books I read were by authors who had cured themselves of illness by introducing living foods into their diet; they were all inspirational.

You have learned so much over the years. What are some of the most important things you have learned?
I have learned that we must keep the body well cleansed and well nourished in order to function properly psychologically, physiologically, and Spiritually, according to the master plan.

Are there any pitfalls you have learned to watch out for on the raw diet?
The mistake that I made initially was trying to sustain myself on salads alone. I had to learn to prepare live, raw foods that appealed to my taste buds.

Weight loss is a big pitfall for many people. Do you have any thoughts about that?
If we eat properly and give the body a chance to find its balance, adjustments will be made in time, and the body will find its natural weight.

What is your opinion of nuts and seeds?
I include soaked and unsoaked nuts and seeds in my diet. I prepare a variety of dishes, such as loaves, patties, cookies, crackers, and pates… Yummy yummy says my tummy!

What is your opinion of grains?
I eat any sprouted grains that I like, even wheat. Unless I experience some ill effect from grains, I shall continue to partake of them, as always.

What is your opinion of eating a mostly fruit diet?
I certainly enjoy whole fruits and their juices, and I see no reason to exclude them from one's daily diet, unless a specific condition dictates otherwise. I choose variety over leaning to-

wards one particular food—for example my diet includes fruits, nuts, vegetables, and seeds.

What is your opinion of sprouts?
Because I grow and eat sprouts in such abundance, I call myself a living foodist. These tiny, succulent morsels (sprouts) continue to grow even after harvest and refrigeration; therefore, when we eat them, we are eating living foods. Isn't that wonderful?

What is your opinion of the Natural Hygiene Diet (eating food in its most natural state as found in nature)?
I support the Natural Hygiene philosophy, but I do not practice it religiously. However, my journey continues, and I do not know where it will lead me.

What is your opinion of supplements?
Vitamin pills or capsules as supplements are not a part of my diet regimen.

What is your opinion of eating seasonally?
Of course it is best to eat foods in season, but, alas, I am guilty of seasonal deviation. Salvador Dali said, "Have no fear of perfection; you'll never reach it."

What is your opinion of fasting?
Fasting is a great way to give the digestive system a rest. I fast every Thursday. It just seems like a good day.

What is your opinion of food combining on a 100% raw diet, and is it necessary?
Since different foods require different enzymes and different lengths of time to digest, it stands to reason that proper combinations are conducive to good digestion. Nevertheless, I believe that a 100% raw diet offers more advantages and gives more flexibility than an omnivorous diet. For example, waste matter passes more quickly through the system on a raw diet. When one eats foods in their natural, raw state, perhaps not as

much harm is done to the system as when one eats an omnivorous, cooked diet. The foods I am careful not to mix are melons; I always try to eat them alone. It is important to include predigested foods such as fermented dishes. Also, it is important to avoid overeating.

What is your opinion of physical exercise?
In my booklet, *Journey To Health*, I advise readers to find an exercise that they can enjoy such as sports, walking, dancing, or whatever—just move that body! Physical exercise is a must, but make it fun.

What are your age, height, and weight? Has your weight changed, or are there any other changes your body has gone through? How did you handle it?
I am sixty years young, five feet six inches tall, and I weigh one hundred and ten pounds. People frequently ask if my waist has always been so small (18 inches). I have always had a small waist, but when I entered the living-foods' realm (live and raw), it got even smaller. Obviously, my weight balanced out to where it should be. I never experienced any ill effects like some people do, and the good effects include mental alertness and mental acumen. I never experienced a downside during transition, so I cannot personally relate to the bad detoxification issue. I have read about people who experienced problems during their transition, but those who made it through the unpleasantness were grateful in the end.

Do you eat 100% raw foods, and if so, for how long? If not, what do you eat that is cooked, and why?
I have been 100% raw for seventeen years. A few years ago I tried to reintroduce some fired (cooked) foods into my diet, but my body would not have it; I felt weighty, bloated, and ill at ease.

What is your average daily diet like? What do you eat,

and how often?

I eat as many times a day as hunger dictates, and that varies depending on the season, the month, or the week. Appeasing hunger, rather than appetite, is my goal. As a rule, I do not break the fast before afternoon, because that is the point at which I have evolved. I like to begin my first meal with juice or fruit, but if I desire something else, I eat it.

What is your favorite food?

I do not have a favorite food per se. My food is ambrosia (food of the gods); my drink is nectar. My favorite food depends on my mood.

Out of all of the foods, which one do you think is the most important?

The molecular structure of chlorophyll is similar to that of hemoglobin; hence, it is sometimes called green blood. There are therapeutic properties in chlorophyll as well. Therefore, greens get my vote as the most important foods, if I must choose one.

How are your health and energy?

I have the blood pressure of a child. There are no cholesterol problems, since there are no animal substances in my blood. Although diabetes is prevalent in my family history, it has spared me. I dislike using definitive terms such as "always," "never" and similar expressions, but seldom do I have any ailments. If anything ails me, I know how to remedy the problem without resorting to traditional, conventional medications or invasive treatments. I joke that if I could bottle and sell my energy, we would all be rich.

How much sleep do you get, and how much do you think is necessary?

I get as much sleep as my body tells me I need; I really do not count the hours. I go by how I feel when I awake. I believe the amount necessary is an individual requirement.

What mental changes have you noticed?
I have always possessed a good memory, but my mental prowess increased on the raw diet. I am keener in thought, more alert, and more of a profound thinker. In other words, the light shines brighter. This shoots down the theory of memory loss due to aging.

Many people just beginning a raw diet have problems because their mates do not want to change. Do you have any comments or suggestions? What are your thoughts about relationships?
We should not try to coerce others into our way of living. We should set an example and hope that we will influence others to at least investigate our lifestyle. When I became a vegetarian, I cooked two separate meals for eighteen years—one for my family and one for me. People of different religious and political persuasions can manage to co-exist, so why can't people who have different food views do the same? It is understandable that when one discovers anything of worth, there is a natural tendency to want to share it with others; nevertheless, we must allow each individual the right to choose his or her standard of living.

Has your opinion of sex changed over the years?
I was a sensual, sexual being before; now, I am a sensual, sexual being living in the raw, on a more heightened level.

Do you think it is harder for a woman to eat a raw diet than it is for a man?
I do not believe that gender is a factor; it depends on the individual.

Do you think there are more raw men or more raw women? Why do you think that is?
I think there are more raw women. I think that machismo may play a part in it. Some men may think that in order to be strong and muscular, they must eat cooked animal flesh. Some

men do not think that raw food will satisfy their taste buds; they do not think raw food is filling. Of course, some women think the same way, but I think more men than women have those thoughts.

What are your thoughts about the female menstruation cycle? Do you think it is natural for a woman not to bleed when she is on a raw diet?

Although I have read that women on a raw food diet bled little or stopped bleeding completely, that was not my experience. I do not think women should feel they have a problem because they continue to menstruate. I think more research needs to be done in this area. Women were designed to bleed periodically until completion of menopause. If this natural occurrence is interrupted, there may be cause for concern.

What is your view on menopause and the raw food diet?

I have no set answers, but I shall tell you about a personal experience with menopause. One day some years ago, I realized that I had not had a menstrual period for two or three months. My cycle had always been like clockwork. I could count on it, the same time each month. I thought to myself, "I hope that I am not pregnant, because I do not want to have anything come out of me that I am this much older than." After a negative pregnancy report, I concluded that it must be menopause knocking at my door. I never had any other indication, such as hot flashes, memory loss, weight gain, crying spells, or other symptoms that many women claim to have. I attribute my lack of symptoms to my raw food diet.

Thank you for giving this interview. Is there anything you would like to add?

I extend an invitation to all to feast at the royal table of life, where you can drink in the beautiful sights and taste of the delicious cuisine. I hope that your experience will leave you enlightened and ready to enhance your existence through living foods.

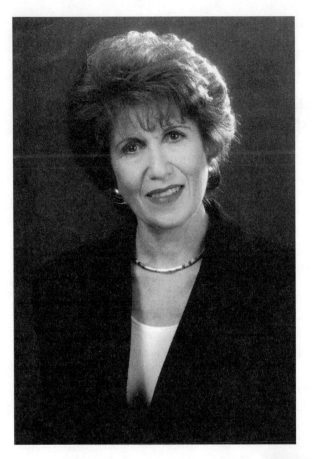

You may contact Célène at:

PO Box 171
Highlands North 2037
Johannesburg, South Africa
Web site: www.healthseekers.co.za
E-mail: celene@healthseekers.co.za

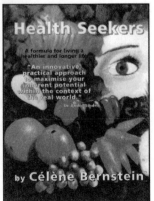

Célène Bernstein

C élène is one of the nicest women I have ever spoken to. She has more knowledge about health and the raw food diet than most people do in this world. She worked many years to obtain this knowledge, and her book *Health Seekers* explains her message of how to make a successful transformation to a healthier diet in an excellent format. She shares many of her ideas in this interview, and I recommend everyone read her book for a full understanding of how the human body works.

Célène has been interested in the field of alternative health for the past twenty-five years. She has a B.A. degree in remedial teaching from the University of the Witwatersrand, Johannesburg and taught retarded children for many years. Subsequently, she taught normal children in the local government schools where she came across many learning problems which might have been overlooked but for her experience with retarded children. She began reading books by Adelle Davis and realized the great urgency to change the eating habits of these children.

Célène pursued her knowledge by studying Health and Nutritional Science at the American College of Health Science, known as the Life Science Institute in Austin, Texas, USA, now relocated to Winnipeg, Canada.

She is the principal in South Africa of the same Health and Nutritional Science Correspondence Course and has over 120 students. She works in conjunction with medical doctors, where she is first and foremost a teacher who assists in the re-evaluation of an individual's eating patterns and lifestyle. In addition, she gives lectures and runs seminars on health-related educational issues at various institutions.

She is the author of a great book titled *Health Seekers*. For more information about her book or to contact her, please visit her website at: *www.healthseekers.co.za*

What got you into the raw lifestyle?
I am a remedial teacher, and I taught retarded children for many years. I felt it was absolutely essential for me to help parents cope more easily with their children. With the help of my reading and research, I decided I would change these children's eating habits to more raw and healthier choices of food. As a result, their behavior improved, and it was much easier for their parents to handle them.

I then left the school for retarded children and transferred to the normal government schools. There I taught many children who were on Rityalin, a psychoactive drug. I made up my mind that I was going to get these children off Rityalin through a correct eating pattern. Without doubt, I received incredible results from these children. They had better concentration, their work improved dramatically, and they all dispensed with the Rityalin. The parents were very grateful for what I had done for their children, and of course I felt a great sense of achievement.

That is when I decided to take the Life Science Nutritional Course through correspondence. At that time, it was in Austin, Texas. (It is now called Feeling Fit for Life Sciences Institute and is stationed in Winnipeg, Canada). I needed to learn more and, of course, I wanted a certificate of recognition. I also received a professorship, in an honorary capacity from the Institute.

How was your health when you started the diet?
I had to change my eating patterns as I suffered severe constipation and had pleurisy. I was aware that taking laxatives for my constipation was not the answer as I was only treating the symptom and not the cause of my problem. I also had a hysterectomy, which I now realize was Mal(E)practice. To date I have had no pleurisy or constipation symptoms. I am glad that I made changes to my initial eating pattern.

Did you make the change to a raw food diet overnight,

or was it a slow transition?
I did not start off on total raw food. I decided first to cut out meat, fish, and chicken. I decided to become a vegetarian with occasional eating of mozzarella cheese.As the years went by and I obtained more information about diet and health, I became stricter in my choice of foods.At the time of my studies, through the Life Science Institute, it was emphasized that one should live mainly on fresh fruit, raw vegetables, very little cooked, and no supplementation whatsoever. However through my own further research I realized that the way food is grown today, the soil does not contain all the necessary nutrients, so correct nutritional supplementation is ABSOLUTELY NECESSARY. In South Africa, it is not very easy to obtain organically grown fruit and vegetables, and if one can get such, there is very little variety. I am glad that I began THIS roller coaster of better health. I feel so well and have lots of energy.

Do you eat a 100% raw food diet? If not, what do you eat that is cooked?
I eat raw food 99% of the time. I am a total vegan.The cooked foods that I eat occasionally are brown rice, baked potatoes, sweet potatoes, and steamed vegetables.

Is there a reason why you eat cooked food?
Here in South Africa, we do not get those wonderful raw foods that the raw food bulletins advertise. So we are really at a disadvantage.At times our raw diet can be rather boring, I only like to eat fruits and vegetables in season, so it is not very easy to always eat total raw foods and keep it exciting. Nothing I eat comes from cold storage.This gives me the opportunity to look forward to the new season's fruits and vegetables, etc. I do not insist that people only eat raw foods.We are definitely not living in Utopia. But because of the diseases manifesting so rapidly, there is a great urgency for people to look to their

existing eating patterns and make the necessary adjustments to gain better health.

Who are some people who have inspired you to do this?
The person who inspired me to change my eating habits initially was Adelle Davis. Then I started reading *Fit for Life* by Harvey and Marilyn Diamond. I must also mention the Natural Hygiene Course, that I studied through correspondence at The Life Science Institute in Austin, Texas. The course really set me going on a change in my eating patterns and lifestyle.

Is there any one person, book, or program that has inspired you the most?
Fit for Life made a lot of sense to me. Harvey Diamond obviously had also done the Natural Hygiene course through The Life Science Institute. I really was inspired to continue with this new eating plan from the Natural Hygiene course because of the improved results I had with my health problems.

You have learned so much over the years. What are some of the most important things you have learned?
I really believe that everyone has to look at their existing eating plan and lifestyle if they are not experiencing optimal health. I have learned through my counseling of clients that eating is a social activity, and it is not very easy to take that away from people. I always advise my clients that it is not what you do now and again that will create the problem, but what you do continuously and habitually that will bring on degenerative diseases. I always make my clients ask themselves three very important questions; the answers will make them decide how necessary it is to change their eating patterns and lifestyle. The three questions are:

1) What are the real roots of YOUR problem?

2) What can YOU do in general to aid your recovery?

3) What can YOU do specifically that medicine, surgery, and

physicians cannot?

When I ask my clients to answer these questions, they come up with the answers: They have to make the change. They have to take responsibility and not push this responsibility totally onto their physician. We are the architects of our own misery. We can create our own destiny.

Are there any pitfalls you have learned to watch out for on the raw diet?

I wouldn't like to look at the completely negative side of a raw diet, using the word "pitfalls". I would rather concentrate on the positive aspects of eating raw and make clients aware that there are certain rules one can follow to eliminate certain reactions they are experiencing. I cannot impose my rigid way of eating onto my clients. I must say that in time, many have become more radical and feel totally safe in what they are doing. For that I give myself a pat on the back!!

Losing too much weight is a big pitfall for many people new to the raw food diet. Do you have any thoughts about that?

I think it is a positive. Everybody needs to lose a few extra pounds. However, if weight loss continues, I as a nutritional consultant would introduce some unadulterated cooked food such as steamed vegetables, brown rice, millet, etc. After a few weeks, I would introduce a total raw food diet depending on how the client was feeling. I would offer him the choice, provided that his health problems had improved. I would also insist that people do weight resistance exercise so the body will build bone and muscle mass.

Teeth problems also seem to be a big pitfall for many people on a raw food diet. Do you have any thoughts about that?

I see this problem if citrus is eaten in abundance. I have made a rule in my book *Health Seekers* that whenever any citrus is eaten, one should rinse one's mouth thoroughly after eating that fruit. This is because citrus fruits tend to make our teeth lose enamel. I do insist that people eat a variety of fruits and not stick to one kind in abundance.

What is your opinion of mercury fillings?
Mercury fillings can play a big role in the illnesses people are suffering. The problem is, you have to find a very good dentist trained in the removal of mercury fillings, and of course some mercury could leak into the system when being removed. I feel that removal of mercury fillings should be a last resort. I would rather let the client change his eating pattern and lifestyle and note the improvements in his health. I believe a 20% change in a person's eating pattern and lifestyle will bring about an 80% improvement in his health, especially if the client is not very ill to begin with.

What is your opinion of nuts and seeds?
Provided that both the nuts and seeds are unsalted and un-roasted, I definitely encourage my vegetarian clients to add these to acid fruits. Doing this helps slow down the metaboliz-ing of the sugar found in fruit. This goes well for clients who tend to be hypoglycemic. I often encourage my clients, who are new to this program of better eating, to eat unsalted and unroasted macadamia nuts with sub-acid or sweet fruits, or even add them to cooked brown rice, millet, etc. This is really for traditional changeover eating patterns. I like my clients to have nuts or seeds at least three times per week. They are a very good form of protein and essential fatty acids. Almonds are the most alkaline of the nuts. Tahini sauce made from pulped sesame seeds is an excellent source of calcium. I am not in favor of people snacking on nuts. They can overdo the eating of nuts if they are eaten alone, and nuts often make peo-

ple very thirsty if eaten alone. I only allow half cup per day, correctly combined with the correct food, three times per week.

What is your opinion of grains?
They have to be unrefined. Examples are brown rice, millet, quinoa, and polenta. I am not in favor of eating these grains every single day. I do find that my clients enjoy these dishes in the wintertime. I do however encourage them not to have them more than once a week. If they like something cooked, I would rather they had steamed vegetables. Grains can be very mucous forming.

What is your opinion of an all fruit diet?
I feel that doing so for only a week is acceptable, if you are not feeling well. Eating this way gives the body a lot more energy for healing. If one wants to go on a detoxification diet, eating fruit only in correct combinations works wonders. However, I would not like my clients to do this for more than one month at the most. I do find, if fruit only is eaten for a long period, cravings for the wrong foods definitely manifest. If the fruit is not organic, it should be peeled, and of course I suggest one should only eat fruits in season and definitely not choose imported fruits, since they are highly sprayed.

What is your opinion of sprouts?
This is a wonderful food, alfalfa, mung beans, etc. They are delicious sprinkled over a salad.

What is your opinion of the Natural Hygiene philosophy?
I do promote this philosophy, but with some changes. We are not living in Utopia, and also the media does not make it easy for us to purchase organic fresh fruit and vegetables. The Life Science course is in the process of having new information added to the original course. I have been asked to add to the course.

What is your opinion of supplements?
This is a very important issue. Natural Hygiene says no supplementation. We have to understand that the soil in which food is grown today does not contain all the essential nutrients, so without doubt, our food is lacking in essential nutrients. One has to choose natural whole food concentrates. I have done a great deal of research regarding the right whole food concentrates, and I have used them with great success in my nutritional practice.

What is your opinion of eating seasonally?
This is very important. Eating this way gives our body a great variety of raw fruit and vegetables, and of course we can look forward to the new fruits of each season. I will never ever eat fruit that has been in cold storage or is imported. Here in South Africa they have grapes throughout the year. They are also very expensive. I just say to myself, "You cannot have them—just look and shut your mouth."

What is your opinion of fasting?
I definitely believe that fasting heals the body ever so much quicker. When one fasts, one should do it under supervision. I have written a special chapter on fasting in my book *Health Seekers*. I do believe that we have to give the body a rest every now and again.

What is your opinion of food combining on a 100% raw diet, and is it necessary?
I do believe in correct food combining, especially if one is eating cooked meals. I feel it is not that necessary on a raw diet. I do suggest, however, that melons should not be combined with any other fruits, only with each other.

What is your opinion of physical exercise?
It is very important. It is part of the non-nutritive factors we

have to take into account to enjoy better health.

What is your age, height, and weight? Has your weight changed, or were there other changes your body went through? How did you handle it?

I am fifty-nine years old. I am five feet tall exactly. My body fat is 17% and I have no cellulite. I have a well-toned body. I have never really had a weight problem. I do find, however, that I waver between 44 and 45 kilos (97 and 100 pounds). The extra kilos (pounds) occur in the winter when I eat more cooked food in the form of grains and gluten-free bread. When I stay on raw foods, I can drop two kilos. So weight loss seems to be a problem with me. So every now and again, I will eat some steamed vegetables, brown rice, or millet, etc. I have not eaten dairy products for five years. When I eat at a restaurant, I only eat a raw salad with cold pressed olive oil. If there is no oil, I will have an avocado. I do believe in fasting, but for me it can create a great weight loss, so I only fast for three days. I don't mean to sound vain about my looks, but eating this way has given me the cut above the edge with regard to my peers. I can see the difference when I look at their appearance.

Have you ever had a really bad detoxification, or were you ever really sick?

At the age of fifty, I woke up one morning and had blurred vision. That really scared me. I was eating so well; why should this happen to me? I then decided to look at areas of my life that I had not paid attention to. At that time I was busy writing my book *Health Seekers*. I realized I was not getting enough sleep and fresh air and sunshine at the right time of day. I went to a regular medical doctor who sent me for a MRI scan and a lumbar puncture. They could find nothing. They wanted to do further tests, but I refused. They wanted to give me cortisone, and I refused. I went home and phoned Dr. Joel Robbins. He suggested that I add some cooked food to my eating pattern to slow down the detoxification going on inside my body. He also insisted that I have ten hours of sleep every day and only go to gym every other day. I added steamed vegetables and baked potatoes every other night, once a day. I used a pair of glasses with a prism and within two weeks I could see. I did get better without invasive therapy or medication.

What is your average daily diet like? What do you eat, and how often?

I wake up in the morning at about 4:30 a.m. I take acidophilus. Then I go to gym at about 5:30 a.m. When I return, I drink a huge glass of boiled water with some fresh lemon, and one hour later I take barley green. I do not take the barley green for long periods at a time. I do give the body a rest. At about 11:00 a.m., I eat a lot of fruit. I keep eating fruit all day until one hour before supper. At about 1:00 p.m., I add lettuce or celery to my fruit. I make sure to combine my foods correctly. I might have almonds with my acid fruit or avocado. If I eat avocado, I do not eat nuts. At supper, I have a huge raw vegetable salad with avocado, provided I haven't had nuts or avocado during the day. I will then just add olive oil and lemon juice. I do not season my food with any condiments. I do not drink tea, coffee, or cold drinks. I do not drink fruit juices during the day. If I do have the fruit juices, I have it sometime in the early morning, homemade of course, and only one glass. I also add dried fruit to my sweet fruits. I do this occasionally. I live on fresh fruit, dried fruit without sulphur dioxide, raw, unsalted, unroasted almonds, pecans, cashews and macadamia nuts. I eat a lot of avocados, and I really enjoy tahini sauce made from only natural pulped sesame seeds. I do add cold pressed olive oil (extra virgin oil) sometimes to my raw salads with some freshly squeezed lemon juice. I never ever add seasonings to my salads or cooked vegetables, rice, millet, quinoa, etc.

What is your favorite food?
My favorite food is avocado and tahini sauce.

Out of all of the foods, do you think one is most important?
The most important thing when on a raw diet is to get a varied diet, preferably organically grown, and enjoy what you are eating. By eating a varied diet and only eating foods in season, you are assured of getting maximum nutrients. But remember, one might need correct nutritional supplementation if organic food is not available.

How is your health and energy?
My health is excellent, and my energy is unbelievable. I have not been on any form of medication since 1979. I am also not on hormone replacement therapy.

How much sleep do you get, and how much do you think is necessary?
On average I get about seven hours. I go to sleep whenever I feel tired at night. I can go to bed at about 8:00 p.m. if I have done a great deal of counseling and interviews on radio that day; otherwise, I usually go to bed at about 9:30-10:00 p.m. and sleep until about 4:30 a.m. The body is really an intelligent organism. I do not need an alarm clock to wake me up. I automatically wake at 4:30 a.m. If I go to bed very late, say about 11:30 p.m., I might only wake at 5:00 a.m.

What mental changes have you noticed?
I have a very clear mind. When I skip a meal in the morning, drink purified water, and eat only at about 2:00 p.m. (fruit only), I have such a clear mind, it is unbelievable.

Many people just getting into a raw diet have problems because their mates don't want to change. Do you have any comments or suggestions? What are your thoughts

about relationships?

If your spouse doesn't share your beliefs and eat like you, there can be problems. My husband loves food. I have made some rules for him: fruit only in the morning and a raw salad before something cooked. I will not spoil anybody's fun when it comes to food. Eating is a social activity. However, when we go out for a meal, I make sure my meal is raw. I arrange with the restaurant to give me the food I want, and there is never a problem.

Do you have any suggestions for people new to this raw food lifestyle on how to deal with other people who are not into eating this way?

You can only advise, you cannot insist. I never discuss eating patterns with other people or pick them out on what they are eating. The funny thing is, they always ask me why I eat like this, and I give them answers. However, I do not pick them out on their choices. We all have choices in life, and it is up to us to choose, unless we are asked an opinion.

Do you think it is harder for a woman to eat a raw food diet than it is for a man?

No, I think it is harder for a man to eat a raw food diet. Women seem to be more committed than men, especially when it comes to weight loss and health problems. Men are very involved in business lunches, etc., and I feel that men cannot stay on a total raw diet for more than two meals per day. I have had a lot of success with women going on a total raw diet for at least one month at a time.

What are your thoughts about the female menstruation cycle?

I have found when I change a woman's eating plan to include more raw foods, her menstrual cycle takes less time to finish and it is not as heavy as a meat-eater's, etc.

182

Do you think it's natural for a woman not to bleed when she is on a raw diet?

I do believe one bleeds less on a raw diet. In fact some women do not bleed, yet they still ovulate. This I have noticed with my clients. I can't comment on this, because when I changed my eating patterns, I'd had a hysterectomy (at the age of thirty-five). If I had known then what I now know, I would never have allowed the doctors to perform the hysterectomy. I have prevented many a client having such, through correct eating.

I am not a doctor and cannot give an adequate answer to this question. A woman has to ovulate, but she does not need to bleed. I have had women clients who have not bled but are still ovulating. Women on a raw food diet do find that their periods are much lighter in color, and they do not bleed for more than two days.

Do you have any comments about the effect of diet on hormonal cycles?

I do believe that eating animal protein in abundance does affect one's hormonal cycles. Animals today are fed with an abundance of hormones, and eating animal protein in abundance definitely affects one's hormonal balance. There definitely is estrogen dominance, and this creates problems with menopause as well PMS, etc. Cutting out animal protein and processed foods, sugar, etc. will definitely give a woman a much more painless menstrual cycle as well as better moods, etc. If anything, I suggest women go on a total raw diet one week before their period and while they are having a period. It definitely works. Women have told me that it has made a huge difference in their moods as well as cramps, etc.

Do you have any comments about pregnancy on the raw food diet?

I definitely do not advocate a total raw diet for pregnant

women. It can be very dangerous, especially if they have not been eating well before conception. I do however put my pregnant clients on a three-day detoxification diet, but no longer than three days. The body goes into detoxification on the third day, and I do not want my pregnant women wallowing in their own toxins and causing miscarriages, etc. A pregnant woman has to eat very well to have a healthy fetus. She can definitely do this by eating two raw meals everyday and having one cooked meal at night. I also suggest whole food supplements. Our food here in South Africa is not grown in soil that contains all the right nutrients. Also, we do not get enough organically grown fruit and vegetables, etc.

Thank you for giving this interview. Is there anything you would like to add?

Through my counseling sessions, I have found that many people cannot stay on a total raw diet, and I can understand why. It's not easy in wintertime, and there are other psychological reasons. But a person who eats mostly raw throughout the day and has one cooked meal at night and makes better food choices will definitely achieve better health. I have advocated this to my clients with tremendous success. I give them a choice and support them in whatever they choose to follow. They have all made radical changes, eating only one animal protein per day and choosing animal protein without hormones and antibiotics, etc. They are all reading labels on bottles, etc. I do find that with time, they are definitely making better choices and are experiencing better health.

Remember, if you have been eating a total raw diet for a long time and you start eating bad foods, your body will react very violently. That is the price one has to pay. This is not a bad thing, however, as it makes one aware of how quickly the body can heal itself if given the right conditions and what can happen if one reverts back to one's old eating patterns. Everything in moderation!

Choosing better foods is not the only thing that will give a person optimal health. We also have to look at non-nutritive factors such as adequate sleep, sunshine, exercise, emotional poise, and belief in God, etc. We have to take a total holistic approach to improving our lifestyle and our health.

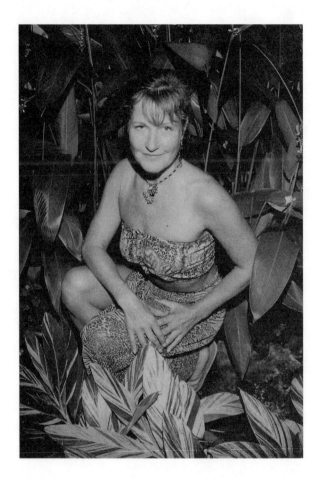

You may contact Rozalind Gruben at:

USA
E-mail:
Healthyunlimited@aol.com
Web: rawmatriark.com
609 North Jade Drive
Key Largo FL 33037
Tel: 305 852 0214

UK
E-mail: Rozgruben@aol.com
Web: rawmatriark.com
1 Cassidy Place Storrington
West Sussex England RH20
4EY
Tel: 01903 746572

Rozalind Gruben

R ozalind has helped me so much, not only in health, but also personally. At first I thought maybe she was just going out of her way to help me and make me feel great about life, but then I met many others who said they got the same feeling from her. Rozalind has helped many people improve their lives. Her wisdom and knowledge are helpful, but most of all, her compassion is what makes her the amazing person she is. In this interview you can read her words, but I highly recommend that you do your best to see her and hear her speak in person. Her energy will move you. She is a real "raw angel" helping the lost souls find the light.

Professor Gruben is an international speaker, writer and consultant in the areas of health, nutrition and fitness.

For well over a decade, Rozalind was Senior National Course Director and Assessor for Exercise Professional Teacher Training in the UK. During this time she was also moderator and verifier for the Royal Society of Arts Fitness Instructor Teacher Training Program. As co-creator of the first European post graduate course in Exercise Prescription for Older Adults, Rozalind specializes in health and fitness advice for the elderly. Other areas of specialization include helping people heal from disordered eating, rehabilitation programs for the severely deconditioned and women's issues. Part of Rozalind's mission is to be a voice for the women of the raw food movement. She leads many women's circles across the globe committed to empowering through education.

Founder of EarthSave UK, Professor Gruben is also deeply concerned with the impact of dietary and lifestyle choices upon the planet and all the creatures with whom we share it.

A long-term Natural Hygienist, who truly practices what

she teaches, Professor Gruben has gained recognition as a highly respected consultant, lecturer, and inspirational keynote speaker. She is a board member and Agenda Coordinator for Healthful Living International.

Rozalind appears on international television and numerous radio broadcasts as well as at conventions for fitness and nutrition professionals worldwide. Her clients include: The Royal Navy, The Reader's Digest, Middlesex University (London), The London College of Naturopathic Medicine, Fitness Professionals UK, and The World, North American, and European Vegetarian Congresses.

How many years have you been on the raw diet, and what got you into it?

I began to wake up to raw foods seventeen years ago. My transition lasted for four years, during which time I continued to include significant quantities of my regular, cooked vegan fare. I have been eating exclusively raw for thirteen years now. The path that led me to the raw lifestyle was paved with both a desperate desire and a profound need to seek out the truths about health. I had been suffering from the distress of intensely disordered eating since the age of sixteen, accompanied by the resulting intestinal challenges and daily battles with catarrh.

How was your health before you started the diet?

Abysmal. I was severely over-fat, depressed, and constipated. My body's toxic state was revealed by its heavily blemished skin. Every joint in my body ached. Lying face down on the floor after almost every meal in order to ease the pains of dyspepsia was a way of life for me. My tissues were sodden with edema, and cellulite was my constant companion. Mucous poured out of my nose at the mere mention of physical exertion. Migraine headaches rendered me nonfunctional, at least once every two weeks. I was a pathetic sight indeed, and I felt twice my chronological age.

Who are some people who have inspired you to do this?

I have been fortunate enough to spend time with many great teachers through their writing, such as T. C. Fry. However, it was Harvey Diamond (*Fit For Life*) and Leslie Kenton (*Raw Energy*) whose writings first introduced me to the raw diet.

Is there any one person who has inspired you the most?

Although I had already sunk my roots well into the soil of eating raw by the time we met, my partner, Dr. Doug Graham, continues to inspire me each and every day in a way that no other person can. Doug is a treasure beyond measure in my life.

You have learned so much over the years. What are some of the most important things you have learned?

This is, in and of itself, an exciting question. It brings to mind a diverse and powerful array of issues. One thing I have learned, which saved my life and enables me to help others tremendously, is that cooked food is unquestionably addictive—especially grains.

One of my work's greatest rewards is observing people get well—people whose quality of life was reduced to a state of constant despair as a result of disordered eating. It is wonderful to watch self-esteem rekindle within these people as they realize they are not gluttonous, weak-willed or inadequate, but simply suffering from a physiological addiction. I have learned that the simpler I make each meal, the better I feel. It also means that I experience a greater variety of tastes and textures over time. This has been of great value.

Are there any pitfalls you have learned to watch out for on the raw diet?

The most common mistake people make is to rely too heavily

on vegetable matter and not enough on fruit. As a result, they constantly feel hungry and overeat on concentrated fats and proteins, such as nuts. The consequence is they experience an array of symptoms, ranging from fatigue and constipation to digestive problems and excessive thirst. The adult human body requires about 75% of its total caloric intake to be composed of simple carbohydrates. The natural way of providing the body with carbohydrates is via breast milk for infants or fruits for those beyond the age of nursing. The other mistake that I often see people make is relying heavily on supplements, elixirs, 'superfoods', refined oils, spices, and other nonfoods. These are toxic—irritating and stimulating in quality. Such a reliance reveals a misunderstanding about what constitutes a natural diet and an obvious vulnerability to the dictates of marketing, disguised as education.

Weight loss is a big pitfall for many people. Do you have any thoughts about that?
The majority of people who start out along the raw path have a history of insufficient exercise. As a result, they have underdeveloped skeletal muscles. This lack of muscle tissue is often hidden under a layer of fat while they subscribe to a cooked diet, and it only becomes apparent once the excess adipose tissue is shed. People then find they have no muscle underneath. The answer is not to regain the burden of excess fat, but to develop strong and attractive muscles through the application of strenuous, physical exercise.

Dental problems are another big pitfall. Do you have any thoughts about that?
Any over-proliferation of bacteria within the body is the result of compromised immune functioning. If gum disease is a problem, then steps should be taken to establish a superior level of health by evaluating all aspects of diet and lifestyle involved in its creation. In some individuals, constant grazing or

190

snacking on acidic fruit throughout the day can damage dental enamel.Therefore, to avoid tooth decay, the habit of simply rinsing out the mouth with plain water after each meal goes a long way in ensuring that teeth and gums remain healthy.The aggressive use of brushes and other tools of dental hygiene can often be the cause of many problems of both gums and teeth. Unfortunately, the combination of destructive dentistry and past eating habits render some individuals vulnerable to experiencing all sorts of problems with their teeth and gums.

What are your thoughts about mercury fillings, and what would you replace them with?

Mercury fillings have been associated with a frightening array of serious health conditions. My advice is to avoid having them. If you have some, be sure to have them removed by a dentist who is trained in their safe removal.The 'ideal' replacement has yet to be discovered. I advise people to seek out an educated dentist who runs a 'non-mercury' practice and follow his or her advice. Different alternatives are appropriate, depending on the individual and the specifics of the cavity to be filled.

What is your opinion of nuts and seeds?

Nuts and seeds are a useful addition to the diet in moderate amounts. It is common for people new to the raw food diet to overeat these foods in search of the familiar, narcotic effect of cooked foods. Nuts and seeds do not contain the toxic qualities of cooked foods, but their consumption results in similar feelings of lethargy and emotional dullness.This is due to the high quantity of fat and protein contained within them that places a heavy burden on the nervous system in order for the necessary processes of digestion to be conducted.

What is your opinion of grains?

The human body is not designed to consume grains. Doing so results in a serious compromise of health. Grains are highly addictive due to the opioids they contain and the stimulating effect they have upon the body's production of serotonin (the 'feel-good' neurotransmitter). These undesirable qualities are not negated by sprouting, and I do not recommend their consumption, in any form, to anyone.

What is your opinion of an all fruit diet?
Very few people are able to sustain long-term health on a diet composed exclusively of fruits. Vegetable matter is required in the diet as a rich source of minerals, phytonutrients, and amino acids.

What is your opinion of sprouts?
To find a few sprouts in our natural environment is possible, but to secure a sufficient quantity to make a meal is highly unlikely. For this reason, their inclusion as a 'natural' part of the human diet has its limitations. Legumes are, in any case, challenging for the body to digest due to their almost equal ratio of protein to carbohydrate. Sprouting does little to solve this problem.

What is your opinion of The Natural Hygiene Diet?
Natural Hygiene is not an alternative approach to health, but a name given to describe the laws of nature under which our organic existence is governed. It is natural law that dictates the development from a fertilized egg to an independent living entity. Natural law is demonstrated by cause and effect; as an example, the absence of food eventually leads to starvation. Natural Hygiene is simply the name given to practices that support life. It is therefore pro-biotic. All approaches to health that do not identify and respect natural law are correspondingly destructive to life, or in other words, anti-biotic. To question whether Natural Hygiene is an intelligent approach to the creation and securing of health is tantamount to questioning whether love has a role in world peace. Natural Hygiene is comprised of over twenty-five different components that need to be considered in order to create, and maintain, a state of health. A raw vegan diet is only

one of those components.

What is your opinion of supplements?

Supplements are refined, fragmented, and perverted substances. They have been introduced into the vocabulary of dieticians and the general population to create monetary revenue for manufacturers and allow people to continue eating unhealthy foods with less guilt. They are 100% unnatural (regardless of their source) and have no place inside the human body. There are, however, some very rare cases where ingestion of a specific supplement may be appropriate.

What is your opinion of eating seasonally?

It is great if you live in a location where the human body's natural foods are available throughout the year. However, for the majority of the population, this is not the case, and reliance upon imported foods is preferable to feeding on cooked foods and local animal products.

What is your opinion of fasting?

Fasting is probably the most misunderstood and improperly implemented aspect of healthcare practiced amongst 'health seekers.' Undertaken correctly and under the supervision of someone who is educated and experienced in the science of fasting, this physiological rest can be life saving. It is a highly valuable tool in the re-establishment of health. Practiced indiscriminately and improperly, it can result in a variety of health problems or even death.

What is your opinion of food combining on a 100% raw diet? Is it necessary?

The natural human diet is almost devoid of food combining, since each meal consists of a single food type. If foods are combined at one meal, their digestive compatibility needs to be considered, even though the foods are eaten raw.

What are your thoughts about physical exercise?
Use it or lose it! Without sufficient physical movement, almost every system in the body is rendered less functional. It is natural for humans to move in order to obtain their food at each meal. Developing the habit of enjoying exercise prior to each meal is supportive to your health. It is a useful tool for maintaining healthy body composition. There are five ways in which the body is designed to be challenged physically:

1) Demands for the heart, respiratory and vascular systems, to take in and transport oxygen.

2) Demands for the muscles to overcome resistances that challenge its maximal strength.

3) Demands for the muscles to endure continual bouts of repeated contraction in the overcoming of moderate to light resistance.

4) Demands for the muscles to stretch and accommodate full ranges of joint movement.

5) Demands upon the nervous system to conduct neuro-muscular communications that demand balance, co-ordination, and reaction time.

What is your opinion of wild foods?
A clear distinction needs to be made between stimulating plants that are favored for their intense flavors and natural plants that, in and of themselves, can be used to form an entire meal. The former are not supportive to health. To secure nutritional needs for free from the countryside is both an economically and environmentally sound practice. However, many plants are highly toxic, so it is very important to learn which wild foods are appropriate for human consumption.

What are your age, height, and weight? Has your weight changed, or are there any other changes your

body has gone through? How did you handle it?
My chronological age, physiological age, and spiritual age are all very different. I consider chronology to be the least important of the three. I was born in 1959, and I am five feet six inches tall. My weight is 130 pounds, and I currently have a body fat percentage of 15%.

Do you eat 100% raw foods? If so, for how long?
I am 100% RAW with NO exceptions. I have been thriving on exclusively raw vegan foods for over thirteen years.

What is your average daily diet like? What do you eat, and how often?
I take my first meal of the day after I have exercised (usually running). By this time, it is late morning. This meal consists of an abundance of one type of fruit. I frequently enjoy a banana smoothie for this meal, which I make by simply blending bananas with water. Late in the afternoon, I usually have one type of juicy fruit before my dinner, which is a giant salad. My salad typically consists of a vast amount of green leaves and often tomatoes plus avocados or occasionally raw nuts or seeds. Tahini is a useful food to carry with me when traveling to places where my dietary needs are not easily met.

What are your favorite foods?
Mangos, durian, mamey, bananas, avocados, lettuce, and tomatoes.

What is the most important consideration when it comes to foods?
It is important for them to be of good quality and eaten in a state of emotional poise.

How are your health and energy?
Superb, vibrant, and continually improving

How much sleep do you get, and how much do you think is necessary?

I sometimes have challenges with insomnia. Due to my current lifestyle, I frequently subject myself to traveling through different time zones. I identify this as a weak link in my heath care practices. Generally, I manage to secure eight hours of sleep per night. The amount of sleep required varies from one person to the next, according to the demands upon their nervous system and the quality of their sleep. If sleep is to be of a quality depth, it needs to be entered into in a relaxed state of mind. When alarm clocks or other methods of artificial awakening are implemented, there is always a sleep deficit.

What mental changes have you noticed?

Clarity of mind, joy of life, exuberance of thought, an increase in creative ideas, and heightened cognitive abilities.

What are your thoughts about relationships? Many people just beginning a raw diet have problems because their mates do not want to change. Do you have any comments or suggestions?

Personal relationships provide us with enormous opportunities for learning and growing. The purpose of their existence is not to endure, but to teach us important life lessons. When a relationship has served its purpose for both parties, there is an opportunity to lovingly release it and move on to more advanced lessons with another spirit. Relationships that last for a short duration can be as beautiful and enriching as ones that last for the entire lifetimes of the individuals involved. The intimate unity of two people that remains constantly enriching for a lifetime is, indeed, a wonderful thing. But to remain within a relationship for the sole purpose of proving the ability to endure in the face of disservice is not the soul's purpose. To attempt to change a loved one in order to make them adopt practices congruent with your own beliefs and preferences dishonors their unique spiritual path. This leads to resentment within both parties. In circumstances where there is a significant conflict in lifestyle practices, it better serves both individuals to create the space needed for each other to grow through the manifestation of his or her own experiences. The possibility of harmoniously remaining in a relationship where lifestyles are dramatically opposed is possible, but each partner must authentically accept and support the other's chosen path.

Do you think it is harder for a woman to eat a raw diet than it is for a man?
No, it is possibly easier for a woman. Women are more likely to be experienced in making dietary changes, due to constant battles with their weight while on a cooked food diet; and because they are pressured by the media to conform to the perfect body size. Also, women are usually the food preparers, while the diets of many men are influenced by the women who prepare meals for them.

Why do you think there are more raw men than raw women?
The majority of raw food teachers and gurus are men. Therefore, men have a vast number of role models to choose from. In addition, many men who live alone and are not skilled at cooking welcome the no-cook convenience.

What are your thoughts about the female menstruation cycle? Do you think it is natural for a woman not to bleed during menstruation when she's on the raw diet?
The absence of menstrual blood is not an indication that a woman is not ovulating. However, if a woman's body fat percentage falls below healthful limits, a discontinuation of the monthly cycle and infertility will likely result.

Do you have comments about PMS?

PMS is caused by hormonal disturbances and the presence of toxins within the body. Specifically, the consumption of animal fats and cooked fats lead to hormonal imbalances. A raw, vegan diet will result in the removal of these substances, as well as a massive reduction of body toxicity. As a consequence, fewer PMS symptoms will be experienced. In the majority of cases, they will vanish altogether.

Do you have any comments about pregnancy?
It is vital for a pregnant woman to understand that her blood is also circulating throughout the vessels of the baby within her belly. Therefore, her diet, and the consequent toxicity or purity of her blood, will be feeding or intoxicating the cells of the developing baby as well as her own cells. If it is the mother's desire to provide her baby with the very best start in life, then the consumption of a raw, vegan diet while she is pregnant is a necessity.

Thank you for this interview. Would you like to add anything?
Adopting a raw food diet has implications that are much further reaching than simply reducing uncomfortable physical symptoms. By eating natural living plant foods, we raise our vibrational rate on an energetic level. In so doing, we are able to realign ourselves with the pulsation of the earth's rhythms and, consequently, can return to fulfill our symbiotic role within the tapestry of all life. True ahimsa begins with not harming our own body temple, which includes not poisoning it with cooked and deranged foods. Without that starting place, without authentic self-respect and self-love, all efforts to demonstrate extrinsic lovingkindness are rooted in the soil of fearful intentions.

It takes courage to go against the tide of mass perceptions and embrace a lifestyle that is considered 'extreme' by others around you. It can be helpful to realize that they see it that way through the eyes of ignorance and a belief that security is to be found embedded in that which is familiar. Simply because something is commonly practiced does not make it the best choice available. A seeing-eye dog can, at best, lead its owner to safety. Regardless of how much it loves its master or mistress, the dog cannot give them sight. Those who have the raw vision, and are committed to spreading its truths, would do best to invest their energies in leading the way by the demonstration of their own habits.

The power for you to do this lies in your next meal.

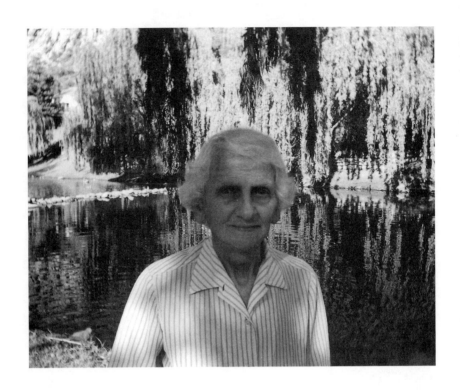

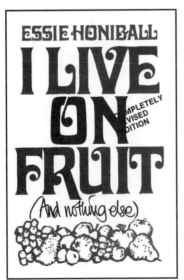

You may contact Essie Honiball at:

Essie Honiball
P O Box 675
Kleinmond 7195
Republic of South Africa

Essie Honiball

E ssie Honiball is an amazing woman and a true pioneer within the raw food movement. She has much to teach about how to eat a raw food diet and stay healthy and happy by sharing her own experiences. Her book, *I Live on Fruit*, is a classic for anyone serious about learning how to eat a raw diet. Once you read this interview, you will know why she is a true trailblazer.

What are your age, weight, and height?
I am seventy-seven years old. I was born on April 12, 1924. My weight is 110 pounds. My height is five feet three inches tall.

How are your health and energy?
My health and energy are exceptionally good. I have scientific backing for this statement.

How many years have you been eating a raw food diet?
I have been eating a raw food diet without a compromise for fifteen years, and with a slight compromise for another twenty-eight years–a total of forty-one years, from 1958 to 2001.

How does your life today compare to your life before you started on this journey?
There is no comparison between my life today and my life before I started on this journey forty-one years ago. Looking back, I realize how I neglected my health. I got very little sleep and no exercise; and I did not allow myself the nutrition that was necessary for good heath.

Do you eat 100% raw foods? If so, for how long? If not, why not?
For fifteen years, I ate a diet of fresh fruit and nuts, rarely eating raw salads and vegetables. I could have gone on eating this way forever, experiencing the kind of health I never realized

existed. My body was functioning like never before. My mind was clearer than ever. I was vibrantly healthy and enjoying life at its best. But then I became a scientific phenomenon and I ran into some problems. Keep reading.

Why did you first become interested in eating this type of diet?

In 1958, my life reached a very low point, caused by a total collapse in my health. A period of trauma and stress, accompanied by a very heavy workload, resulted in my getting tuberculosis. I was only thirty-four years old. Finally, that same year, I decided to give up my omnivorous lifestyle and switch to the fruit diet, also called *The Eden* or *Genesis Diet*. It consists of fresh fruit and nuts (some seeds), complemented by an occasional raw salad. My life was at stake, and the diet was simply the last straw of hope I had.

How bad was your health before you started this diet?

My health was in a desperate state of deterioration. I suffered a loss of weight. Sleep was nonexistent. I struggled to get out of bed. I had sores and ulcers all over my body. I could not breathe properly. I could not lift my feet from the ground; they were like lead. I experienced a total loss of appetite. I fainted often. In fact, I was a hospital case, but something in me refused to continue taking medicine. Too much medicine taken over a long period of time was already part of my problem, and surgery was not necessary. My body was nearing a total collapse, and slowly but surely, I was dying.

Were there many people eating this *"Eden Diet"* (natural raw diet) back in 1958?

At the time, I read two books, one by Arnold Ehret, and the other by Johanna Brandt. They were both early pioneers in this movement. I had no knowledge of anyone else interested in this diet.

Who are some people who have inspired you to do this?
After trying almost everything, I still had no answers. Destiny stepped in and brought a man into my life. He solved the problem for me. Without his knowledge and guidance, I was totally blind to the answer to my problems. That man was Cornelius Valkenberg de Villiers Dreyer. He was one of the very early pioneers of this lifestyle. He was a picture of vibrant health and youth. I happened to fall into his hands at the right time, and my circumstances forced me to adhere to the rules. At last, Cornelius had found his guinea pig, someone who was willing to contribute to the hypothesis that a fruit diet was the answer to man's imbalances, diseases and deterioration. That guinea pig was me. He was the one and only person that inspired me so much that later I married him.

How did he help you?
Right away, he put me on a three-day water fast. I did not have time for a gradual adaptation, like some people do today. It was do or die. My health was in a bad state. I could not tolerate more than three small pieces of fruit per day, taken seven hours apart, with only water in between. There were no compromises. This period of eating very little lasted for weeks.

How did it affect you?
It affected all aspects of my life. The bottom of my old lifestyle, literally, fell out. As time marched on, I fit in nowhere. I was confronted with insurmountable social pressures and psychological problems. After all, I was living ahead of my time. I was subtly rejected. I faced a life of isolation that every pioneer knows only too well. Physically, my weight went down, and instead of looking better, I looked worse.

Is it better for people to make a change in their diet overnight, or should they ease into it?
The transition is a slow process. The body will need time to adapt. Presently, the majority of people on a traditional diet

203

may not progress beyond 30% raw foods in one lifetime. That does not have any impact on me. Everybody moves at their own pace, according to their unique circumstances. No two people are alike, because all our bodies are built differently. Getting from the old body into the new body calls for research over a long period of time, using human guinea pigs, not animals. That is yet to come. Today, all people on this road are pioneers braving a new fruitarian way of life. The point is not how fast we can withdraw from traditional structures, but how we can move in the right direction and build firm foundations. One must move in body, mind, and spirit as a whole; therefore, adaptation must include all aspects of one's life.

If you were to do it all over again, would you do anything different?

Nature did a wonderful job on me while I ate this diet. I have not experienced any of my old complaints. It seems like they have been completely wiped out forever.

During your transition, you lost a lot of weight. Weight loss seems to bother many people new to this way of eating. What are your thoughts about your own weight loss? How did you deal with it?

My experience has proven to me that the body loses only what it needs to lose. On this diet, weight loss should not be feared, but accepted as a blessing in disguise. I was underweight when I started on this diet and my weight kept going down, until I was skin and bone. But I felt better everyday. I had more energy and fewer problems. The elimination of whatever caused my problems continued to improve. There were no more obnoxious smells, constipation, or irregularities, only supreme functioning. My low weight of sixty-nine pounds did not worry me, although it worried everybody else. I stayed with the diet regardless of what everyone else said.

When did your weight start to come back?

One day, after seven months, the miracle happened. My house was in order. I was ready to feed on real building material provided by the Creator in nature's garden of life. My appetite returned and I started eating so much, I was ashamed of myself. I ate half a box of peaches and six avocados in one meal, tiny me! But then the scale started going up, and I returned to my normal weight of 110 pounds, which I have maintained for forty-six years.

Did you ever feel you were overweight?

I did once, when I lost control. My weight went up thirty pounds. I was looking and feeling overweight. I felt awful for putting all that pollution back into my blood. Once I got back on track, I dropped the excess weight the natural way, and I felt fine! After a year, I was back to my normal weight. I have maintained this weight for four decades. I have never looked back. Nature has done a very good job. I have not experienced any of the symptoms of my omnivorous life.

Do you have any advice for people dealing with weight loss issues?

Derailment is not unusual on this diet, but weight loss is not an issue when you follow the rules. Nature takes time to put her house in order. There is no use feeling frustrated and trying to hurry nature, it will not work. However, fluid intake must be maintained. Otherwise, you are in for dehydration and all its sad effects. Therefore, even if your appetite remains zero, drink pure water. Eat when you are hungry, and eat as much as your body demands. You'll know when it says, "Stop eating, I am satisfied." One thing we can feel happy about is that nature will never allow one to lose more weight than is absolutely necessary for regeneration, especially if we abide by her rules. At first, I was underweight, but after seven months, I started to regain the weight without changing my diet. This should be enough proof that if you do not worry about the weight loss, nature's course will allow your weight to become exactly what it should be.

How did the reactions of doctors, friends, and family affect you?

I resisted the ongoing pressure from friends and family who tried to get me back to a hospital, where I probably belonged. I became as stubborn as a mule, because from the start, I sensed that the raw, humble food was already achieving what no other food or treatment had ever succeeded in doing.

How did you resist the pressure from them?

While I was married to Cornelius, we lived in unspoiled nature for more than a year. We were eating live food and camping outside without any noise, hurry, or any obligations other than regaining my health. At the end of that year, I was a transformed person with vibrant health and an uncluttered lifestyle. I was living on fruit and nuts only. My ties to my old life and environment had been severed.

During your transition, did you ever think of giving up and going back to your old diet?

I had help and guidance all the way. To beat death and begin living again was the most difficult challenge I have ever faced. Had it not been for Cornelius's calm nature, discipline, and inspiration, I would have given up the struggle, especially during that first year. It was never a highway to success or easy going at any time. I experienced pains, cramps, weakness, and nausea. But no matter what the symptoms were or how I felt, it called for faith, inner discipline, grace from above, and living one day at a time.

Thank God Cornelius was there. He had the faith, insight, knowledge, and experience to guide me through it all. It was no easy task. My transition demanded much patience, perseverance, and discipline. My return to a healthy life involved not only the purification of my blood, but also of my soul.

How was your soul purified?

The new lifestyle is no fashion to be changed again and again. It is a supreme adventure of conscious living. No matter how healthy the physical body is, if the body does not house a sound mind and is not guided from within by the spirit of Christ, it means nothing. Rebirth and regeneration of the physical, mental, and spiritual self requires responsibility that revolves around the Creator, our fellow man, and all life on earth.

Do you think it would have been easier for you to make this change of lifestyle in today's times?

It was difficult for me to stop eating omnivorously and transition into eating fruits and nuts, but it is far more challenging to function as a strict fruitarian within the duality of our time.

Thanks to the efforts of every pioneer, this lifestyle has caught on and opened new vistas in today's society. Natural eating is not such a strange phenomenon anymore. It is accepted and practiced in growing numbers.

When did you start to see results in your recovery?

After one month, my skin was clear. My health was improving. My suffering decreased, and my symptoms started disappearing slowly but surely. After seven months, my natural weight returned. This meant only one thing: my body had entered a new phase of rebuilding. From then on, my recovery was much easier.

Was diet the only factor that contributed to your recovery?

It was the main factor, but not the only one. The spiritual angle is always contributory to health. So are breathing exercises, movement, rest, and sleep. Fruit eating or becoming an Eden eater is not a matter of following rules and regulations, but a matter of a total transformation.

You have learned so much over the years. What are some of the most important things you have learned?

When I started on this path, I was a product of book learning. I was a lecturer in health. I taught biological subjects at a teacher's training college. Later, I became the vice principal of a school for physically disabled children and adults. However, the knowledge that I obtained did not help me when my life almost ended at thirty-four years of age. I had to start looking at life from a totally transformed angle.

The new lessons I learned contradicted the lessons I had learned in the past. I began adapting to a lifestyle that led me away from my old lifestyle. I became transformed by shedding the artificial layers I was once enslaved to. I had to learn how to live naturally, and in doing so, I was forced to escape civilization and its hold on me.

· Living the natural way is like a journey into a new day, a new life. It is a supreme adventure, where you never stop learning new lessons. As you adapt physically, mentally, emotionally, morally, and spiritually, a vision opens and expands from within. Transformation is not a matter of learning, but of becoming conscious of what you were unconscious of before.

It sounds like you had all the answers and were doing fine. What happened?
Had it not been for the fact that I was living ahead of my time, I would have been fine, but I was totally out of step with the outside world. This did not bother me while Cornelius and I were living in paradise. I never dreamed of a more enjoyable way of life, camping together in unspoiled nature. That was by far the most joyful period of my life. Unfortunately, society viewed our lifestyle as unrealistic. After Cornelius passed on, I was on my own, and I had to become part of civilization as I knew it before. After three years of fruitarian eating and withdrawal from society, I realized that my life of isolation was gone forever.

Getting back into a traditional life was a big challenge. I fit in nowhere. In those days, I was considered a fanatic. It took many years to adjust, and I was rejected slowly and surely by my fellow men as not being one of them. I became a loner on an island, completely out of step with my environment, a catastrophe. No man can function on an island alone for an extended period of time. We are all part of a human body and we cannot function without the balance from day-to-day interaction among people.

How did you survive?
Although I was rejected scientifically and socially, I felt I had to carry on. I was obsessed with expressing this truth I found from within, and I continued to do so, against all odds.

What was the next step for you?
For some years, I was part of a research study to scientifically justify my diet. During the study, the leading professor reacted to my complaints that I was suffering from aches and pains that could not be explained, and he told me I had psychosomatic problems. He ordered me to go back and eat with my family again. I did just that. I refused my plate of fruit and asked for porridge. Used to my fanaticism, my family was stunned! "What? You're asking for porridge?" They could not believe it. But that is what I got, and that is what I ate. Believe me, at that moment, I experienced the warmth that I had longed for and craved for years. I finally felt accepted. I was in heaven! I felt I was back in the human body.

However, after fifteen years of fruit eating, my body could not handle this sudden change in diet. The cooked food was tasteless, and I could not enjoy it. Eventually, the symptoms of sore throat, constipation, etc. came back, and I quickly returned to a fruitarian diet. But this time, I was willing to compromise as circumstances demanded. I chose to be less strict with myself, and that is what saved me.

Can you elaborate on that?
I started all over again. This time, I did not abide by forced or strict rules of my isolated laboratory life. I was back in the fold

and moving along with the human body, not as an island but an integral part. This meant I was back in the world again.

So now that you are not as strict, what is your average daily diet like? What do you eat, and how often?
I eat like the birds: I eat when I am hungry. I do not have rules or regulations. Sometimes, I feed once or twice a day, and sometimes, more often. I eat mainly fresh fruit. Occasionally, I want a change, or the fruit is lacking in taste, so I will I eat a fruit salad or fruit porridge (liquefied). When the fruit is tasty and freshly obtained, I eat one kind of fruit per meal. Sometimes I eat a variety at one meal. My body guides my intake, so I do not worry about combinations.

I still compromise on cooked, traditional food for many personal reasons. It is a matter of choice and being able to balance my physical, emotional, and spiritual life. By adapting the best I can to the new lifestyle, I have lost my taste for almost all animal products. I have forgotten what meat, fish, etc. taste like. I rarely eat chicken, except on very specific occasions. Sometimes I eat raw salads, but I do not really care for them. At times, I would eat a meal of steamed vegetables, but rarely now. I still eat whole wheat bread, but fruit and nuts seem to be my main food. I also enjoy seeds, such as raw corn on the cob or peas, when in season. My compromises vary according to my particular circumstances. I eat about one half dozen to a dozen fruits per day. The amount of food intake varies continually from year to year and day to day, as one adapts to this diet.

I have a feeling for what I should and should not do at any moment. Without any rules or regulations, I simply move towards the inner vision of tomorrow's world and adapt to that.

Do you think the raw diet can cause dental problems?
Fruit eating will loosen and discard teeth that are not sound. Fillings will loosen and fall out. This is Nature's attempt to get rid of any foreign matter.

I lost most of my teeth before my fruitarian days and many could not be saved. I have had teeth problems for as long as I can remember, and I lost all of my teeth in the 1960's. In the end, I opted for dentures. They are not as good as having your own teeth, but they are better than nothing. Teeth should not be discarded. Healthy teeth are a valuable asset, and it is very important to take care of them.

Although my dentures are not a supplement for healthy teeth, they are of great help. I hope today's youth realize that once the human body is neglected, it cannot be replaced at random like the worn out parts of a machine. The artificial crutches help, but nothing can ever replace the natural sense of chewing and crunching with natural teeth.

What is your opinion of eating seasonally?
The fruitarian diet stretches over twelve months comprised of spring, summer, autumn, and winter. There is natural food provided in every season. I believe seasonal eating is important. It keeps the human body healthy because there is a twelve month recipe providing all the nourishment needed to replenish cells, keep us warm, and supply real atomic energy.

What do you think about raw vegetables?
Raw or even steamed vegetables are not an ideal food for man. However, I do believe they are a very valuable food during the transition period from an omnivorous diet to a fruitarian diet.

What is your opinion of fasting?
When my body was very polluted, I needed fasting. But as I became detoxified, fasting became unnecessary because I was replacing toxic matter without adding more.

The human alimentary tract and blood are a wonderful feeding ground for bacteria and all kinds of parasites. Fasting helps free the body of these obnoxious parasites and problematic matter. Fasting is very beneficial when it is done correctly.

What is your opinion of food combining on a 100% raw diet, and is it necessary?

Once the human body reaches a certain stage of development, I do not believe food combining is as important as it believed to be in today's time. I never worried about combinations. I went from an omnivorous diet to a 100% fruit and nut diet overnight, and I stayed there for fifteen years. In the beginning, I could not eat very much. I would have three small portions of fruit, seven hours apart. I never mixed anything. As time went on, I ate whatever I could obtain. Sometimes, I would enjoy a variety of fruit and nuts in one meal. I found eating this way to be easy, without experiencing any discomfort.

My problems start when I combine live food with cooked, prepared food. I have learned by trial and error to eat one of the following alone: fruits and nuts, raw vegetables, stewed veggies, or whole wheat bread. I do not mix too many foods in one meal if I can help it. I have no eating rules, only a vision to which I adapt the best I can under everyday circumstances.

In today's time, there are all different stages of transitions, from omnivorous eating to fruitarianism. I believe everybody can benefit from the available knowledge of proper food combining. However, great pleasure is eating frugally and enjoying fruit by itself. Each piece is a special creation with a unique taste. Sometimes, I would eat only one kind of fruit for days on end, depending on what kind of fruit was ripe and available.

What do you think about the quality of food today?

Mass production and chemical spraying have destroyed the exquisite taste of fresh fruit and vegetables today. It is very sad. It is a miracle to find fruit that has the supreme, heavenly taste which fruit is meant to have. Once you taste it, you cannot stop enjoying that particular fruit. There is little eating pleasure in the fruit you buy today. I always hunt for tasty fruit (which is often the least attractive to look at). If you are lucky enough to be able to discriminate, you become a selective buyer and you'll manage to survive!

212

What is your opinion of physical exercise?
It is very necessary, especially natural exercise. Exercise that is creative and productive, such as walking to work, climbing stairs, cycling, and hard labor in the house and garden are great.

If I have time, I exercise by walking wherever I need to go instead of driving. I cycle sometimes. I like to visit caves near my house, and I easily climb 300 steps up the mountain to get to them. I swim, and sometimes I go to a gym. I also work in my home and garden.

What is your opinion of supplements?
I have taken some supplements on and off. I do not know whether it was good or bad. Taking them is not a normal part of my ongoing good health.

I do not agree with what people are doing today. We are robbing our food of its nutritional value and trying to put back the same value in the form of supplements. This process is not natural at all. However, with our poor soil, expensive food, polluted water, polluted air, and bad habits we may need supplements at times.

What is your opinion of overeating?
We have forgotten what it feels like to be hungry. In the west, eating and overindulging has become a way of life, with regretful results. It is important to wait for hunger before eating, because your body will receive the food better and the meal will be more enjoyable.

What is your favorite food?
My favorite food is fresh and tasty fruit. There was a time when I used to enjoy steamed vegetables and pasta, but I rarely eat those anymore.

What are the most natural foods for man?
I believe fresh fruit, nuts, and seeds are the most natural foods for man.

Other than fruit, what do you feel is the best food for man?

I feel that green leaves are the up and coming modern medicine for man. Nothing in the fruit tree leaf is harmful to man. The green drink I consume contains a handful of green leaves from fruit trees. I am convinced that these leaves have very important factors that contribute to the healing process. The fruits help build the new body, while the leaves of the same tree help heal the body. This is my belief, and it is a subject to be investigated, I would say.

What are your thoughts about sleep?

The hours before midnight are by far the best sleeping time. This is when nature has the opportunity to cleanse the system and the body is revitalized. I wake up very early, at 4:00 a.m., and I do not sleep during the day. I like the early hours, because I can go for a swim, etc. In the evenings, I may read or perhaps watch TV, but I am in bed as early as possible. My day ends at dusk.

Have you noticed any mental changes on the raw diet?

When eating a raw diet, you are more alert. I think the greatest benefit derived from this diet comes from the spirit working through our consciousness.

What are your thoughts about relationships?

When living the new life, led by spiritual inner forces, you do not go hunting for company. You join forces with whomever is sent your way. When God joins man and woman, and they love as a whole, there is no need for another partner; they are perfectly filled in body and spirit.

Do you think there are more women or more men on the raw food diet?

I do not know if there are more woman or more men on the raw diet, but if I were to guess at it, I would say I think that men on the whole are not all that interested in food. They have their favorite foods and stick to them; they eat what is given to them by the wife or the cook. Women are more dependent on health and beauty and work harder at it. They also have the responsibility to tend to the family's needs and have to think about what they are doing to their children and husband. That is just my guess.

What are your thoughts about the female menstruation cycle?

On this cleansing diet, the menstrual flow stops. Blood is never to be wasted. Blood is life; it nourishes and replenishes the body. Why would nature want to spill blood? There is no reason for bleeding when the body is pure.

Do you think it is healthy for a woman to stop bleeding during her monthly cycle?

This is a question to be answered by science, whose work it is to prove things. Our answers are subjective and cannot possibly be objective, taking all variables into consideration. But they have value in the sense that they keep the conversation going and interest growing until science investigates what is being done by more people who not only believe that this is the road to tomorrow, but also prove it by getting better results healthwise than they did on an omnivorous diet.

Many women tell me they feel it is more difficult for a woman to eliminate cooked food and eat a raw food diet because of emotions they have to deal with around the time of their monthly cycle. Do you feel it is more difficult for a woman to eat a raw food diet than it is for a man?

I do not feel gender has anything to do with this. It is a matter of choice. It is a matter of motivation and need. A lot of research will have to be done on human guinea pigs willing to subject themselves to the strict rules of the laboratory before

215

we will have the correct answers. My guess is that if a woman with polluted blood switches to a raw diet overnight, she may have a difficult time coping with the stimulated elimination and cleansing that is already part of menstruation because her body is not being prepared for it. But it can only be beneficial even if she suffers more discomfort. For someone used to a raw diet, it should cause no suffering or difficulty.

Is it healthy for a woman to eat a raw food diet when she is pregnant?

I can only speak from what I have seen. Yes, many have tried it and many did not find it wanting. Of course, I have seen only a limited number of people going on this diet when pregnant. They were healthy anyway, but they felt even better. One had severe arthritis, and her baby was born on a fruit diet that she stuck to because her arthritis improved so much for the better. Her baby was extremely healthy and was given fruit from the time it was weaned. It thrived. But nothing about this is a matter of simplicity; therefore, it will take many generations before we have the real answers.

Thank you for this interview. Is there anything you would like to add?

In today's time, no one is anywhere near the Eden life. Our planet is simply a long way from being the proverbial paradise. We are just awakening to the horizons of a new day, but nothing is as exciting as taking that courageous step towards the transformed world of tomorrow. It is a world where God is in charge, and man accepts and honors His law, order, and creations in word and deed.

This is a one man's game. Everyone must live his or her own unique life. We all need to have compassion for life. We need to be tolerant of those people still in darkness, suffering from our enslavement to sin. We all need to be aware of God's protection and guidance and Christ's salvation. We also need love in our hearts. Then we can hold hands and move together as one unit, a human body, expressing its supreme life, like a real jewel in the crown of creation.

My conclusion to is all is:

Drinking pure water, breathing pure air, and keeping a positive attitude are all things that make up a healthy and youthful life. We must continue with our task of recreating our planet and its habitats, as well as recreating our own habits and outlooks on life!

The Eden Diet is the solution to most of man's problems. We cannot hang on to the old civilization; it is over. Why not leap forward towards a new day, in a new life? There is nothing to lose, but everything to gain, by adapting to a natural way of life.

I have gained insight from this way of life for over four decades. I have seen the promised land of tomorrow, and I have touched the fringes of life in birth. I am thrilled to have chosen this path for myself. No matter what the challenges were, they were more than worthwhile.

Life is more than beauty. It is more than physical, spiritual, and emotional health. Our body is a temple in which the Son of God resides. Our temple must hear His voice and be able to express life. But at this stage of our development, it is yet a hidden vision.

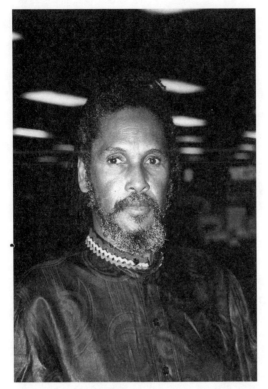

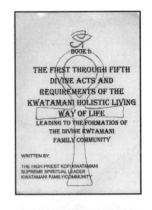

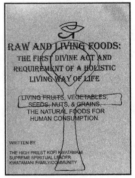

The High Priest Kofi Kwatamani is the author of many books and has made many CDs.

You may contact The High Priest Kofi Kwatamani at:

Kwatamani Private
Organic Gardens
and Spiritual Retreat
PO Box 706
Chipley, FL 32428
Ph: 850-258-9684

E-mail:
kwatamani@hotmail.com

Web Site:
www.livefoodsunchild.com

Kwatamani Holistic Institute of Brain, Body and Spiritual Research and Dev. Inc. P.O. Box 11079, Atlanta, GA 30310, Tel: 404-808-8466

The High Priest Kofi Kwatamani

High Priest Kofi Kwatamani's words have moved me so much. His energy is felt even when I just think about him and his powerful message, which is why I asked him to write the foreword in this book. I think everyone should make the time to visit him and feel his amazing energy. I am sure you will be moved just as much as I was.

The emergence of the High Priest Kofi Kwatamani on this planet in 1946 was heralded by his spiritualist/soothsayer Grandmother Essie. He was identified as a soul-seer and spiritual healer during childhood and began cultivating the fundamentals of a raw and living lifestyle at an early age despite opposition and external pressures.

His diverse and extensive background includes formal education at UCLA where he received an undergraduate degree in history, and he further completed graduate studies at UC Irvine. He served in the Air Force during the Vietnam Conflict in the late sixties where he continued a major struggle to maintain the necessities of a raw-and-living diet and a holistic living lifestyle. His responsibilities as a personnel administrator and affirmative action officer in Orange and Riverside counties in California accented his exceptional interpersonal and communication skills, which he has re-directed towards the divine science of holistic living.

His travels have carried him around the globe, serving as a research lecturer at the University of Lagon in Accra, Ghana. The High Priest has acted as CEO of holistic health enterprises and served as a healing consultant and guest speaker in various countries in Africa, Europe, Asia, and the Americas. His message has consistently focused on holistic living, featuring raw and living foods as the primary component. As a Grand Master

Chef, his years of experience and exposure to the numerous cultures and culinary styles have added an exquisite range to his recipe repertoire.

In the 1970's, the High Priest Kofi Kwatamani orchestrated the First Innercourse in Philadelphia, PA, the first raw and living-foods center of its kind in the United States. The High Priest continues to serve as an authority in the field through the various publications and productions of the Kwatamani Holistic Institute, a non-profit organization dedicated to promoting mental, physical, and spiritual development.

Major media appearances on local, national, and international television networks and radio stations have distinguished him as an expert on topics related to a holistic living way of life and self-healing. His lectures have inspired many from every walk of life, regardless of their age, race, creed, color, sex, disability, religion, or national origin to begin making fundamental changes in their attitudes and behaviors as major steps to holistic living health.

How long have you been on a raw food diet?
Over a quarter of a century. After you get past that, it is no fun remembering anymore. It makes you begin to think you are analyzing age, instead of realizing the most important thing is eternal continuation, and that is what I am upon right now.

When did you start eating a raw food diet, and what got you into it?
I came to the planet to inspire divine community. I am very clear on that. Immediately upon my deliverance and as a young child, raw and living foods were a natural to me, being a breast-fed baby. From there, I took to raw and living foods as most divine children will do, if given the opportunity. My parents were a bit headstrong because they came from the old school of thought; you need three square meals a day. 'Square' meant dead and devitalized. I couldn't take to that. At an early age, I became very ill

when consuming that stuff they call 'food.' On at least three to five occasions, the medical field told my parents, "Sorry, there is nothing else we can do. He won't live through the night."

The wonder woman, as I like to call her, who helped me was my grandmother. She would bring me apples and other fresh fruits from the farm. As I would consume them, my strength would begin to come back and after a period of time, the medical field started to realize this was a real unusual case. They would say, "We don't know exactly what is wrong with him, but we do know if he eats certain things, he gets better. So, we'll include those things in his diet."

That was a struggle, as far as my parents were concerned, because they had a different philosophy. On many occasions, before I could get total control of my own life, we would have tremendous battles. When I was a little child, it is not fair to say 'fights,' but 'struggles' against the deceit energy that dead and devitalized foods would create in them. Thanks to the Most Supreme Spirit of Love, the raw living foods of the mind, the body, and of the spirit won out. As I gained greater control, I became fully concentrated on raw living foods, the divine way of living.

Do you have any siblings besides your brother Aris who have followed this path and are spreading the word?
No, with me being the elder, and from the point when my spirit, as the essence of life, started to take greater control of the body and mind, my focus became more intensified on aggressively setting divine examples.

At a particular point in time, my brother Aris and I made a strong commitment to go forward to perpetuate the divine example of raw and living foods as the first divine act and requirement of a holistic living way of life. The idea was to spread the raw and living foods vibration throughout the country and throughout the world. Even though it may have seemed like a childish or young man's challenge, what was our objective is ex-

221

actly what has occurred. That was the first phase, the raw and living foods. The remaining phases include the establishment of a divine, social economic family community, because the best is yet to come.

Why do you think it is so hard to convince other siblings to eat a living foods diet?
The mind needs to surrender to the spirit. Again, understand that there have to be divine examples set throughout one's aging process through the institutes and so forth. However, you will start to realize that it is extremely difficult to cause change agents to occur, especially if there is a tremendous economic situation going on, where billions of dollars are being spent to perpetuate the death industry.

What advice would you give to somebody who is raw but whose loved one is going through a health crisis and will not oblige to a raw food lifestyle. How would you suggest the person deal with it?
I would tell that individual to give his or her loved one fresh juices and to get him or her to do a little bit of meditating and relaxing, and the results will come. But the challenge comes after getting the results. That is the most difficult challenge for friends, family, or loved ones, because once the results have been accomplished, they begin to think, 'Okay, I am better now,' and they go right back to the death industry's products.

Now, when I encounter any being, I go directly to his or her spirit and past the mind of thought, because his or her mind thinks from only what it knows, from the root of its behind. If it does not have the knowledge of raw and living foods, it cannot think about raw and living foods. If you can get into the spirit, into the core of the foundation of the individual, you can get that individual to have a new experience, and that means you must use examples, divine examples.

We take our living foods and herbs which we have worked

on for well over thirty years and prepare them in such a way that it becomes something difficult to resist. We have encountered individuals from all walks of life, in every space, from the ghettos to the wealthy neighborhoods. These individuals when consuming the foods, have nothing to say except, "What is this?" We then have the opportunity to come in with the strength and the power of Supreme Love. We say, "This is raw and living food, unadulterated, live, and in living color, prepared with love. This food is fresh fruits, vegetables, nuts, seeds, and grains. If you consume these foods, your body can rid itself of various illnesses." One of the first things the individual encounters is that he or she has quicker bowel movements, and those who have been congested start to realize, "Wow, it must be doing something, it is moving my bowels!"

Of course there are those who become afraid, because they are used to having bowel movements only once, twice, or three times a week. They become fearful and think they have diarrhea. But that, in itself, has been one of the major elements that can cause change. Once the individual has had some kind of example of raw and living consumption and the individual takes that consumption in and it starts to be pleasing and palatable to him or her, then he or she has the ability to change.

I have maintained a divine principle of never consuming anything dead or devitalized, regardless of the influence of any individual, even an attractive female. It does nothing. Most of my family and friends say, "You can't convince him to eat anything cooked or of that nature. He doesn't even know what it tastes like anymore." Or they will say things like, "He doesn't sacrifice life; he doesn't want to eat meat. All he eats is fruit!" Of course to them, eating fruits and fresh vegetables is considered as not eating. As time passes, they begin to realize and respect you for the principles that you live by, even though they look upon it in a very critical way. But if you hold strong, firm, and tight to those principles, they will come to give you that respect and realize you are very serious about your way of life. You begin to set a good example, because they see the foods you eat. They see you living a set of principles with a strong and whole way of life. Finally, those individuals will begin to say, "Well, let's try," and once you can put the proper supreme love energy together and get them to take the first step, there is a possibility of change.

Are you saying no matter how long it takes, stay strong and focused on your own goal and eventually, they will come around and then is the time to really make your move?
Actually, that would not be a bad statement. What I would say is, stay focused on your own goals, objectives and mission. Also, live a holistic way of life, maintain strong principles, and yield for no one, whether they are family, friend, girlfriend, foe, cousin, regardless. Stay firm and strong, and if they do not decide to step forward, that is their ball game. You must make sure you adhere to the divine laws of the universe. That is the example that you must make as a being. If you hold firm to the divine laws of the universe, then the universe will work for you. If that individual has any spiritual consciousness or strength, you will see that individual come around.

If you see that individual deciding to sacrifice, then that individual's existence upon this planet is really his or her business. There is really nothing you can do, because force is a contradiction to the laws of the universe.

What should people do when a spouse or mate will not change? Should they stay in the relationship and respect their partners' choice to eat devitalized foods, or should they find somebody else?
Let me take my son, for example. He decides that he is going to disobey the divine laws of the universe. Regardless of what I say to him, the most important thing that I can do is not to attempt to use force on him. You must allow that particular person to

224

take his or her own course, even if it is a course of self-destruction and you realize it. I have an obligation to put forward before my son the holistic living truth about Supreme Love. However, if I put that before him, and he takes it and throws it in the garbage can and says, "This is not for me!", then I get out of harm's way. Now, that is as personal as I could get.

I recognize that a mate, wife, or spouse should be considered even closer. Therefore, if they decide to maintain a death-oriented way of life, then they have declared that we are no longer mates, spouses, or any other thing of that nature.

We must realize if we come together as spiritual mates, then that takes care of all the rest of us. If we are not unified in spirit, there is no bond except some physical intercourse. The relationship will be empty. Anyone who has encountered that knows that it is one of the most frustrating things. Therefore, if you become spiritual mates, your spirits are going to unify and move forward.

On many occasions, a person will not be eating a raw diet, and later their spirit leads them to the raw and living way of life. They begin to discover the theme of life, but at the same time, their mate is not raw and living. At one time, they used to eat death together, Big Macs. They would do all the other elements that support the death industry as well. But all of a sudden, one spirit decides that enough is enough and moves forward with that urge and surge of divinity. There is nothing that should stop him or her from moving forward. The other person may decide, "Well, I am not ready for that." You must understand what you put in, is what comes out. What comes out is what you will draw back to you, and misery loves company. As a result, the individual who chose to eat raw and living foods has drawn an individual to him or her who is not whole and complete in and of him or herself. As the person eating living foods becomes more aware and complete within him or herself, he or she must begin to realize that unless they are spiritually bonded or it is a mutual choice, there is really nothing there, except the physical mind-oriented relationship. Be aware that any relationship that is not whole of the mind, body, and spirit has no way of being divinely successful. The best that one can hope for is peaceful coexistence.

Today's society brainwashes people into believing that they are doing something wrong if they only eat raw and living food. What important tips can you give to people who are new to this?

First, there are billions, trillions of dollars spent to perpetuate the death industry. Anyone who does not make a firm, 100% commitment to a holistic living way of life—consuming mentally, physically, and spiritually of raw and living foods—will have absolutely no way to continue on a divine, evolutionary path.

Billions and trillions of dollars are being spent to influence your existence, to become a part of the continuation of the death industry. It is a very serious type of program that is going on, and you must realize you are part of the program from birth. The hope is you maintain and perpetuate the programming from birth until the grave. Therefore, breaking away from this status quo means you become a part of the divine energy of the universe, a resistor to death and the death industry.

What are some common pitfalls people who are trying to eat a live food diet should avoid?

First, playing percentage games has to be one of the most devastating acts that can occur. Once you begin to play percentage games with yourself, you are not actually playing a percentage game on how raw or how living you are. You are actually playing a percentage game on how un-raw and how un-living you are. As you play the percentage game, you begin to measure the degree of raw food you are eating, not necessarily how many toxins you are putting into your body. You begin to weigh it based on if you ate one apple, and then you ate something cooked, then you are

226

fifty-fifty (50% raw and 50% cooked). If we understand simple mathematical equations: +9 and -9 = 0. Therefore, saying you are 50% raw means you are actually 0% raw and living foods.

The other pitfall is this 'fad' concept. This present time is a divine window of opportunity. To think, in any matter of degree, that consumption of raw and living foods is not the most supreme and holistic living act of the Most Supreme Spirit is a great pitfall. When you begin to think it is a fad and you want to be on the bandwagon, because you see all your friends doing it, you're actually feeding into the death industry. It may look like a popular thing and it looks like an economic adventure, but you are really becoming an agent of the death industry. You are becoming an adversary to yourself and the universe, and there is no way for you to maintain a holistic living way of life, because you have not even started it. You are talking about consuming another commodity.

Furthermore, you can consume anything, at any point in time, and this is where people fail. They start to consume cooked foods, and they say things like, "Well, I will only eat a little." Once you do that, it is no different than being a drug addict. You are definitely addicted to the drugs of death and the death industry. You are actually an addict to dead and devitalized foods. The addiction is so powerful, you begin to create rationalizations and justifications, just as a drug addict or smoker would do. You take yourself to your own fatality of spirit, because you never truly got in touch with your spirit holistically of mind and body.

What is your opinion of a diet of just fruit and nothing else?

If you decide you want to live a holistic way of life of mind, body, spirit, divine consciousness, and divine harmony with the Most Supreme Spirit of Love, Righteousness, and the Holistic Living Truth about Supreme Love, you are going to eat your fruits, vegetables, seeds and nuts. Also, you are going to eat your grains properly, and you are going to be fine, wholesome and healthy.

At this present time on the planet Earth, you are being exposed to a lot of environmental toxins from aerosols, pesticides, exhaust fumes, and all manner of contaminants. If you do not consume the proper fuel, you are going to become very, very weak. You will become very thin of mind, and you will become ill. You can't reason, and that proves you have not taken in the proper divine fuel. You need the herbs to heal and you need the fruits to cleanse. You should enjoy your fruits plentifully, particularly if you can get them in their fresh, whole, and natural state; however, if you do not repair continuously and consistently, you will be knocked down with some sort of illness. Over the years, whenever I have been exposed to, or felt the effects of any type of toxin, I have immediately sought out vegetables to consume for healing and repair. If you eat spiritually, you are going to eat according to your environment. Presently, the planet Earth is simply not in its pure, whole, and natural state, and as you look back to a certain time, you will see that the fruits were given to us as our meats, and that the vegetables were given to us as our herbs so that we might dwell in the house (the temple of the body) of whole health forever.

Are you saying that consuming a variety of foods is better than consuming just one, because focusing on one type of food causes confusion and may lead to poor health?
Absolutely, when I organized a raw and living foods center in Philadelphia, the first of its kind to deal with raw and living food preparation, I started to say, "raw and living foods." The reason why I would say "raw and living foods" over just "raw foods" is that there were individuals who were asking, "Are the nuts raw?" and I would say, "Yes, and living!" If you take a microscope and look into them, you will see living energy.

Many things people identify as nuts are not even nuts. The mass majority of things identified are seeds. The most powerful one we talk about, the almond, is not a nut; it is a seed. Those who have scientifically categorized it as a nut, didn't even know what almonds looked like on a tree. The almond is a fruit and the seed of the fruit is the almond seed that we eat. Therefore, if we consume the fruit and the seed, then we have gotten the whole nourishment from that food.

I look for organic produce and eat it all. I eat the in and the out of it. I have eaten this way for many years in Africa. I had no question whether my produce was organic or not because it was right there on our plantation. I would go out and get a mango. I can't imagine peeling the skin off of a mango. There is one called libero, and I can't imagine peeling the skin off that. There is something else amazing, the seeds! Many seeds we don't imagine eating, like olive seeds, are actually very delicious.

What is your opinion of nuts and seeds?
Nuts are one of the basic foods you can store in a whole and natural state. Actually, it is within a divine universal order to store them as a food.

When I say, consume raw and living fruits, vegetables, seeds, nuts and grains, it is unquestionable, we should eat nuts and seeds. I did not go to the university to find that out, I went to the jungles to find that out.

In the jungles, I watched how trees grow. I noticed fruit trees grow such an abundance of fruit; it only takes one seed to grow a whole tree back again, just one. If you let a bunch of seeds lay there, not all of them will grow a tree. Most of them will not even get a chance to sprout again, because the other creatures will think, 'Here are all these smart and intelligent human beings, and if they are so intelligent, then why are they going to leave all this food here? We are going to take it and eat it then.'

I decided to sit with the creatures and eat with them. I have been very familiar with such creatures as squirrels. We know squirrels enjoy nuts to no end, and they pack them away.

Nuts can get dried become dehydrated when stored for too long. What is your opinion about that?
If nuts are kept a long time, there is no question that soaking

them puts back the liquid. I am totally opposed to any mechanical dehydration of any sort. Putting them into a dehydrator is absolutely a contradiction to raw and living food consumption. Dehydration is a mechanical cooking device. Sun dried is different, that happens naturally. The sun does more than dry it. The sun adds another dose of life to it. If nuts, seeds, fruits, and vegetables have been stored and dried, add liquid to them. This will help to activate the enzymes.

What is your opinion of sprouts?
Sprouts are an excellent food for human consumption. A sprout is the first growth of life to burst out of a seed. It is the embryo of life of the plant and houses a tremendous amount of whole nutritional value. Sprouts that are known to be very powerful as whole wellness foods are wheat berries, mung bean sprouts, soy bean sprouts, lentils, almonds, and many others. Let's explore the almond seed. When you eat seeds in their fresh, whole, and natural state, they are entirely different than when you eat them from the store. If you eat almonds in their fresh, whole, and natural state, they are so soft and tender. Once removed from its shell and left for an extended period of time, the seed begins to oxidize, because it is exposed to the air, and it creates an outer, protective shell to preserve the life force within. In order to reactivate the life force, it needs to be re-liquefied.

If you are in an almond environment, you should consume them straight, raw and natural from the tree. You do not need to soak them coming out of the shell, because nature has already prepared them for easy digestive consumption.

It is when man decides to cook them, preserve them with chemicals, or maintain them for extended periods outside of their natural home (their shell) that harm is done to the life force within the seed.

All raw and living seeds contain stored whole life energy. It needs to be reactivated for life. Today, this is known as sprouting. If you can't get seeds in their fresh, whole, and natural state, I would say you should definitely take them and soak them up to, and including, that phase we call sprouting and consume them with the delicacy we call Supreme Love.

What is your opinion of juicing?
The reason why we juice is probably what needs to be understood. We realize our bodies have become so depleted, generation after generation, over and over again. Therefore, we should get the optimum fuel in us as quickly as possible. Juicing does just that. It also gives the digestive system a chance to rest while the rest of the body works to correct the total madness that has taken place in our temples. Animals also juice. They find the juice of fruits, suck it out, and drink it.

What is your average daily diet like?
I definitely do not have the stomach to consume large amounts, because that has never been my way of life. I consume until the spirit says, "Okay, that's enough." It usually speaks kind of quickly. The old saying is, "Your eyes are bigger than your stomach." Because raw and living foods can be so delicious, you want to eat lots of them. Upon eating, there comes a point where you feel you have been nourished and you stop. That is the most important thing, you eat to live, not live to eat.

Do you eat every day?
If my focus is on some type of spiritual evolution, with my children, someone within my community, or an important spiritual presentation, then there is no consumption. There is no desire to consume, because I am being fed from the fuel of the spirit. That can occur two or three days at a time. Some people call it a dry fast. I call it, no desire to consume.

Have you done many long fasts?
Yes. So, I hear. Those who have known me over a period of time have said that there are times when I have fasted for entirely too long. Bear in mind that fasting is when you abstain from con-

sumption—chewing, swallowing, or intaking additional foods into your system. Therefore, if you are juicing, you are consuming foods, foods that are more quickly and easily digestible, however, foods nonetheless. I've heard people use the word "fasting" very loosely. There are individuals who say that they are fruit fasting. There are individuals who say that they are vegetable fasting. There are individuals who say that they are juice fasting. There are individuals who say that they are fasting on raw and living foods. There are individuals who fast from sunup to sundown while indulging like a starving person before and after. Sounds like what they are saying is that fasting means consuming, or breaking consumption for a brief period of time during the day, like break fast (breakfast).

There was a particular point in time in West Africa when many of my associates swore that I would die, because people were only supposed to be able to last three days without consuming anything at all. I won't tell anyone how may days I fasted, but I did exceed the three days. It was not a desire. I did not plot it out. I didn't scheme to do it. I didn't want to impress anybody.

The body was obedient to the spirit, and the mind had no choice but to humble itself. I consumed nothing at all, just fresh air. Finally, I switched to the consumption of maybe a cup full of cucumber juice. This consumption of strictly limited amounts of cucumber juice lasted for an extended period of time that went into months. It wasn't a situation where I was deciding that this is what I was going to do. I was on a spiritual vibration and movement of energy of foresight, seeing the path ahead. It was beyond this body and totally beyond this mind.

How did you feel? Did you loose a lot of weight?
I became very frail. People would say there was a skeleton walking around with a slight layer of skin. But I felt wonderful. I have never felt a vibration like that before in my life! The energy, the zeal, the vibration was so powerful, it was beyond me. The whole experience was a beautiful, positive, divine meditation.

On average night, how much sleep do you get? How is your energy?

The higher your energy intensity, the less sleep you can actually indulge in. On occasion, if we are working on a CD or a book or preparing some type of healing with someone, people say to me, "Do you know that you haven't slept for the last three or four days?"

Sleep is not a real thing anymore. I am just so energized. There are occasions where the most sleep I get is fifteen minutes. That's almost too much! Those fifteen minutes are more like a nod. I get to a point where I lay there and I am not really asleep, because I am fully conscious; but it is enough. Sometimes when we are on the road, I will literally lay there consistently for three or four hours. Then, I will feel like I need to get up and move around.

We often sleep at a certain time of the day, after sunset or before sunrise. As I am lying there, the spiritual energy starts to waken me, the spirit refuses to lay there dormant any longer, and I get up.

I think it is nonsense to have the mind conditioned for eight hours of sleep. Even if you are conditioned, once you consume the optimum fuel, you can forget about sleeping that long. When you hear people say they need a lot of sleep, it is very obvious and clear they are consuming badly.

If you eat only live foods, the digestive process takes place smoothly and quickly. The body, brain, and spirit want to get up and get going.

On average, I would say I have gotten four hours of sleep a night. The rest of the time is spent in meditation or just vibration.

Do you think it is natural for a woman to bleed during her monthly cycle? Is it natural for other animals?

When you recognize what happens with the feminine body, you understand that if the egg is not fertilized, it has to be released. That egg is created from the whole system, the feminine energy.

Therefore, when it passes, it will pass with blood. That doesn't mean she should be sitting at home through this long bleeding process. Some women talk about their cycle lasting for seven days or longer. That is totally against nature.

Women who have been very clean in their diet and environment start to go through a whole different kind of a cycle. All that heavy bloody stuff starts to disappear after a period of time. Also, I have seen animals in the wild have spotted mucous. Take note that domesticated animals tend to have a longer menstrual period, probably something to do with their unnatural way of consuming. This subject gets much deeper in scope than what I am able to speak of in this interview.

Is there anything you would like to add?
Clearly and obviously, I have absolutely no question as to why this spirit is upon this planet. Regardless of race, creed, color, sex, physical handicap, religion, or national origin, this is the time for divine gathering of the Sacred Few. This is my spirit's mission. Also, this spirit has come to recognize, we are really only one. As I say in some of my CDs, regardless of being blonde or bald or natty, natty dread, we must come into divine alliance with the universe, and the first divine act and requirement of a holistic living way of life is the consumption of raw and living foods.

We have a holistic institute called the Kwatamani Holistic Institute of Brain Body and Spiritual Research and Development. We also have a divine, social, economic family community, the Kwatamani Holistic Living Family Community. These two entities actually act as one. The Institute is for individuals who are working towards change. They want an alternative lifestyle and an alternative way of healing. Usually they have encountered illnesses where everyone else rejected them. After healing, if they decide they want to take it a little further, they can stay at the Institute and study. Eventually, they will graduate from the Institute and begin to live in a divine, social economic family community setting. For those who are interested in extensive rest and recuperation in a whole life venue, the Kwatamani Holistic Living Family Community houses the Kwatamani Private Organic Gardens and Spiritual Retreat', tucked away on over 21 acres of pristine woodlands in the lush rolling hills of northwest Florida, just miles from the beautiful white sand beaches of the Emerald Coast as well as many natural springs.

The spiritual message is that we must all develop divine, social economic, family communities. It is my desire, wish and hope that the masculine and feminine energies will come into divine oneness and recognize and honor the basic laws of the universe; divine consumption, divine humility, divine social economics, divine sisterhood and brotherhood relationships, and divine marriage; as the basic necessities for divine, social economic family community. That means the total abstention from the use of leather or any products resulting from death or murder, therefore moving into greater alignment with the laws of nature and Supreme Love, Righteousness, and the Holistic Living Truth. When we take that course, it can take us anywhere on this planet. But wherever it takes us, we must go into supreme alliance with the Most Supreme Spirit of Love, Righteousness, and the Holistic Living Truth about Supreme Love. There is no more time for deceit. Actually, deceit has died. It is just the ghosts and goblins that live in our heads that follow us to work and to school and to bed. They keep us on the program developed by the death industry. We must resist the death industry with every divine means available and necessary. We must honor the sacred and blessed spirit of self and the Most High, the Most Supreme Spirit of Love, Righteousness, and the Holistic Living Truth. Once we have done that, we must focus on the children. Because if we don't, we are laying a path of confusion, death, and deadly destruction for ourselves and those yet to come. Life is eternal, and death has been created in the mind. When we cease to perpetuate life, we are perpetuating death and we have become a vital part of the death industry.

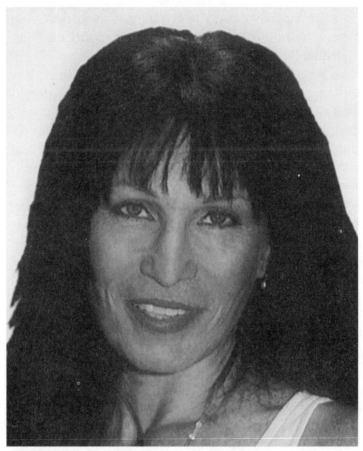

Youkta 2001. Photo by Jennifer Girard, Chicago

You may contact Youkta at:

Youkta
P.O. Box 1556
Mount Ida, Arkansas 71957

Ph: 870-867-4521
Web: www.youkta.org
E-mail: youktaspiritdance@yahoo.com

Youkta

I have never had the opportunity to meet Youkta, but after speaking with her on the telephone, it seemed as though I had known her for a very long time because I felt comfortable asking her anything. She is a great person with so much knowledge to share about living a healthy lifestyle. I believe that her information in this interview will help many people.

Youkta, under the tutelage of many world-renowned teachers, has studied, practiced, performed, and taught dance, yoga, and fitness for more than twenty-five years. Youkta has been dedicated to the living foods lifestyle for twenty years and will soon be releasing a book.

Youkta, a grandmother in her fifties, remains dynamically and passionately inspired in Dance and Yoga Kinetics, utilizing movement as an evolutionary tool and inspiring personal growth, joy, and the celebration of sharing. She is the founder and director of the "International Woman's Festival of Healing Arts." She also operates a dance and yoga studio in the Hot Springs area and partners with Viktoras Kulvinskas in All Life Sanctuary, the holistic lifestyle resort camp school. Youkta is available for group and private instruction, workshops, and performances.

How long have you been eating a raw diet, and what got you into it?
I've been eating a raw diet for at least twenty-five years. I got into it for health reasons. After years of researching many different approaches, the outcome was raw foods.

How was your health when you started the diet?
I was very old at age thirty. I had symptoms of all kinds. If I had

237

not changed my ways, it is questionable whether I would be here today.

Where did you first hear about a raw food diet?
I first heard about it from books. I have read many books. The book that really made the difference was *Love Your Body*, by Viktoras Kulvinskas.

Who are some people who have inspired you to do this the most?
At that time, no one I knew was dealing with the same health issues. Inspired by what I had read, I persevered by myself for five years.

How did you and Viktoras start working together?
After being alone for those five years, I asked Viktoras to come and lecture near me, and that is how we connected. I went to his center, and I knew I needed to be there because I wasn't getting support anywhere else.

You have learned so much over the years. What are some of the most important things people should know about the raw food diet?
I think the most important thing is making a gentle transition that makes sense. If you don't understand what's happening and you feel that the process of evolution you're attempting is too challenging, it usually means you've skipped a step or two, and that often leads to failure. It's important to go slow and steady, letting the body's chemistry shift, instead of trying to live what is perceived as an ideal. Shift your life towards improvement by slowly making little improvements, until they settle and make sense. Then you will have intuition as to what the next step is.

Are there any pitfalls you have learned to watch out for on the raw diet?
Sometimes people perceive what is optimum and try to obtain the ideal - an all raw diet - without taking all the necessary steps on the ladder of success within dietary means.

What people do not realize is that they are shifting on a cellular level as well when they are changing their diet, and that takes time. For instance, if a person who has been eating a very dense diet of meats and breads and things like that starts eating living foods all of a sudden, he is likely to starve because his cells really can't make the exchange of nutrients with the bloodstream because his cells are so dense. That is why people who are not used to eating fruit claim that eating a particular fruit makes them go into a stage of diarrhea. For example, they eat a lot peaches and all of a sudden, their body goes into a cleansing mode and they reach the wrong conclusion. There is no need to do anything so radical.

There are many different types of raw food diets. Which one do you feel is the best?
I don't feel that one diet is necessarily any better than the others. I think it's a personal choice. It is a matter of what you feel you need and what you want to do in life. Whatever the diet is, I think the most important consideration is whether people feel whole and have the energy they want and feel good and are doing activities they enjoy in life. I know that a lot of people are absolutely not interested in the raw diet because it's not convenient. All their friends and most people in the world are into cooked foods. I feel that having the knowledge of how raw food affects the body will sooner or later help people move their diet in a direction where they will have more energy and will feel better, as well as knowing what to do during a health crisis.

What is your opinion of nuts and seeds?
They are important concentrated foods - a source of complete protein, essential fatty acids, and especially calcium.

What is your opinion of grains?
Grains are very important for long-term fire energy and stamina. They are our complex carbohydrates. When I started the raw diet, I didn't have any grains in my diet. I read a lot of information

239

that claimed that grains were acidic, mucus-forming, and definitely something to stay away from. About ten years into this diet without having any grains, I ran into a wall. I didn't have any stamina or long-term energy. Basically, I had to question the diet and ask what I was doing wrong; why was I feeling this energy loss? I knew the raw food diet made a difference in my life. It made such a dynamic difference, I didn't want to give it up. But I had to find the missing link. By integrating a meal of sprouted grains every day without changing anything else in my life, my whole body changed. My muscles filled out, I stopped having bone loss, and my whole body just looked a lot fuller and a lot healthier.

In your opinion, could someone eat a raw food diet without including nuts, seeds, or grains?
Without them, the body will break down prematurely. I've heard many fantastic stories, but I have yet to meet anybody who practices such a diet for over a decade who looks strong and healthy without them.

What is your opinion of an all fruit diet?
If you look in the dictionary, it says that "fruit" is anything which bears seed. People think "fruit" means apples and oranges and produce like that, but fruit actually consists of much more. Fruits include some of what we know as non-leafy vegetables, nuts, and the fruits of grass, which are the grains. To understand what fruitarianism is, a person would benefit from looking up that word first because it could broaden one's view. All the other foods which do not fall under this category are the leafy greens, roots, and tubers, which are the true vegetables.

Do you think it is important to have leafy greens as part of the diet?
Each season provides different foods. If you observe monkeys, you'll see that during the winter, they have a diet of tubers and barks. However, during the spring, they usually eat leafy pro-

duce, when there's not much of anything available except for lots of tender vegetables and leafy greens.Towards summer, they begin to eat more fruits as they become available. Basically, I am saying that it makes sense for us to have leafy greens as part of our diet.

What is your opinion of sprouts?
Sprouts are like children: they have lots of energy and enzymes for growing.When you eat, you optimally eat for fuel.Therefore, if you integrate sprouts into your diet, you are eating foods that are a high source of enzymes and lots of energy. However, I wouldn't eat a diet of just sprouts. I think some mature foods are very important, as well. I think it's good to arrive at a balance and really understand and feel the experience of your diet and journey.

What is your opinion of supplements?
Before taking supplements, it would be good to make sure that they are based on whole foods, preferably enzymatically active. If a person is deficient, or if the body is not making something, then supplements are a good way to help, heal, strengthen, and balance out the body. But I don't feel that living on supplements is optimal; I think they merely serve as a Band-Aid. It is, however, a matter of whatever a person needs to balance his energy.

I think we are so compromised these days.The genetic code of each generation is breaking down more and more as each generation becomes more nutrient-deficient.The more this happens, the more the human body is unable to produce certain essentials in adequate quantity or quality on its own naturally. I think that people need to do whatever it takes in order to balance their chemistry and make it work optimally now and in the future.

What is your opinion of eating seasonally?
I think it makes sense.

What is your opinion of fasting?

If the body needs a rest or cleansing, fasting is absolutely the best.

What is your opinion of food combining on a 100% raw food diet? Do you think it is necessary?

Yes. It's all about eating for easy digestion. The stomach balances the alkaline-forming and acid-forming foods for digestion. If you eat grains, they need an alkaline stomach. If you eat protein, such as nuts, they need an acid stomach. If you're mixing grains with proteins, you've got your stomach trying to figure out which way to go. If you have grains in your stomach and you eat protein, it's going to dump some acid in there, which is going to sour the grains, which will slow the digestion of the grains. It can be very uncomfortable.

What is your opinion of exercise?

I think the body's circulation depends on it. As the old saying goes, "If you don't use it, you lose it," so in order to build muscle and keep bones strong, it's important to do some activity. As you age, you'll remain comfortable and relatively free in your form.

What is your opinion of wild foods?

If you have the privilege of understanding them and knowing what they are, I'd say that eating them is optimal. I think they were the original diet. That's what I call "a divine diet", because they are provided by the creator.

What are your age, height, and weight?

I'm in my mid-fifties, and I weigh 125 pounds. When I first started this diet at the age of thirty, I was five feet four inches tall, and I am now between five feet six and five feet seven.

You have actually grown taller?

Yes, because I opened up my joints. Earlier in life, I felt a lot older than I physically was. I was very sedentary in my body and I was a lot heavier. Now the joints are open and I have grown.

Has your weight changed, or are there any other changes

your body has gone through? How did you handle it?
I was overweight as a teenager because I grew up on the diet that most of America lives on. I always had a weight problem. I was one of those people who are afraid to eat. If I smelled food, I felt like I was going to gain weight. Because of that fear, I ate like a bird. When I shifted my diet towards raw, the weight balanced out and the energy went up.

During your transition, did you ever get really sick or have a really bad detox?
I didn't feel my body, and I think I was very fortunate because of that. Many of us grow up denying our bodily sensations, so we don't even feel them. We are taught to do what we have to do in life and act as if the body doesn't exist - until, of course, it breaks down and goes into pain. I was very ignorant when I shifted my diet. I think it was by divine grace that I found my way. As I experienced it, I slowly woke up and realized it was a magnificent journey. I went from being a zombie into something new and alive. I was healing and growing. I was becoming more youthful.

Over the years, have you eaten a 100% raw diet consistently?
For the first ten years, it was very much like a roller coaster ride. I just didn't have all the information. Even though I stuck with it pretty well, I always felt very hungry. I was starving my cells.

Over the years, there were periods where I was 100% raw for many months. Then I'd go back and forth by eating some cooked food, especially when I went to visit friends. I relaxed a little bit. There was a phase in the winter where I'd have some cooked food occasionally. If I was in a restaurant and they didn't serve anything I needed, I'd have rice or a baked potato. If I did eat cooked food, I ate whole foods. I could get a salad just about anywhere, so that was not a problem. Sprouted breads or anything like that was definitely not available. However, I always ate what was considered healthy by average means. But for me, I needed to go more toward the optimum. Nowadays, I do eat

99% raw foods.

Currently, what is your average daily diet like, and how often do you eat?

I developed my personal diet choices by paralleling my diet with that of an athlete. I took the same measures, but I converted it towards the raw.

I try to eat small meals. Your stomach is the size of a clenched fist; therefore, ideally, you don't want whatever you put in your stomach to exceed that. At the same time, you want to eat enough food to meet your energy output. If I'm going to be dancing for six hours, or taking part in any other physical activity like that, I'm going to need high power energy. But if I'm going to have a day where I'm more relaxed, being in my house sewing or engaging in more quiet activities, I'm going to eat a lot lighter. I eat the proper type of fuel to support that physical demand.

Does food take energy from the body, or does it give the body energy?

Aloe and the fruit juices will provide the immediate energy people need to get through physical activity, whereas the grains or carbohydrates you eat at night are really fuel for the next day. If you eat a grain meal in the evening, the body will store its energy within to give you power for the next day. I'm usually on top of my diet when it comes to the amount of energy I'll need the next day. But in a circumstance where I didn't get the proper fuel the day before, I would probably eat cereal in the morning, like most people. However, that's not something that I usually do, because it takes longer to digest and its energy is released more slowly.

What is your favorite food right now?

I am eating a lot of fresh produce from my garden right now, and I love it. I really like all fresh raw foods, and I have a passion towards my food.

What is the difference between eating a cooked diet and a raw diet?
A raw diet has many benefits. People need to understand that any meal made with cooked foods can also be made with raw foods. The difference is, with the raw foods, you're eating something that is vital and alive. Because the food is raw, it is enzymatically rich. You're getting the energetics and the prana within the live foods and exchanging that within the body.

Out of all the foods, do you think one is most important?
Not really. A balanced choice of food, appropriate for your immediate energy demands and long-term health, is the best direction. The chemical balance of blood is more complex than any one food.

How are your health and energy?
Excellent. When I was tested, I was off the charts. I was in what they call a "superior" category. It's not that I don't have room for improvement, but under average circumstances, I'm considered well above average.

How much sleep do you get, and how much do you think is necessary?
The amount of rest a person needs depends upon the individual and what he is doing. There have been times in my life when I naturally slept two hours at night and two hours during the day. I did that for a long time, and the experience was very vivid. Everything was really clear, and people remarked how good I looked. It was something that was fine for that time in my life, but I wasn't living in the average everyday world; I was living more within the cycles of nature. There was also a time when I lived outdoors in the jungle for many months. I was really resonating within nature. When the moon was full, there was so much energy and activity throughout the jungle that my eyes adjusted to it. It was like daylight, except it was blue light from the light of the moon. In this natural rhythm, a long night of rest was not nec-

essary. However, during the new moon, there was silence and darkness in the jungle, which called for a long night's rest.

I recognize that a constant eight hours of sleep per night is typical within our average world, which is so removed from nature. We have so much stress during the day, some people really do require eight to ten hours of sleep to balance out the stress and just be able to move on to the next phase. So it depends on the circumstances. When I'm living in the everyday world, I definitely go for the eight hours.

Have you noticed any mental changes on a raw food diet?
I used to be very depressed unless I was on some sort of stimulant. I was like a zombie, always dragging my feet and feeling very lethargic. I felt heavy in my body and in my mind. Now, all that has improved. I don't think I'll ever be brilliant, because there might have been some possible brain damage, but I'm definitely a lot more awake in my body and in my mind. It's as though a light bulb has been switched on and I feel more inner-connected with life. Before, I didn't feel that way at all.

When it comes to relationships, many people new to the raw diet run into problems because their mates do not want to change. Do you have any comments or suggestions?
Human beings are creatures who need companionship. We are tribal by nature, to varied degrees, of course. Some people are happier in a more isolated situation, while others are happier when they are really close to another. I think it is very important to understand what your personal needs are before you can attempt to interact and co-create with someone else. In the case of Viktoras and myself, neither one of us has lost ourselves in the relationship. Instead, we are one another's absolute, solid support. We have history together and we have a great understanding of each other and compassion for one another. We're completely different, but Viktoras lives his life fully and I live my life fully. Even though we both live our separate lives, we are

both raw foodists, so we kind of meet in the kitchen. That is our common ground. We appreciate each other's differences, and we really appreciate the support we give one another. I think that's what relationships are about. It is a matter of what you're connecting with. It's the willingness to accept the differences and feel comfortable with them. For some people, it's not important to meet in the kitchen or eat together; they can each do their own dietary thing and that is their difference. Just as important, they connect with each other in a different area. It's really an individual thing, but I feel the more support you have, the easier it is.

Do you have any suggestions for people with unsupportive mates or family members?
If these loved ones are creating obstacles by not accepting your differences or not being supportive of your choices, then I don't think they really care as deeply for you as it may appear. There are a lot of things where I don't agree with Viktoras, but I understand that it's his choice and I respect him, and he respects me and my choices as well. I think we can equally compare our differences while giving caring support. That's a very powerful healing source, and it is what we all really want. So it doesn't matter if one perceives one type of a diet as better than another. It's a matter of what are you willing to accept, understanding where your boundaries are, and what choices you make. It is an individual choice on how you prefer to exist or be.

Do you think it is harder for a woman to eat this way, or is it harder for a man, or do you think it's a personal thing?
I think it's personal. I don't think it's any easier or more difficult for one or the other.

What are your thoughts about the female menstruation cycle? Do you think it is natural for a woman not to bleed when she is on a raw diet?

From what I have observed through the years, some blood is natural and it's meant to happen. But the chemistry does fluctuate radically and the duration of flow will be very short. Basically, it's more of an intuitive experience, where you observe your body going through changes. There shouldn't be pain and discomfort and there shouldn't be lots and lots of blood. Having no blood at all is usually a sign that there's an imbalance or deficiency of some sort. This is what I have learned from talking with healthy women over many years.

In our society, men try to keep weight on, while woman try to lose weight. This obsession with the 'perfect body' image affects many of us through our food choices and often leads to problematic relationships around food and distorted eating behaviors. What is your opinion on all this?

Many times when the body is not totally connected with itself physically, mentally, emotionally, socially, and spiritually, the inner intelligence tries to balance out the body. If you're trying to gain weight and eating a tremendous amount of food and you have tension behind it, the tension is going to eat up all that food, so you're not going to put on weight. Women put on weight more easily because they have a natural layer of fat; so it's easy for them to go in that direction. Even if the body is balanced, naturally, women still have a higher fat count than men. I think we need to understand the balance of each gender and honor that instead of trying to balance the body through diet alone. It's important to tend to the other aspects of self. Eventually, an inner harmony will surface, and you will experience food as just fuel. Then you can do whatever you want to do and you won't think about the weight issue.

Do you think it's easier to eat a raw food diet today than it was years ago?

I think it's easier today because there are many more people following this path. Twenty to thirty years ago, there were very few people who tried it, and most ended up falling apart because they did not know what or how to do it. Because of that, they either went to a macrobiotic diet or back to their old traditional way. In today's times, I think there's a greater understanding of what the diet needs to consist of. There are many more culinary artists (raw chefs) working within the raw foods community making lots of raw palatable, transition dishes. I think because of that, people getting into the raw diet are not going to feel hungry and deprived. I feel these culinary artists are sort of bridging the gap between divine creation, from where you pick food off a tree or from the ground, to making things like pizzas, nut loaves, and ice creams. This is good, because the average person can taste it and connect with it and feel satisfied enough to move in that direction. So I think the success rate is going to increase and more people will stick with it.

Where do you see the raw food movement in the future?
Because there are so many more people doing it now, I think there will be another cycle that will come along in another twenty years and the success rate will go even further. Many people design their lives around convenience. Therefore, I think there will be more people working in culinary services making palatable raw dishes and meals. More raw foods will be available, and there will be more people involved in the movement.

Thank you for this interview. In closing, is there anything else you would you like to add?
Basically, I think that the greatest issue for most people is the transition and support. My feeling is that there is so much dietary information, it is easy to become confused. Eating is a natural process. I think if we can realize that from the divine creation the raw food was the original diet, it could lead us to a wider horizon of healthier choices. Choosing to eat more natural foods, from a balance of food groups, will help people to move in a direction that will be more satisfying and more successful.

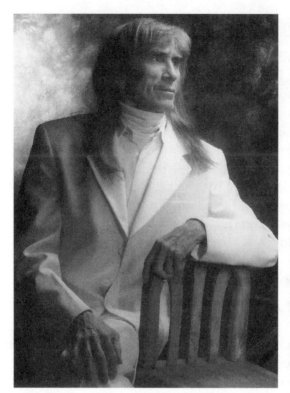

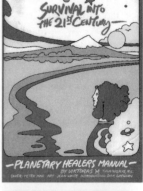

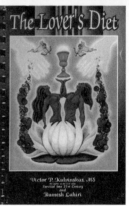

Viktoras 2001. Photo by Jennifer Girard, Chicago

Viktoras has written several books about the raw food diet and lifestyle. You may contact Viktoras at:

Viktoras Kulvinskas, MS
All Life Sanctuary Retreat Center
P.O. Box 2853
Hot Springs, Arkansas 71914

Ph: 870-867-4521
E-mail: viktoraslive@yahoo.com
Web site: www.youthing101.com

Viktoras Kulvinskas

O f all the people I have met, Viktoras is one person who I never thought I would get an interview with because he is so well known within the raw food community. I thought that even if I ever did meet him, he would not have time for me; I was wrong about that. Not only did he give me the time I needed for a great interview, but we also became good friends. He is without a doubt one of the nicest people I have ever met in my life and one of the most knowledgeable. Now I am happy to pass along his knowledge to you in this interview. Enjoy.

Viktoras was born in Lithuania before World War II. While growing up, he lived in displaced person camps in Germany. He graduated with an MS in Mathematics. He taught college and was a computer consultant for decades with Smithsonian Astrophysical Observatory; Apollo Project, Harvard, MIT, etc.

His personal health was failing and he was becoming more disabled. He researched alternatives and became involved with the well known healers Walker, Warmbrand, Christopher, Jensen, Wigmore, Szekely, Howell, and Murray.

Viktoras co-founded the *Hippocrates Health Institute* with Ann Wigmore now in West Palm Beach, Florida, where he continues to give workshops. He wrote a bestseller, *Survival Into the 21st Century*, with a Peter Max cover. He has been a practitioner in the holistic field for thirty-five years. He was Nutritional and Educational Director of Dick Gregory's Obesity and Substance Abuse resort for two years.

Viktoras is a senior executive with Cell Tech, Inc., provider of Super Blue Green Algae - raw, wild, complete food - the choice of many top athletes.

Viktoras is a natural healer, Essene minister, worldwide lecturer, and Live Food Chef.

When did you first change your diet and experience the benefits of detoxification?
When I was a child, when my family moved from Lithuania to Germany during World War II, we were forced to eat a semi-vegetarian diet. We foraged from the forest - berries, mushrooms, and nuts. We grew cabbage and made kraut. We traded the belongings in our horse-drawn covered wagon for whatever edibles that were available. We had to live on a lot of simple foods - mostly turnips, potatoes, cabbage, or corn bread - no cooked milk or gluten products. On such an improved diet, I had my first cleansing experience. Boils broke out all over my body for well over a year. I had fevers, colds, and skin eruptions. The remnants of mucus and incompletely metabolized cooked milk and cooked grains that I had consumed as a child in Lithuania were being released from my body. Also, I began having fewer migraine attacks. That was my first approach towards a semi-vegetarian diet. Within five years, I became relatively healthy, although at that time I was not as wise or as healthy as some people who have had a similar path such as the raw family of today, the Boutenkos.

After that, when was your next attempt to eat a healthier diet?
At age ten, after coming to United States, having no understanding of what took place in Germany, I found myself degenerating on the rich SAD (Standard American Diet) diet with the return and/or development of migraines, frequent colds, allergies, dandruff, sciatica, stiffness, and fatigue. I started drinking coffee and colas for stimulation. I tried to be vegetarian again for a short time in high school and again in college for a whole year. I was looking for a meaningful philosophy and experimenting with meditation. Being alone in my experiments, I easily drifted back to the behavior of my associates.

How was your health at that point in your life?

By age seventeen, I had bleeding ulcers and bi-monthly migraines, I was tired often and drank a lot of coffee, my skin showed pimples, my tongue had a crease in the center (indicative of digestive disorders), my nipples were swollen and enlarged (due to all the hormones in the milk and poultry that I was eating), and my knees were severely enlarged from pasteurized milk calcium build up. I had a very low level of concentration, and I was held back three grades in grammar school. Under the same circumstances today, a child would be diagnosed with ADD/ADHD.

What happened then? Did you find what you were looking for?
I responded to stress by consuming rich foods and stimulants. In college, the scholastic demands, my manic-depressive personality, and my bleeding ulcer led me to crave the sedation of ice cream and rich foods followed by the stimulating effects of coffee to help me be scholastically productive. I used medication for pain and ulcers quite often. Eventually, I lived on burned toast, ice-cream, and as much as twenty cups of coffee per day.

Following the loss of an important relationship, I felt empty. I took up smoking (over three packs per day) as well as some drinking. Within a year, I quit cold turkey. My ongoing level of concentration was sporadic. To escape the insecurity of the last semester of graduate school, I was lured into the sedation of emotional eating. I gained over fifty pounds. I had a triple chin and a 200 pound body. The fear of failure and the shame on behalf of my family led me, three weeks before finals, to stop all of it and go on a fast and study ceaselessly, which culminated in six days without any sleep. My concentration returned with almost photographic memory, and I was empowered by the psychic support of my guardian angel. I practiced mindlessness, silencing all doubts and concentrating only on the task at hand. I passed some of my exams and excelled in others. I graduated with a Master of Science in Theoretical Mathematics. I worked that summer for the graduate school, designing software for the administration, and I hung out with the hackers' new computer cult. I was obsessive. I worked around the clock, sleeping only when I was exhausted and eating only when I was starving. My weight dropped to 145 pounds. Then I left for Cambridge, Massachusetts to join a consulting firm.

I lived alone and worked around the clock, seven days a week. For entertainment, I designed furniture, did portrait photography, and studied foreign movies. My eating habits improved. I ate animal organs, fish, oriental foods, and some salads. In spite of this, I was very acidic and enzyme-exhausted and I had daily indigestion. By my late twenties, I was severely calcium arthritic petrified. I had excruciating pain shooting down my legs as well as my lower back. I had kidney pain, my legs had edema, and I had to lie down every two to three hours to reduce my lower back pain and to offset the leg edema. My health was being challenged by my behavior and eating habits. I started seeing doctors, but they found nothing wrong with me physically, outside the fact that my stomach had migrated to the pubic area, I had an ulcer, and I was depressed.

Only when my body became disabled did I look for alternatives. At a health food store, I discovered Dr. Walker's books. I called him. He gave me a lot of inspiration and suggested that I visit Ann Wigmore, who was only a few miles away from me.

I also connected with a naturopath doctor named Dr. Warmbrand in New Haven, Connecticut. I ended up visiting him and becoming a client of his. He encouraged me to eat simple, vegetarian foods, three meals a day, and to do some exercise. Under his guidance, I ate both raw and cooked foods, with two to three different foods at a meal.

When did you meet Ann Wigmore?

After meeting Dr.Warmbrand and getting back on a vegetarian diet, I finally went to the Ann Wigmore center for a visit. It was the Spring of 1968.At the church, twice a day, everyone drank wheatgrass as a healing sacrament. The meals served were a mix of simple raw foods, kelp powder, and protein seed/nut dressings and cooked stew or grain/legume loafs. I ate small amounts and chewed it well. I was really surprised to see how agreeable the food was. I bought Ann's book, *Why Suffer*, and read it in four days. It was just what I needed. I decided to quit my job in computer consulting and spend a few weeks with Ann Wigmore.Afterwards, I planned to take a long sabbatical, to study and travel. I was even considering going back to college to get a Ph.D. in Mathematics.

How long did you stay with Ann Wigmore?

I only planned on staying a few weeks, but I enjoyed the service and the excitement of something so revolutionary and controversial that it fed my soul. Weeks turned into months, and months turned into seven years. I was never paid. I took the vows of poverty and chastity with my creator and devoted myself to serving others and became at one with unconditional love. Ann offered me a place to stay at her five-acre farm.That was the clincher. I was in heaven. It was a return to innocence and nature. We wore cotton and went barefoot, even in the city, and made our work our play.Within a month, I started weekly chiropractic adjustments, which led to the return of feelings in my legs. Later, I attempted yoga and made very little progress due to my rigid structure and muscle stiffness.After a few years, I discovered rolfing and had a year of this painful deep tissue massage, which greatly improved my flexibility. Eventually I got involved in Kundalini yoga for two hours daily for several years. I later got certified as a teacher of Integral Yoga. My best yoga advancement took place during the many years I studied Youkta Yoga.

And you started to work with Ann Wigmore?
When I joined Ann, she was operating under a Rising Sun Christianity foundation, with a mission to teach Biblical truths that are related to health and wellness. I loved her heroic ways. I was dedicated to Ann and totally committed to her. I loved learning, and the next thing I knew, I was gardening, learning carpentry, fixing electrical wiring and plumbing, shopping for food, repairing an elevator... We had hardly any money, and I was the one to try to solve the mechanical challenges. As I studied the natural healing and living works of others, I started lecturing on the subject. The best way to learn something is to teach it. Eventually, I managed to get a pass to the Harvard Medical Library, and I would spend hours a day studying health and the causes of disease, which laid the foundation for my book, *Survival into the 21st Century.*

How much weight did you lose when you started the program?
I started off at 140 pounds and got down to 90 pounds. I lost about fifty pounds.

How was your energy?
Even though I lost so much weight, I was fully active, to everyone's surprise, working twelve to sixteen hours a day. Much of it was hard labor. I was handling crates of fruit and 100 pound sacks of seeds.

You mentioned that some cooked food was served when you started Ann's program. Why did you decide to drop cooked food from the program?
After a year with Dr. Ann, I discovered the live food writings of Professor Szekely and the Essene esoteric biblical teachings within the *Essene Gospel of Peace* (Jesus's holistic teachings on wellness, the live food diet, and wheatgrass), which led me to be ordained as an Essene minister twenty years later. Due to my dedication, Dr. Ann trusted me, and with my encourage-

ment, we gradually got rid of one stove at a time to make more room. Eventually, we were all raw. At that point, we co-founded The Hippocrates Health Institute, which was to become the educational/therapeutic out-reach branch of the church, teaching the live food lifestyle and natural healing.

As demand grew for our service in the Mansion on Exeter Street in Boston, we acquired one floor and then another and another, and eventually we filled up five stories with guests and staff. Ann and I saw much better healing results on live food. However, at the same time, we didn't really have what would be considered a nutritionally complete program. It was great for cleansing, but folks stayed slim, unless they introduced cooked food. But with cooked food included in the diet there was the issue of severe enzyme deficiency on the cellular level that made healing slow and rebuilding very stretched out. Also, we did not place enough value on exercise, rest, or water. We needed a raw food rebuilding and maintenance program. It was several decades later before we had all the components. In spite of that, we saw many folks healing from leukemia, cancer, MS, obesity, diabetes, asthma, chronic fatigue, even AIDS. It was exciting. I was running around the country, as well as running around locally, promoting The Hippocrates Health Institute and Dr. Wigmore as much as I could.

How did you promote the Institute?
When I joined Rising Sun Christianity, Ann had no staff and only a few clients. Ann put out a monthly magazine that went out to several hundred people. After about three years, I was very involved in the promotion of our Institute. I basically did all I could to put Ann Wigmore on the map. After a few years with Dr. Ann, I persuaded Shilo Farms, who were a Christian community and distributors of organic produce, to take me along as a worker on one of their delivery routes. I joined them for several months and took Rev. Ann Wigmore's *Be Your Own Doctor* magazines to about sixty health food stores. All

of a sudden, we started having clients come to Hippocrates. I also went out to lecture at alternative expos and yearly Rainbow Tribe Gatherings and did radio and TV as well as publish *Grass Revolution*. At the Institute, when I first started giving lectures, we would get two to five people. I kept up a weekly lecture series. As I became more experienced, as well as more entertaining, the numbers eventually grew to dozens and hundreds. At one of the NHF Expo's, my audience was well over 5000. I published *Love Your Body*, followed by *Survival into the 21st Century*.

Eventually, I left Hippocrates to help my grandmother, who was suffering from Alzheimer's. It seemed that I had an even more significant effect on the Institute after my departure. According to Brian Clement, who followed me as the director of the Hippocrates Health Institute (now in West Palm Beach, Florida), my book, *Survival into the 21st Century*, was responsible for over half of the clients at the Institute.

You have made many discoveries over the years. Some of them being Buckwheat Lettuce and Sunflower Greens. How did you discover Buckwheat Lettuce and Sunflower Greens?

Dr. Ann already had the baker tray wheatgrass indoor growing system. At one time or another, she had grown other grasses. As many wonderful gifts happen, they seem to be accidental. I had placed an order for sunflower seeds and forgot to ask for the hulled ones. We had no way of hulling them. So I decided to compost them at our farm. We delivered our compost weekly. On my second return, I found the compost pile covered with short-stemmed, two-leaf weeds. I was always looking for new greens for our Institute salads. I tasted them and they were delicious. As I was harvesting, I pulled up the whole plant and found a sunflower seed shell at the root. I was in ecstasy. I bought more unhulled sunflower and proceeded to grow them on trays in the same fashion as the wheatgrass.

Everyone loved it. I proceeded to look for other seeds which could be used as salad greens. The most successful were buckwheat and peas and, to a lesser extent, lentil, mung, alfalfa, fenugreek, and radish.

How did you discover the importance of fermentation?
That was another lucky, divinely guided accident. During the two years when I was chef for our guests, we served protein seed/nut dressings which were 60% fat and high in hard-to-digest protein. The meals were rich and not very therapeutic. I noticed that when the leftovers sat in the refrigerator, they tasted much better on the second day and were easily digested. After much reflection, I saw that I had discovered a seed milk fermentation, analogous to milk yogurt. In creating the ferment, I drained off the acid whey to further remove acid, using a cheesecloth. Seed Cheese was thus born. About that same time, Ann discovered the famous rejuvilac.

Prior to this discovery, I weighed ninety pounds. I stayed at that weight for about two years. I was strong and worked long hours. But no matter what I ate, I could not gain weight. The nuts and seeds felt heavy and gave me gas. I could not digest whole and soaked nuts and seeds. I started eating a lot of fermented sunflower seed cheese with bananas. Within about a year, I put on around forty pounds. I started to look healthier. I think the reason why fermented foods agreed with me so well was because I was so enzymatically exhausted. I was amazed.

In the study of primitive cultures that are noted for exceptional health, two consistent factors are found: (1) the consumption of some form of fermented foods, and (2) the eating of whole natural foods, with an emphasis on a plant based diet.

Did you go through any emotional detox during that time?
I continued to work with juice fasting, using fruit and vegetable juices. The longest lasted six weeks. I got to the point

where I was touching very dark psychic areas. A lot of old emotional stuff associated with the personal pain and repressed feelings of my dysfunctional World War II childhood background began to surface. Every feeling that one holds onto, whether it is joy, fear, love, or anxiety, actually has a unique macro-molecule associated with it. That is the essence of the feeling. If you do not process these molecules of feeling and excrete them, they come to the surface years later when you start cleansing.

As a child, I had a lot of love from my parents, but at the same time, we were immersed in the violence of war. People were killed, disembodied, and shot at. There was a lot of fear and unreality. I was also immersed in the fear-enriched mythology of primitive Christianity and the frightening folk tales of demons and violence. I was afraid of darkness and afraid to be alone. I have no memory of my childhood. I suppressed most of my past memory, as I had a very limited experience with language. Basically, I was silent, with a language development challenge until mid-high school, where I was like a child, trying to learn to speak and carry on a conversation.

How did you deal with this emotional detox?
As I started reliving my insecurities and the fearful past, I started eating more to suppress it. I didn't understand that it was a process that I could eventually be freed from. Instead of fasting, I started eating more and eventually started eating cooked foods and drinking coffee again. I soon started getting migraines again. Emotionally, I was a wreck.

So the emotional detoxification affected your diet in a big way?
Yes. I eventually became bulimic. I started eating and throwing up as a way to control the migraines. It lasted for about ten years in spite of my involvement with the live food movement. One of the good things that I did during that time was to re-

main a vegetarian. I also consumed enzymes after all my purges. That kept my immune system intact, as well as keeping my digestive power at a high level.

How did you eventually get control of your emotions?
I was introduced to an algae product. A caring friend, Show-shawme, basically, through endless pestering, got me to try Super Blue Green algae. It jumpstarted my life. I was one of the 50% of the algae eaters who saw a very dramatic effect within a matter of few days. I started to feel less depressed, I felt clearer and more integrated, and I started to change my life. From esoteric and color therapy, we know that the blue of the algae has a dramatic effect on creativity, concentration, and mental faculty. The purple affects intuition, attitude, and emotional poise. A decade later, much research has been published on this algae, especially its impact on emotional poise, ADD, and total health (see *www.celltech.com*). Within a month, I started taking progressive action to correct my life and diet. The algae jumpstarted my life, but I had a long way to go to maintain it...integrating the holistic lifestyle and exploring the path of the Essene, as well as Yoga.

What else can you tell us about your recovery?
Once again, I was back to eating natural foods, and I felt confident about my future. I started doing yoga and weightlifting. Things were moving along fine. I was working with Dick Gregory on an addiction book.

To get more mileage, I started drinking coffee again. Coffee was my place of comfort. Furthermore, my diet was still too acidic. I started having the migraine attacks again, and eventually they became frequent! My migraines were related to structural problems - too much acidity, failures in communication and judgment, inadequate hydration, as well as poor eating habits. I became sloppy and irresponsible. Youkta was my yoga teacher and counselor. We also shared a friendship at

261

that time. She found that her life was affected in a negative way by my baggage. I had to shape up or ship out. I had to find an answer fast. I prayed for direction, and intuitively, I was guided in the many changes.

I discovered Spinology, which is a form of simplified chiropractic. I started having daily adjustments. That continued for about two to three years. The adjustments allowed me to control and or prevent my migraines. I got into weightlifting as a serious way to build up muscle tonality so I could maintain my posture, which was improved by yoga and Spinology. The enzymes, alkaline diet, Super Blue Green Algae, and water all contributed to my becoming more alkaline. I became more conscious of my rest needs. I still had an obsession with food on an hourly basis. The migraines became less intense and less frequent, only occurring due to some slip-up in my system, such as too many days without adequate rest, poor posture, overworking, excessively large meals, or poor food combinations. My structure improved radically. So did my strength and my attitude towards life. Eventually, I could handle more and more stress without the migraines returning. For over twenty-five years, migraines had often appeared bi-weekly and lasted as long as twenty-four to thirty-six hours; within a matter of about three to four years, the migraines became a thing of the past. I have now been migraine-free for twelve years, which feels miraculous. My diet of live food was working.

What did you do after leaving Dr. Ann?
I helped my bedridden, Alzheimer-affected grandmother to get well within a matter of four weeks through enzymes and whole food supplements. I traveled and lectured and wrote a few more new books. With the funds raised by the bestseller, *Survival into the 21st Century*, I purchased a seven acre farm and started the All Life Sanctuary. We had raw foods, Youkta Yoga, Temple Dance, and a community of about a dozen friends. I lectured extensively, went to many of the Rainbow

Tribe Gatherings, taught live food preparations, started studying numerology and palmistry, and got into lifestyle consulting. In spite of helping many others, I continued to be confronted with my own fears about life. I was very slow in opening up to emotional issues. With the help of Youkta, I finally overcame my out of control food addiction for good. After my recovery, I became involved in super food formula design and marketing and worked with morbid obesity - folks who were as heavy as 1000 pounds - at the Dick Gregory Obesity & Addiction Center. I continued to do research in degenerative diseases and write reports. Youkta and I opened a retreat center, the All Life Sanctuary, in Arkansas - the Natural State - on 90 acres of wilderness. Initially, Youkta ran women's festivals. Now we are open as a retreat center, where people can stay in simple housing, become immersed in study, destress, get counseling, learn by doing live food and indoor gardening, and participate in yoga and dance.

What did you discover when you started working towards maintenance, rebuilding an athletic diet?
Youkta, in her late thirties, was into the most athletic phase of her life. She needed to find a diet to maintain her energy and weight. We both found that overeating was a problem for people who were going to try to get adequate calories from a raw fruits and vegetables diet. Fifteen bananas for breakfast with a six cup fruit smoothie for lunch was just too energy draining on the digestive system for most people. Optimum health requires eating small meals, no more than two cups in size, and eating only when hungry, so we started looking for more concentrated foods.

At that time, many athletes advocated the complex carbohydrate diet. We converted that concept to a live food equivalent. The answer we found was sprouted grains and soaked seeds. At one point, we rejected sprouted grains totally, but we became more open to them. We tried many single sprouted grains. Youkta was having allergic responses, possibly because the wheat and rye were hybrid and not like the more primitive grains. Also, I think that was more of a genetic condition. I found no such problems with my own response. We started mixing oat, barley, buckwheat, millet, rye, amaranth, wild rice, quinoa, kamut, etc. We sprouted them for two to three days and soaked an equal weight of a mix of sesame, sunflower, and pumpkin seeds. We found that this mix worked wonders for us. It has been part of our diet for well over ten years.

We have muscle tested such combinations, and they tested strong. Such meals lead to plenty of power. We were very pleased that we could eat small meals and gain lean muscle mass with resistance training. Our food obsessions disappeared. That was the first time I really felt no concern around food. I felt that I had really found a "safe zone." However, I did not care too much for the taste, and it was too much of a challenge for my poor quality teeth, so I stared innovating. I tried creating blended soups and salad dressings with the sprouted grain and seed mixture. The best results came from the food processor. We eventually designed a whole range of simple and extremely tasty food preps, especially the Essene RAW breads and patés. I found something that was satisfying and worked for us. The other foods that played a major role were soaked nut smoothies, sea vegetable salads, raw olive oil, and avocados.

How many years have you been eating raw foods?
I have been eating raw foods many years. For about ten years, I have had a high level satisfaction and consistency. I started the raw food experiment over thirty-five years ago, but due to the pitfalls of pioneering, the severe toxicity, the emotional and mental garbage arising from isolation, and no one to guide me, it took much longer to find a way that works for me. Best of all, I survived my own ignorance. Today, there are many experienced raw foodists, books, and health care professionals

to guide people in the upgrade of their lifestyles.

Do you have any problems eating raw food while on the road?

When my wife and I were on the road, there were times when we would use sprouted Manna or Essene bread, but overall, we travel very well with one appliance - a blender. We take seeds, sea vegetables, and olive oil and eat foods that grow locally. In tropical environments, we place a high emphasis on fruit and have one meal of grains and sea vegetables. Our diet is at least 20-30% fruit, depending on the season. We also eat algae, which is rich in all known minerals and Vitamin B12, five times higher than wheatgrass in chlorophyll, and very rich in small chain amino acids that facilitate mental and neurological activities. It is a gold mine of essential fatty acids, especially Omega-3 and a wide range of nutriceuticals and phytochemicals. Millions of people have tried it with beneficial results.

When did you notice your recovery to health, and what did you attribute it to?

With chiropractic help and an alkaline vegan diet, most of my symptoms disappeared. Other important aids included Super Blue Green Algae, enzymes, and probiotics. Doing daily reflexology during the first few years was helpful. Massage and rolfing made a big difference and continue to be an important part in my life as do the teachings of Yoga and the Essenes and my relationship with Youkta the many friendships within the Cell Tech family and all the great teachers of natural living that proceeded me and all the new ones that have evolved. As long as I kept on studying health, looking for inspiration and integrating more of the wholistic principles, I was improving yearly. I also noticed how much my judgment of others disappeared, as well as accepting others as they are.

I was seeing miracles all around me. People who had cancer were getting well in a matter of three to four months. I saw a man whose arm had been paralyzed fifteen years; within four months on the program, it was back to normal. I saw a lot of people get well who had tried the medical approach, which failed them. Every Live Food Health resort is rich in stories of miraculous cures. It should make some people wonder why these miracles are occurring there so frequently.

How did you know that their health recovery was due to diet?
When clients left the Institute, those who regressed back to their old eating habits had their illnesses come back.

Why do you think they went back if the diet helped them?
Because when they returned home and went back into society, they had very little support. At the center, they made diet changes, but they did not work on a mental, emotional, and/or consciousness shift. As a result, their home environment had a striking impact on them. If one is out of harmony on an emotional level, carrying toxic thoughts, one will regress to a diet that matches one's emotional and mental states. This principal was well understood by the Ancients (see Baghavad Gita and the Essene writings by Professor Edmund B. Szekely). One would be helped greatly by having a buddy system such as local or virtual cyberspace groups, or within one's family, where we grow together. Working on the detoxification of mental, emotional, physical, and social levels, it would help to create a local support group and start potluck monthly gatherings, avail others with books, videos and tapes, have fun the live food way.

How is your health today?
I have not seen a physician or a doctor for over thirty-five years. Basically, I got rid of my insurance forty years ago and I have not had to use medical service. I continue to have

monthly chiropractic spinal alignment, or as needed. Every day, I do my personal yogic spinal adjustments, as well as inverse hanging. I frequently use massage and self reflexology. I maintain a balance of different energy fields on myself as a way of enhancing my overall physical, mental, and spiritual health. I know that I will continue to upgrade my life, as the age demands. Being a healthy raw foodist is the most revolutionary thing you can do for yourself and others. You have no use for drugs, fast/processed inorganic produce, animal farming, synthetic clothing, doctors, psychiatrists, or the military... Life becomes more joyous, simpler, and more natural.

What is your age?
I am sixty-two years young, and getting better. I know that we age chronologically, but biologically, we can get younger. With better integration of health principles, I feel that we will see the teachings of the Essenes made flesh - you live as long as you desire, in a young body.

Do you have any health challenges now that you would like to overcome?
I want to correct my eyes. I have been spending a lot of time researching this subject. One of my eyes is legally blind, and I feel that it can be corrected with a combination of eye exercise and eyewashes, as well as reflexology. These are the kind of treatments that bring energy and will clean up that area of poor circulation. I would like to get more rest and have a consistent yoga and bodybuilding program. I would like to have a much more balanced life. As with many innovators, they are not keeping up with all their desires and insights.

Other than that, how do you feel?
I feel much healthier than I have ever felt before. I find that my levels of concentration have radically improved. My strength and flexibility have also increased dramatically.

How much sleep do you feel you need per night?

My sleep needs vary with physical activity, diet, and the associated recovery times. When I eat heavier meals, such as a meal of sprouted grains, two or three times a day, I end up needing between six to eight hours of sleep. When I eat lighter, and when I'm involved in intellectual work, I find I do quite well if I get between four and six hours of sleep. At home, I find myself sleeping four to five hours per night, but I also take a nap during the day. Taking a nap makes for a good balance for me. I feel refreshed, and I feel able to get two days into a single day, as far as work goes. The cat nap or doing "Savasana" (the corpse pose), whereby one de-stresses the spine, relaxes the muscles, and reduces pressure on the legs, is a very powerful practice. Within the animal kingdom, all creatures take many naps and sleep very little at night.

When it comes to water, some people claim that there is no need to drink any water when eating live foods. What is your feeling about this?

I think that in early stages of cleansing and detoxification, water is extremely important, especially for the more acidified people. Personally, when I was growing up, I hardly ever drank water; I drank cola and other carbonated drinks and lots of coffee. Distilled water or low mineral water is best. The body cannot use the inorganic minerals effectively. Upon rising, or at any time when the stomach is empty, you may drink one to three glasses of water. Wait at least half an hour before eating solid foods. During the day, you can drink half a glass every hour. Gradually reduce water intake towards bedtime, especially if it interferes with sleep. Water is best when it is warm. The necessary level of water intake will depend on activity, environment, and other liquid/live food intake.

Tell us about migraines. What do you think causes them and how did you cure your migraines?

My decades of indulgence in acid oriented diet, cola, and coffee was changing my body. Because of the rush of adrenaline that caffeine gave me, I slept very little and always felt like I was on speed, and it led to a high lactic acid buildup in my body. The acid reached supersaturated states and crystallized all over my body, leading to a painful irritation of nerves. I am convinced that is why I had all those migraines. As a matter of fact, research indicates that over 85% of migraine sufferers have lactic acid intolerance, and ingesting a few extra acid foods leads to the onset of a migraine - which means that they have such an internal excess, any further intake threatens all of their metabolic systems. All of the acid excess due to inadequate sleep, acid coffee and carbonated drinks by the gallon, cigarettes, an acid diet, stress, and acid air contributed to my state of acid crystal induced pain and acid uptight thoughts.

On an alkaline cleansing vegan diet, the periodic healing crises, which on a superficial level felt like migraines, appeared bi-monthly and sometimes more frequently with the meltdown of the stored acid (lactic, uric, ascorbic, fermentative and protein rot). This led to the acid being in my blood and circulation, and it challenged my life. Some of it was excreted via urine; at times, it was excreted by the skin (sometimes I had to wash myself six or more times per day to flush away the acid skin itch), and quite often, it was excreted via the internal skin (the stomach lining). If the metabolic processes were not excreted fast enough, my blood pH could have been compromised and I could have died. There were times when I was close to that, due to exhaustion.

There were times when friends revived me. Migraines were the sign that there was excess acid in my blood and it was rapidly being excreted into the stomach (which is a natural acid place). We initiated stomach washes. In yoga, it is called "Vamana Dhauti", and it is the equivalent of a colon cleanse, except it is done for the stomach. I drank about a quart of water with some salt or baking soda to neutralize the acid as well as filled my stomach, then did deep breathing and mixed the stomach contents by pumping my stomach rapidly with my fingers, then tickled the upper back of my mouth and pulled up the stomach rapidly and forced myself to regurgitate. On a few occasions, I tested the regurgitated liquid, and it had a pH of 4.5. Sometimes I would have to add extra baking soda in order to neutralize this high acidic condition, which was burning my throat. The crises period varied. Sometimes I would have to do this procedure four times an hour, for twenty or more hours straight! If I did not, the migraines pain was unbearable. Eventually, bile would come up; according to yoga, I knew I was done. The crises were over, with no more migraines. I felt wonderful. I fasted for few hours, drinking mint tea or unpasteurized warm miso, then rested and waited for normal hunger to return. I followed this with blended green energy soups. The crises occurred for more than two years. Initially, I did not fully understand what was going on. However, I always felt better after it was over. I knew that I was heading in the right direction.

Did you ever feel you wanted to go to a medical doctor or naturopathic doctor to help you?
I did visit a few healthcare professionals. They wanted to prescribe remedies to suppress the cleansing. They failed to understand that it was a healing crises and not a symptom of disease. I trusted inner guidance. Sometimes, you just have to take the risk of personal responsibility. During the last ten years, I have used a stomach wash only on four occasions to address souring and indigestion associated with the few times I ate under stress or excessively. A stomach wash, just like an enema, can give one the most rapid relief. Very few alternative doctors understand the concept of "crises" in the healing. They see the "crises" as a symptom of a disease that needs to be suppressed. For example, I had a fever of 105 degrees for

eight hours, which I controlled by staying in a warm tub. This was followed by a fever of 102 degrees for ten days, whereby I fasted and rested. Doctors want quick results. Nature wants one to rest and drink liquids.

Would you agree that the consequences of overeating and under sleeping are one of the causes of poor health in this country today?
Absolutely. When you fill the stomach beyond its digestive capacity, digestion is incomplete. Major toxemia results from rotting protein, souring starches, and rancid fats. The human stomach is geared for grazing and eating small meals to satisfy hunger. That applies to both raw and cooked foods, as well as animal protein. The toxemia from animal protein is far more severe and the consequences are more devastating. Even with raw foods, you can create fermentation, because if a large meal of fruit stays in the stomach for too long, some of the sugar gets converted into alcohol. If a large salad stays in the stomach for too long, eventually it can end up creating inner kraut or make grains turn sour. The larger the meals, the less conscious one becomes, because so much of the body's energy is used in the digestive process. You can talk to anybody in the theater or lecture circuit - they know how important it is to eat nothing or eat extremely light meals or be slightly hungry, prior to giving a presentation. Otherwise, one ends up being boring or even confused.

As far as rest goes, most people need the overnight fast because of their dietary overindulgence during the day. They need rest from the physical activity, the toxic environment, and the foods they have chosen to eat. During the day, the body builds up more and more toxins, and one becomes unconscious (as in sleep). In a similar fashion, if you are drinking alcohol, you become eventually unconscious from the toxemia. I am pretty sure I am correct in saying that animals in nature never sleep. They just rest. The reason they don't need sleep is because they live on live food and eat small meals. They just keep nibbling on whatever they need, and then they are off to be physically active or they rest. They are always fully conscious. Because of our overall history of not eating live foods our entire lives and coming from many generations of poor eating practices, along with our own poor lifestyle practices, we find that we need quite a bit of unconscious sleep. But during fasting, as an example, we find that we do well on an hour or two.

How has fasting affected your sleeping patterns?
During graduate school, I would fast and not even bother sleeping for as much as seven days. Instead of sleeping, I would lie down on the floor and do what is called "Savasana", the corpse pose. It was a deep level of relaxation. By doing that two to three times a day, I was able to bypass all my sleep needs. I was able to have a very clear mind. I would stay in the corpse pose for twenty to thirty minutes, basically to the point where I felt like I was floating above the ground. It has taken years of mastery for me to do this. At deep enough levels, one enters astral travel as well as total knowledge.

How were your sleep patterns when you were growing up, before you got into fasting?
When I was a child, I was an insomniac due to fear. I was also an insomniac in high school. At the time, I did not realize it, but the large amounts of coffee I was consuming kept me from sleeping. Finally, I decided, if I can't sleep, I'll teach myself to master rest. All night I would work on rest and relaxation.

Have these Yoga techniques helped you in other ways?
I was held back three years in grammar school, and I was a very poor student until my sophomore year. However, once I learned to master the Savasana posture, my Kundalini energy awakened and allowed me entry into knowledge/wisdom. In my freshman year and the beginning of my sophomore year, I was in classes

for the "intellectually challenged." After months of spiritual practices, I reached mental clarity, which changed my academic performance. I was moved into advanced and honor classes, and I received all kinds of awards. It is hard to believe that just by practicing meditation and deeper relaxation, one can have such a dramatic effect. I also practiced mind control – both mindlessness and/or abstinence from any negative thoughts. If I feared something, I did not dwell on it, for I knew that what you concentrate on avoiding is attracted into your life. They are some of the most powerful techniques to master when one wants to take advantage of what the universe is giving to all of us. In college, due to poor class attendance, there were many times when I practiced mindlessness for several days instead of studying for exams, then channeled and automatically wrote perfect dissertations, even in advanced theoretical mathematics courses.

Do you think your diet helped you master these techniques?
At that time, I was not on any great diet. In fact, diet was unknown to me back then, although I did discover that if I wanted to be intelligent and have high performance, I would have to give up eating and practice these aspects of inner silence. The academic results were amazing. If students only knew the value of fasting and meditation during exams, we would have the most intelligent and holistic universe. We would be connected with one another instead of being buffered by fears and mistrust. We would not have a world of war and violence, and asocial behavior would be nonexistent.

What advice would you give to somebody whose loved one is going through a health crisis and will not oblige to a raw food lifestyle? How should the person deal with it?
In general, it is much easier to "jumpstart a life" by having

clients add a few supplements to their diet than to demand that they give up addictive food habits. Once they are on super foods, their mental clarity and energy increase, and often, once the disease is healed, they become more open to upgrading their lifestyles, though not everyone is open to such a change. It is a slow educational process. It also helps a lot, when you are trying to help close friends, for you to be an example of health. When I had to deal with my immediate loved ones, it was an education. I spent hundreds of dollars putting together a three-inch thick document to help them realize I had the facts and the best direction, according to the medical model they believe in. I wanted them to see the information I compiled that could help cure them without any drugs. Unfortunately, my information and facts were not enough to change the misinformation people have been taught to believe.

My own mother had cancer, and she had a successful colon surgery. No medical research gives any indication that there is any advantage for people over sixty in having chemotherapy after a successful colon surgery, nor is it recommended. My mother's doctor didn't insist on chemotherapy, but instead he would say, "Would you like some chemotherapy?" He continued giving her the choice and encouraging her to take it. The doctors make many thousands of dollars for each therapy. My mother has already had six chemotherapy sessions. I initially educated my whole family - my brother, my sisters, as well as my mother. I also asked for my mother's permission to send the documentation I had compiled to her doctor. She refused. In our discussion, she became so stressed, I could see that I was going to do more damage with my forcefulness than I would by taking no action and being supportive. I decided to back off. She was going to have chemotherapy. Her doctor obviously had excellent training in bedside manners, politeness, and kindness. My mother totally loved him and was completely devoted to him. She believed in him. She believed that the doctors had saved her life, and in a way, they did.

I found other ways to help my mother. I already had her on a whole super food supplement program, and I got her on more intense enzymes, more Super Blue Green algae, and more friendly bacteria cultures. The medical doctor was so surprised by the fact that she continued to have her hair throughout the early years of chemotherapy. She continued to have her energy too, except for a few times when they over-chemicalized her and she wound up going through a purging process. Then they stopped the chemotherapy treatments for a while. But she still completely believes in it. I believe tremendously in the power of prayers and the power of love of family. Therefore, I was there for my mother, as well as the rest of my family, with loving support through both prayer and positive encouragement. She was never a water drinker, and I reprimanded her for it. I asked her, "How much liquid is your doctor telling you to drink when you undergo chemotherapy?" She said, "About four to eight glasses." I asked her, "Well, Mom, how much are you drinking?" and she said, "None." I responded, "Well, are you going to listen to your doctor or not?" I just kept hammering that into her. Now she is drinking four to five glasses of water, and it is making a big difference. She is walking, shoveling snow, taking care of a home, and keeping a positive attitude. These are all contributing factors. They are not nutritional factors, but they can still make a difference.

At the same time, this is my premise. While life is good, death is good. Sometimes I say death is better for some people. Basically, I see death as a continuation of life in different energy forms. Families that play together do it in many lifetimes. So if my mother ends up splitting, that's cool. I have no problems with that, because we are going to get together and finish our relationship in our next incarnations. So I do not have any sadness. I do a lot of eulogies, and I really turn them into a celebration. Death is meant to be a celebration with the right attitude. I love my mother. I don't see death in her. I see her as the child she is. We play, we joke, and that is the thing that really works. I will give you another example. My cousin, who is a few years younger, had breast cancer and everybody was pushing her to have surgery. We talked extensively, and she agreed to go to Hippocrates and do a program. Now, she is totally pleased. She found a system that she can live with. Another cousin of mine had severe skin conditions, swollen legs with oozing pus, and a coffee addiction. I invited him to live with me at the farm, and he overcame all of these conditions. He has been in good health for over twenty years. Another cousin also lived with me for six months and was doing well. Then, once on his own, he went back to his old self-destructive way of life.

The Super Foods represent the most promising help for all of our loved ones. It is much easier to get most folks to add a few pills to their diet than to have them give up their self-destructive habits. So, I have all of my family and friends on enzymes, probiotics, green super foods, and specialized herbs, as needed. Many of them ask for further guidance in life upgrade when they experience increased health and energy.

You win some and you lose some, but you are not attached to the outcome. You just do the best you can with lots of love and lots of support, no matter what their decisions are. If you end up getting overly aggressive, you might risk contributing to their early demise. I have tried education and helping, but if it doesn't work, then I back off and do the next best thing. That has been my approach. With some loved ones, you are going to be successful. With others, all they are ready for is the next incarnation, which is okay too, but at least they are going to get that education. Eventually, we all have to go on that spiritual journey.

How dangerous are pollution and poor air quality to

overall health? Should they be a big concern for someone who is eating a raw food diet?

I think poor air quality is a significant issue. It can lead to a buildup of pollutants in one's system and it is very harmful to one's long term health. It is much worse in big cities. In the book titled *Man's Higher Consciousness,* Hilton Hotema says, "The individual living in a polluted city can accumulate one to two pounds of waste of dust chemicals in the first year. The dust piles up into their systems, but it systematically gets pushed through into the cellular level, so that the lungs can continue to function." I once lived in New York City for two years. After being there, I left and went to spend some time in the Andes, visiting the late Johnny Lovewisdom. I was high up in the mountains and sleeping outdoors. After a week, I started having nightmares where I was up to my belly in a sewage system and gasping for air. I woke up and started vomiting all this black soot that I had accumulated in my tissue space. A vegetarian couple I knew who lived in a major city also went to the Alps for a vacation. At that time, they were fasting, and the same thing happened to them around the second week.

However, I have to emphasize that diet can do more damage to our bodies than air born pollutants. A Physicians Committee for Responsible Medicine study showed that the impact of pasteurized dairy products on the incidence of lung cancer was far worse than smoking cigarettes.

What should people who live in big cities do?

If one continues to live in a big city, the answer is basically to have an excellent air filtration system in one's bedroom, office, or wherever one works. Don't jog on the streets. For exercise, do trampoline, yoga, and weightlifting in purified air. This will limit one's exposure to the polluted air. As a result, one can better tolerate the polluted environment. A good organic diet, adequate rest, and time out in the country can further enhance one's quality of life.

How do you account for people who live well into their nineties despite living in a polluted environment, eating a poor diet, and practicing all other poor habits?
They might be living longer, but they are not in better health today than people were in previous generations. It all has to do with their genetic material; which has radically been altered over the last four generations. If you take a look at photos of children fifty years ago, they look very different from today's high school athletes. You'll see that children in the past had long ear lobes. Look at elderly people that are living now. Most have long ear lobes, and more often than not, they have very wide nostrils and a more primitive nose that is close to the head. This is a reflection of strong genetic material. The ears are related to liver and kidney; the nose is related to lungs and heart. My mother and father, as an example, lived in a farming community, and their main crops were grown next to a river that flooded every year. It deposited every known mineral in the floodplains, and these people had unbelievable power. My mother lived on two to three hours of sleep for well over forty years, while working hard physically. She ran a bakery, and she would lift 100-pound bags of flour and sugar. She had long earlobes and a primitive nose. People in the old days had moons on all their fingernails. My mother had moons on all her fingernails until she started chemotherapy. Now they are only on two or three fingers. The moons indicate mineral resources, the strength of recovery, and the ability to adapt to all kinds of stress. Also, if you take a look around today, we all have tiny noses. We have ear lobes that stick close to the head, and it is common to see bags underneath our eyes. You see creases in the ears, which indicate a cardiovascular compromise at a young age. Over 60% of the population is overweight. Obesity affects over 40% of children. Over 80% of the population is addicted to one drug or another,

whether it is caffeine, nicotine, sugar, alcohol, white flour, or street or prescription drugs. So we are talking about two different ages of genetic material. In the past, they had the full spectrum of minerals, or at least a much higher level of minerals. They came from a much stronger genetic stock, and as a result, they could tolerate much higher stress. But with people today, we are seeing old age diseases appearing in children. According to the World Health Organization statistics, 25-30% of our children are sick with incurable diseases, and 45% of them are already degenerating. Each generation is producing inferior offspring to the point where sterility is rampant. It is affecting 50% of people of a reproductive age, if not more. Even people in their twenties and thirties, many of them athletes, are sterile - incapable of reproduction. We have seen the same thing happen within the four-generation study by Pottenger Cats. Basically, we have seen the degeneration occur by the second and third generations, when reproductive ability disappeared completely. Sexual choices become confused and or disappear as well. Basically, males become effeminate. Females become more masculine. Hormones strictly rule the gender issue. All the hormones added to animal feed, insecticides, and pesticides mimic and interfere with natural hormones, causing sexual identity or sexual preferences to become confused. I had nipples and breast development when I was a teenager. My high consumption of pasteurized and strongly hormone-imbedded foods lead to the alteration of my physiology and also the confusion of my own sexuality. It took a few years of a vegan diet before it became normal again.

Are you suggesting that if we continue on this path of overeating, under sleeping, and practicing poor health habits, the average life span will decline?
Yes. It will decline by twenty-five to thirty years, and that won't last for more than a generation, because the reproductive capacity will be lost.

In my opinion, what is going on now will parallel the Bubonic Plague, because our immune systems are so severely compromised. Junk foods place a great demand on the immune system, and over time, if one eats a cooked and/or processed meal without the intake of enzyme supplementation, the white blood cell level can go up by 2 to 400%, equivalent to an infection. Other stressors are the chemicalized environment, medications, lack of sleep, and the emotional turmoil that is going on in most people's lives. Anger and violent behavior are very pronounced among families and children today. It is all related to the toxic blood stream.

What is the answer to stopping this downfall?
To solve this, all we need to do is go vegan and make the transition to a live food consciousness, with green super-foods and enzymatic and probiotic supplementation, at least for the first generation. If that is done, people will turn around in a matter of months, if not weeks. I have seen the reversal of so many degenerate conditions. Through dietary means alone, people come back to who they really are. The salvation is here, and the knowledge must be applied. Then the people can become well, happy, and beautiful.

If anyone is interested, please get in touch with an alternative health practitioner versed in enzymatic nutrition, such as myself, for guidance. As a generation, the live food movement is one of the few oases of hope, offering the world as a direction to go. It is a place of joy, physical health, and youthfulness, never knowing old age.

Basically, by continuing on live foods, our life span will be greatly enhanced. It is all determined by the live food we eat and the fasting practice that we integrate into our lives. With this, we can have a radical increase of life span.

So you are suggesting that if we follow these health practices, the age limit is endless?
We have many desires and dreams. A life of one hundred years is

too short to manifest and express one's dharma. Meditation and prayer will put us in touch with our true nature and guide us in self-realization. We can be the creators of our own future. When one has finished one's incarnation, one will leave behind one's earthly youthful body. Most people leave this earth by destroying their body vehicle and die of old age. The Essenes have a lot to offer us.

As a departure, I wish to share some insight into this next Millennium. It goes way beyond the science of Dr. Roy Walford's plan to live to age 150.

The Future is Here

"And in those days
the children shall begin to study the laws,
and to seek the commandments,
and to return to the path of righteousness."

"And the days shall begin to grow many
And increase amongst those children of humans
Till their days draw nigh to one thousand years,
and to greater number of years than (before)
was the number of days."

"And there shall be no old people
nor one who is not satisfied with one's days,
for all shall be as children and youths."

"And all their days they shall complete
and live in peace and in joy."

(*The Book of Jubilees*, XXIII: 26-30, Vol. II, p 49)

To follow is a special message from Youkta and Viktoras:

Dear Friends,

We are sending you our love. Life is one. We feel the disharmony. Change is hard. We join you and the world in prayer, so that our leaders take wise steps in tune with long-term goals of humanity and Mother Earth. We pray, visualize, and live in the world we create by our unified field of love.

We are happy to share with you our response to these challenging times. We know the healing and nurturing power of nature. Clarity comes through prayer and meditation, immersed in silence and fueled by organic live food and juices. Our retreat center might be the answer you are looking for.

Yes, we are opening our retreat center - a place to lift the spirit, empowered by nature.

All Life Sanctuary Retreat Camp is a rustic 90-acre center surrounded by the Ouchita National Forest. You will be immersed in nature, sharing dormitory-style cabins (or tent sites, individual cabins, teepee), charming out-houses as well

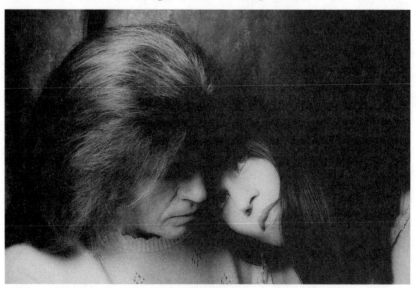

Youkta and Viktoras 2000, photo by Jennifer Girard, Chicago

as nine complete bathrooms with hot/cold showers, with a 2000 sq. ft. open on three sides dining area with an adjacent closed-in large live food kitchen.

The land has a pond, dammed creek for swimming, Ouchita River is within walking distance through forest, nature walks, and many subdivided isolated fields. There are many special spots for communing with nature, contemplation amid the symphony of birds, singing coyotes, hooting of owls, movement of raccoons, flight and song of birds, deer, and many other creatures.

On arrival through the gate, a sense of peace prevails. We encourage the participants to immerse totally into the environment, and limit self to nature, listening to nature sounds instead of the telephone or TV, maintaining the growing inner peace and calm, that won't be disrupted by the outside world. You will have a rejuvenating, empowering, ready to face the challenges of the world experience.

We are looking to the future with hope, peace, and trust that love will prevail. Here is what we are offering you. We hope you will take the opportunity to come and rest, learn, grow, and be empowered.

Love In Service
We are One

Youktoras
Youkta and Viktoras

For details, Contact the retreat center at:

Retreat center
Phone: 870-867-4521
E-mail: viktoraslive@yahoo.com
Web: www.youthing101.com

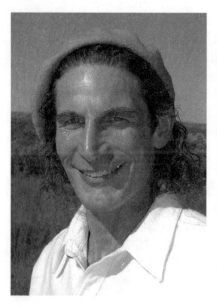

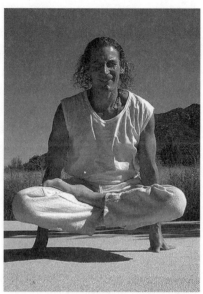

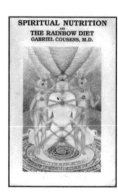

Gabriel Cousens has written several books about yoga, health, and the raw food diet and lifestyle.

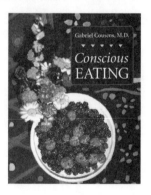

You may contact Gabriel Cousens at:

Tree of Life Rejuvenation Center
Attn: Gabriel Cousens
PO Box 1080
Patagonia, AZ 85624

Ph: 520-394-2520
Email: healing@treeoflife.nu
Website: www.treeoflife.nu

Gabriel Cousens
MD., MD(H) Diploma in Ayurveda

I've met many people in the health field, and I feel Gabriel's knowledge about the human body and how it works surpasses most of theirs. He is also one of the kindest and most gentle persons I have ever met. We covered a lot of important topics during our interview. Of all the interviews I have conducted over the years, this one is of the most informative.

Gabriel Cousens, MD, MD(H), Diploma in Ayurveda, founder of The Tree of Life Rejuvenation Center (www.treeoflife.nu or 520-394-2520) in Patagonia, Arizona, is an internationally celebrated healer, spiritual facilitator, world peace-worker, and author. As a holistic medical doctor, psychiatrist and family therapist, licensed homeopathic physician, and Diplomat in Ayurvedic Medicine, Dr. Cousens uses the modalities of vegan live-food nutrition, naturopathy, Ayurveda, homeopathy, and acupuncture, blended with joyful spiritual awareness, in the healing of body, mind and spirit. A graduate of Amherst College, he received his M.D. from Columbia Medical School in 1969. He is a best-selling author whose titles include: *Conscious Eating, Spiritual Nutrition and the Rainbow Diet, Sevenfold Peace*, and his latest book, *Depression-Free for Life*. He is considered one of the leading medical authorities on live foods in the world.

How many years have you been on the raw diet, and what got you into it?
I started in 1983. In 1975, I had a deep Kundalini* awakening and in the midst of that, a little voice cried out that said, "You should learn to eat in a way that nurtures Kundalini." I was vegetarian at that time, and I began doing research trying to find the diet that best nurtured the Kundalini. Through the process and my research, it became clearer and clearer that a live food diet

was by far the best diet.

Kundalini: The Kundalini is the mystical spiritual healing force within each person, that when released moves throughout the subtle and physical body, spiritually healing the subtle nervous system called the nadis, the chakra system, and every cell in the body. According to Carl Jung, the awakening of the Kundalini is the next evolutionary step for humanity and is a major step toward enlightenment.

How did you arrive at that conclusion?

By observation. I had the opportunity to work literally with thousands of people both here and in India, helping them to adopt a diet best for spiritual life. I learned that the ancient Yogis lived on a live food diet. They did not eat the cooked, Indian food that most people think they did.

Why are live foods best for the Yogic diet?

Live foods do two things, which make them special in the Yogic diet. First of all, they detoxify the body. Second and more importantly, live foods are very high in Prana (another name for energy; it is often associated with breath, but it can also refer to cosmic energy). Prana is particularly important for clearing the nadis (the subtle and energetic nerve channels in the Yogic system). When those nadis are cleared, we become in essence like a super conductor of the cosmic energy.

There are 72,000 nadis or nerve channels in the human body. Where the channels intersect with one another is what makes up the Chakra system. The Prana works to expand the mind by bringing in the Air and Ether elements, which vitalize the system as well as lighten and purify the body.

In essence, live food provides the closest real source of the most vital energy we can have in terms of the Pranic energy we can obtain from food. They help expand and increase the Air and Ether elements, which purify, energize, and increase the Prana in the body, furthermore, bringing enough Prana to expand and deepen the mind consciousness as well. We call this the 'Sattvic state', which is an inward-directed mind into the spiritual.

What I discovered by my direct experience actually became

the foundation of my first book, *Spiritual Nutrition and The Rainbow Diet.*

I observed that live food very clearly brings increased detoxification, strengthened energy, and increased Prana, which is another subtle level into the system. Prana is what makes this whole way of life very exceptional and unusual. By eating this way, one thereby increases the Sattvic mind, allowing one to become a super conductor for the divine energy. That was my direct experience for myself, and I have begun to prescribe it for other people.

How was your health when you started eating live foods?
My motivation to eat live foods had nothing to do with physical health; my motivation was strictly for spiritual purposes. My health was fine, but it is better now.

My experimentation centered on how live foods could help meditation and how they could sustain my ability to eat very little. This is a very important point. When I was in different levels of intensity, I was meditating six hours per day, chanting for three and a half hours, and sitting in silence for another two hours a day with my teacher. I had to develop a diet where I could eat a minimum and get a maximum of energy. Live foods fulfilled those criteria. The diet was the best for my spiritual life. I really did not have an exposure to the live food movement as we know it today. My choice of live foods just arose from my experience and scientific exploration.

To help people who are new to this path, please tell us a few of the most important things you have learned on a spiritual or physical level.
Living a live food lifestyle is a way of healing and nurturing oneself. The whole process should be one of gentleness in the unfolding. For me, I just went on it. I explored it and I kind of moved in certain directions and I decided, "This is it." But unless a person has an immediate health problem like cancer, where they need to go on 100% raw foods immediately, I believe peo-

ple need to transition gently so they don't form any resistances to it. I think the number one advice I would give to people is to be gentle on themselves.

The second point is: there is not one type of live food diet, as I point out in my book, *Conscious Eating*. We all have different psycho-physiological constitutions. So it is extremely important to be aware of what your constitution is and then eat a live food diet that matches your constitution. That way, it is always about success. If you are gentle, you are going to have the right diet for your own constitution, and you are going to be successful. For example, some people need a higher protein diet, with more nuts and seeds and so forth, while other people need lower amounts of protein. At one point, it was very easy for me to be a fruitarian because my body constitution calls for a diet lower in protein. For another example, some people need to eat frequently. I am happy on two meals a day. But there are no rules here. The goal is to learn your psycho-physiological type, season, time of life cycle, and other factors, and then eat that way.

Do you think people can change their psycho-physiological constitution type?

You can modify it, but it is more of a genetic thing one inherits. A lot of people have hypoglycemia today. They end up eating more frequently, but when they clear that up, they can discover what type of constitution they have. If they are 'sympathetic,' which is what I am, then they do not need to eat much. But if they are 'fast-oxidizers', they still need to eat somewhat more frequently in a higher protein diet.

How do people find out what type they are?

It is more than just type. We have to look at your Ayurvedic dosha-type. This is very important. We need to see if you are a fast or slow oxidizer. We need to look at certain implications of blood type. There are a bunch of things we need to look at. In my second edition of *Conscious Eating*, I outline that explicitly.

Do you think that some types of people might need ani-

mal protein in their diet?

In twenty years of working with people eating a live food diet, I have known only one person who needed animal protein. She was from northern Sweden near the Arctic Circle. She was very committed to being vegetarian, but she needed fish. I think it had to do with her genetic diet. But this was before I figured out the slow and fast oxidizer thing, and now I believe she wouldn't need it.

As a scientist, I always look at what is not working. I take the attitude, "If it isn't working, what is not right here? Let's explore this scientifically." This is how I came up with the importance of individualizing your diet. At this point in time, with the technology we have, I believe that eating animal protein is not necessary, no matter what a person's constitution might be. After many years of research, I now understand how anyone can be a successful vegetarian and a successful live fooder, regardless of his or her constitution.

What are some of the common pitfalls people who are trying to eat a live food diet should avoid? What are your suggestions for dealing with them?

One of the common pitfalls is not knowing your dosha-type. In the earlier phases of the wheat grass/ low protein diet fad, people who are fast oxidizers did very poorly and had a lot of imbalances. Many people were very low in oil. They developed Omega-3 deficiencies. That is easily remedied by consuming ground flax seeds.

A second pitfall people often face is not having the right diet for their constitution. Some people need more protein, while other people need less.

The third pitfall is staying too long in the 'cleansing phase' of a live food diet. One of the breakthroughs that I made in *Conscious Eating* and in our new book, which we will probably call *The Rainbow Diet Food Book*, is the whole idea of learning the difference between a cleansing diet and a maintenance diet. People need to learn this difference, because we first need to detoxify initially and then maintain. Most people feel great when they fast. But you do not fast your whole life. You need a maintenance diet which maintains your weight, your health, and your wellbeing. In *Conscious Eating*, I talk about a maintenance diet and eating live foods rather than staying too long on a cleansing diet. For one thing, people's bodies can become too alkaline on a prolonged cleansing diet. There are a variety of people who focus too much on wheat grass. Don't get me wrong; wheat grass is very good when you are treating cancer, and it is very good when you are initially detoxifying because people's bodies are often very acidic. But when you move to an excess alkaline state, you can get all kinds of imbalances in the body. For example, your body can become hyper-reflexive, and you can become spacey. This happens to a lot of people on a live food diet. That is because they have stayed on the cleansing diet too long and they have created literally a physiological imbalance in which they have become too alkaline. They get a lot more muscle spasms. I actually experienced this at one point because my body adjusted to a high alkaline diet. You don't want to be too acidic, but you have to find the right balance so that you do not become too alkaline, either.

What is your opinion of nuts and seeds?

Nuts and seeds are good. I often see omega-3 and omega-6 deficiencies in people who do not eat enough nuts and seeds. Omega-3 and omega-6 are essential fatty acids, and nuts and seeds are the best sources of these. They are particularly needed for protection of the nerves, circulation, immune, and skin systems. A high percentage of these good fats are found in flax, hemp seeds, and walnuts. I do believe it is best to soak the nuts and seeds before you eat them. However, since I wrote about it, people might take it as a religion. You can eat nuts and seeds without soaking them. My point is simply they are a little easier to assimilate if you soak them because they begin to break down and they begin to sprout and they kind of change their energetic field a little bit.

Do you think people can live on a raw food diet without any nuts and seeds if they have a certain constitution?
Anything is possible. People can live on just water, but it is rare. Theoretically, it is possible, although I have never met anyone who lives on air or water. Generally speaking, we need a little bit of protein in the diet. We can get that protein from vegetables. Vegetables are mostly carbohydrate, but they have a certain amount of protein in them. Ratio-wise, spinach has the highest amount of protein of anything, in terms of its calories of protein.

I think it is possible to live without nuts and seeds. But I don't think it should be a goal, because you do not get the Omega-3's without nuts and seeds, and that is one of the big deficiencies that can occur. If people actually get to a place where they are not eating nuts and seeds and they acquire Omega-3 deficiencies, it can really hurt them.

What is your opinion of grains?
I have had almost no grain in my diet. We use almost no grains at The Tree of Life Rejuvenation Center as well. We occasionally use buckwheat. The dried buckwheat is really a seed, as far as I understand. I don't think grain is needed. I have found that grain slows down the flow of the energy in the nadis. But there may be some people who need some grain. The sprouted grains are okay, although it is not something that we do. I have some grain recipes in my book, *Conscious Eating,* but in reality, I don't eat grains and I don't recommend them too much. One of the reasons is because so many people have fungal candida problems and the grains contribute to that because they are primarily carbohydrate. Grains are builders. For babies, I think nuts, seeds, and grains are germinal seed energies that can be very good. We do have some grain porridge recipes in *Conscious Eating*. Live grain porridges have been especially good for people in the transition phase. But once the body balances, I don't see grains as part of a maintenance, long-term raw food diet.

What is your opinion of an all fruit diet? Do you think some greens are necessary?

As a scientist, I look and see and I use a dark field microscope. I also use a dry field approach. It is very clear to me that a generally fruitarian diet at this time in history is not a good idea. I say this because as I have been doing research and it is very clear to me that most people are suffering from mycosis. Mycosis is a general fungal infection that creates a "rotting" composting situation that can turn into many diseases, including cancer. It comes from too much acid, acid food and junk food, excess sugar, and low oxygen. A high sugar diet including dried fruits and high glycemic fruits significantly contributes to problems.

In the last few years, I have done much research on this topic. It is very clear to me if one goes on a diet primarily of vegetables and a few nuts and seeds, one can significantly reverse the rotting, composting situation that even live fooders have to a lesser extent. It can be reversed quickly, within a matter of three months. I am not talking about cancer necessarily, but in some cases, there can be amazing reversals of cancer.

What is your opinion of sprouts?

I think sprouts are terrific. They are incredible, biogenic foods.

What is your opinion of the Natural Hygiene diet?

Even though it is the purest diet in the sense that it is the highest in raw, whole fruits, vegetables, nuts, seeds, and grains with no processing, I don't think it is the most functional and practical diet. We live in such an upside-down world. I believe you ought to be able to grind flax seed or use a blender to make certain things. If you have the time and that is your focus in your life, I think it is a good thing. But for what I teach and what I see in the movement, practically speaking, I feel that Natural Hygiene is a diet that would be very hard for most people and would limit the movement to a very exclusive number of people.

Theoretically, the Natural Hygiene people are saying you shouldn't juice or use a blender. At the Tree of Life, we put people on green juice fasts, and I do like to use certain appliances. There is no question about it, juicing results in incredible positive effects. Look at Norman Walker and so forth. I like the general idea of doing as much as you can in the form of Natural Hygiene, but I do not think it is as functional. By eating only whole fruits and vegetables, I don't think you can obtain as many nutrients as you do when you do a little bit of processing.

What is your opinion of juicing?
I think one of the greatest health things we can do is juice. I have been supervising spiritual juice fasting retreats since 1988 with phenomenal results. I find that juicing is far superior and far safer than water fasting. I think by juicing, you get maximal nutrient concentration, nutrient quality, high enzyme energy, and high micro-electric energy, as long as you drink your juices almost right away. I think it is good for everyone's diet. I do not do that much juicing. I do have one fresh juice a day. It is more of a way to keep myself hydrated.

What is your opinion of fasting?
Fasting to me is one of the greatest health things we can do for our bodies. It enhances the vital life force. I have been leading spiritual fasting retreats since 1988. I have completed a variety of fasts. I have done fasts that lasted as long as twenty-one days on water and some up to forty days. I have explored different things on our spiritual and juice fasting retreats. These consist of seven day cycles, which I consider the minimum for a juice fast. It takes about seven days to clear out all of the bowel toxins out of the system. I have scientifically monitored people. I checked the blood and urine and so forth. On average, by seven days, most people's toxins are cleared from the bowel. People really get great results.

When people are fasting, should they be resting, or can they move around?
Fasting means withdrawing from food and mental, emotional, and environmental work toxins. It is a complete rest. The pur-

pose of fasting is to rejuvenate and reactivate the vital life force in the body. When I am talking about fasting, I am talking about juicing and water, not a dry fast.

Juicing is a big part of it, but complete rest is what we do. When people come to the Tree of Life to do this, we give them that total experience. Plus we do pranayama (breathing exercises), yoga, and meditation. We help people reconnect to their spiritual essence. I supervise people on long fasts such as seventy day fasts and things like that. We do this mostly for people who have serious health problems. They still do best with complete separation from the world so their bodies can rejuvenate and re-organize. However, for some people, that is a whole chunk of their life, and it can be pretty hard. In those cases, they can do it at home. You can get minimal effects from a fast if you continue working. You get a body detox effect. But the real power of a juice fast lies in the whole rejuvenation of mind, body, and spirit. It is a mystical death and rebirth that you cannot obtain by working while you fast. I know this sounds unusual, but for fun, I had no water, juice, or anything for five days and I still worked. I don't recommend this to anyone, but I was just seeing how that felt. It is not the same experience or the same effect on the body. To truly fast, you need to fast from the world.

Do you see a big difference between water fasting and juicing?

There is a big difference between water fasting and juicing. Water fasting has a higher chance of problems, because you have more mineral imbalances and cardiac irregularities. People are not as happy, and they are often really weak. However, during my twenty-one day water fast, I still did 100 pushups on the last day. Most people don't do that; it is a stress on the system. Juicing brings in the bioelectric potential that we need to really activate and heal our bodies. That is something which doesn't happen with a water fast. You get the cleansing part, but you do not rebuild. You do not bring in the alkalizing elements that you get on a juice fast. So those are some very big differences. I tend to dilute the juices in half. There is something about the bio-electric potential Dr. Bercher-Brenner talked about that I believe is absolutely true. Most of the clinics in Europe that I visited liked juice fasting better than water fasting because of all the greater rebuilding and healing qualities of the bio-electric potential in the juices. I think vegetable juices are best. Fruit juices concentrate the sugar too much. The result is more of a fermented problem.

What is your opinion of supplements?
Depending on a person's health, I think there is a role for supplements. Viktoras Kulvinskas and I spent a long time thinking about this issue. I think it is good to take digestive enzymes to build up your enzyme force and to keep from depleting your enzyme energy. Enzymes are depleted when you eat cooked food. You still tap into enzyme reserves when you eat live food, but you continuously replenish your enzyme reserves. I also think there is a role for certain supplements because the environment is so toxic. Sometimes we need higher amounts of anti-oxidants that we cannot obtain from a live food diet alone. For example, when we fly in an airplane, the amount of radioactivity we are exposed to is ten times higher. So if I fly, I will take anti-oxidants. I have actually taken a meter with me on the airplane. At 30,000 feet, you are exposed to ten times the amount of radioactivity. We were not designed to fly. We live in a modern complicated world, with positive and negative things. I think we should always adjust to our environment. If you are doing something abnormal, like flying, then you need to do other things to balance that abnormality.

What is your opinion of eating seasonally?
I think it is the correct way to eat. In the Ayurvedic system, you always eat to balance your personal dosha and the dosha of the season.

What is your opinion of food combining?
I think there is a role for it. I think there is less of a role for it

when you are eating live food and you are not eating too much. If you are eating too much, you should always focus on food combining. If you are eating cooked food, you should be aware of food combining. If you are eating live food, it is not as important. I generally do follow the rules of it, but not as a main practice.

What is your opinion of physical exercise?
I am a strong advocate of exercise. There are two things that have been scientifically proven to create longevity. One is eating less, which naturally happens when you eat live foods. The second thing is exercise.

I exercise all the time. Each type of exercise has a different purpose. I do yoga for the flexibility aspect. I do Pranayama (breathing exercises). I do a little bit of weights, but not much, for toning. I do rebounder. Rebounding with a trampoline helps the lymphatic system, and it has a whole anti-gravity effect and it helps the body rid itself of toxins. I also do fast uphill walking. Research shows that at least thirty to forty-five minutes a day of up-hill walking, five to six days a week, gives you 90% of an effective Olympic workout. I do a fair amount of exercising, but I do a whole variety of different things. I just did the Sun Dance. This is my fourth year of it. This year I did the Eagle Dance, which is a little bit more intense. I stood from sunrise to sunset as well as dancing the whole time.

What is your opinion of wild foods?
They're the best. They are my highest choice.

What is your opinion of Urine Therapy?
In this country, I can't legally recommend urine therapy. When I was in India, where it was legal, I used urine therapy a lot, and I had a certain amount of expertise, but I don't do it anymore. I actually used it to inject people. Once it had been filtered, as an injection, it would get rid of the allergies almost immediately. It was miraculous.

As I began studying Ayurvedic medicine, they said, "Don't

take the three malas: urine, feces, and sweat." Ayurvedic medicine does not really support urine therapy. The Yogis will do it. They do it when there is nothing else around and it's clean. But then I began to study heavy metals. Heavy metal toxicity, pesticides and herbicides, is another problem we face in our world today. These toxins come out in the urine, and this is the downfall to urine therapy, because it will reintroduce the heavy metals back into your system, along with pesticides and herbicides. It is good for skin and hair, but again, the heavy metals are absorbed back into the body. If you clear your body of heavy metals, then I think urine therapy is okay. I think more than okay; I think it is a good thing. I have already cleared my body of heavy metals. But I actually do not recommend urine therapy.

With all the pollution in the air, can we ever clear ourselves of heavy metals and stay clean?
To a certain extent, yes. A lot of the heavy metals come from the mercury in dental fillings, fish, or other things. But if we are living a fairly organic life, we're in pretty good shape. People are so toxic, it's a problem. So the rules are not always the same for everybody. People who have heavy metals in their systems may have to take certain supplements to get the heavy metals out. Because we live in a toxic environment, eating a strictly fruitarian diet is not optimal anymore. Instead, a live food diet would optimize our position in the world today.

What is your opinion of mercury fillings?
Get them out. They are associated with immune deficiencies, all kinds of neurological toxicity, Alzheimer's disease, and heart and kidney problems. They are potentially a very serious problem.

What is the best material to replace them with at this time?
A lot of people feel that composite is good. Some people feel that pure gold is good. It depends on the electricity in your teeth.

What do you have to say about weight loss on a raw food diet?

I tell people they will naturally have weight loss. They will go down to their normal healthy weight. Normal healthy weight is about twenty pounds less than what the insurance people call your "optimum" weight. I have been at my normal, optimum weight, which is a lot less than when I was a football player. Once you get to your optimum, healthy weight and physiology, you basically gain or lose weight to get there. Once you eat a live food diet, it helps to reset and bring you back to your normal, optimal healthy weight.

What are your age, height, and weight?

I am fifty-nine, 5'10" and 150 pounds.

Do you eat 100% raw foods right now?

Yes, and I have since 1983.

What is your favorite food?

I don't really have one. The live food diet is a part of my life. My goal with this is to find a live food diet that fits in with the rest of my life. It is not the center of my life, but one of the pillars that makes up part of my spiritual life.

Out of all the foods, do you think one is most important?

The most important food would probably be flax - ground flax. It provides the essential nutrients we don't get from all the other fruits. It is all about balance. Fresh ground flax contains lots of fiber and lignans, which have a lot of anti-cancer qualities, and it is far superior to flax oil. Flax seed oil is good, but it gets rancid very quickly and it is processed. I recommend going to the freshest level - the least processed level. If you ground your flax each day, you'll have fresh flax.

What kind of flax is best?

Golden Flax.

What is your average daily diet like?

In the morning, I have one apple and two tablespoons of ground golden flax. I have bee pollen and mix with water. I mix them together. Lunch consists of salad, with avocado, tomato, greens, and raw Nori sheets. At the Tree of Life Café, our food is so incredible. I have a sprout salad with some nuts or seeds and our entrée, which is usually some extraordinary cultural international cuisine event. In the evening, I usually have a green drink with a little bit of Vitamin Mineral Green or Pure Synergy. That is basically it.

Do you think people can consume too much flax?
I think people can overconsume anything. I think two to three tablespoons twice a day is the maximum.

Currently, how are your health and energy?
Around the time of my fifty-eighth birthday, I did 520 push-ups. I expect to do 600 when I am sixty. I would say I have superior health and energy. There are very few people who can really keep up with me.

How much sleep do you get, and how much do you feel is necessary?
Sleep is one of the most important things that I have had to struggle with personally because, until recently, I did not get enough sleep. Between college and medical school and so forth, I just got used to sleeping less. I think most people probably need a minimum of seven hours per night. I struggle to get that much.
I have found that inadequate sleep is a common deficit in terms of people's health. I know we say that we need less sleep on a live food diet. That is partly true, but there is a whole regenerative process and a whole immune system thing that happens between 10 p.m. and 2 a.m. It is very easy to get into a cycle of sleeping five or six hours. You can do that, but it is really not good for your health. It actually speeds up the aging process. It weakens the immune system, and it upsets the endocrine system. The research really supports that statement. It decreases

creativity, memory, and clarity.

When it comes to sleep, is the time of night during which one sleeps important?
Yes. I have observed that if I can get to bed by 10:30 p.m., it is better than getting to bed at 12:30 a.m., even if I sleep the same number of hours.

Have you noticed any mental changes on this diet?
It is hard to say. It has been over twenty years. I would say I am clearer and stronger and more sensitive to the sacred. My energy is steady and strong all day long. In other words, I can go non-stop. I can work a twelve or fourteen hour day. I can handle all kinds of things, and I am fine.

Many people just beginning a raw diet have problems because their mates do not want to change. Do you have any comments or suggestions?
I am a family therapist, and this is a common issue. There is no problem if the other person isn't opposed to what you are doing. First, there has to be an agreement between both people. One partner respects the live food, spiritual lifestyle, while the other respects the non-live food lifestyle. Second, they must have patience or tolerance. Those are the two most important things. Furthermore, neither partner may proselytize the other person; both partners should simply support the other as much as they can.

What are your thoughts about the female menstruation cycle? Do you think it is natural for a woman not to bleed when she is on a raw diet?
When we use the word 'natural', we have our theories. My observation of women who are really healthy is that they only have about a day of light bleeding. That's it. That's how my wife is. If a woman is not having a period, then physiologically, she does not have enough body fat, and it probably means a deficiency of some sort. Some female athletes stop menstruating; they acquire

an imbalance. I find that the healthiest women still have their period, but they have a very light period that really doesn't have any affect on them. Unhealthy women stop their periods. This is nature's way of protecting women and the species.

Do you think it is more difficult to eat a live food diet today than it was in the past, or is it easier?
I think it is a lot easier today, because we have more technology and we have more knowledge. When I started, there was no support. Ann Wigmore existed, but I did not know who she was. Dr. Szekely existed. People in this country have been eating live foods since the 1820's, but I did not know about that. There was no information out there. There was not any technology. Now, the path is made very easy. In *Conscious Eating*, I lay out all the pros and cons and make it very easy: how to find out your right constitution, how to individualize your diet, and how not to get caught in the theory. Because of all this, it is much easier today. We have a lot more equipment today, so if you want to start eating a live food diet, it is easier. My feeling is that people intuitively know what the best diet is. There is overwhelming research showing that the live food diet is the healthiest of all diets. People intuitively know it, but many of them use all these other theories and things to make an excuse not to eat a live food diet.

Where do you see the raw food movement in the future?
As the society's rotting potential increases, more and more people will intuitively turn towards a raw food diet as a way of reversing the rotting cycle.

Is there anything that you would like to add?
It is pleasing to watch people who are eating live foods become more open to the spiritual reality in their life. The live food diet helps them do this naturally, because it is a more Sattvic diet. They become more sensitive to the sacred and more open to the spiritual purpose of life. To me, that is one of the most exciting and relevant things about the live food movement.

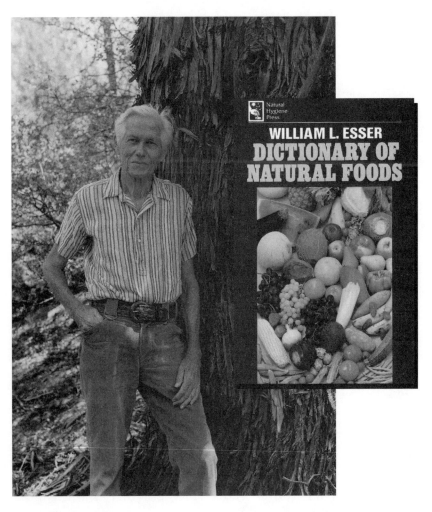

Dr. William Esser is the author of the book *Dictionary of Natural Foods.*

Dr. William Esser had a raw food fasting retreat called Esser's Ranch, in South Florida for many years. Dr. Esser recently sold the retreat and is enjoying his life in the sunny state of Florida. I have been unable to get contact information for him at the time of printing this book. I do plan to add his contact information to a future edition if I get it.

William Esser

I have had the great opportunity to meet William Esser several times at his ranch in South Florida. His energy surpasses most people half his age. If you want to be the best, model the best. I don't know anyone else who looks as great as William Esser does at 92. He is doing something correct. When I am his age I'll be very happy to have the amount of energy he has. The information he shares in this interview is very basic and simple. Keep it simple, use sense and you will be fine.

William Esser has been an active practitioner of Natural Hygiene since 1935. He has helped thousands of people regain and maintain good health the Natural Hygienic way.

How did you get started in the raw food life style?
The Natural Hygiene program was more or less inherited from my father. I have been practicing principles of Natural Hygiene throughout my entire life.

Who are some people who have inspired you to follow this path?
I was very good friends with Dr. Herbert Shelton, the great professional Natural Hygienist. Also, I went to school to study Naturopathy and Chiropractic skills, and Natural Hygiene simply became part of my life.

For people beginning this lifestyle, what is the most important thing they can do to help themselves, and what should they watch out for?
First of all, I think people should have a general knowledge of health and their bodies, with the positive aspect that the body is a living organism that repairs itself. Knowing those fundamentals, they should automatically alter their lives and avoid negative causes. If they do that, they will avoid illness and dis-

ease, and instead experience worthwhile and valuable results, keeping themselves vital.

Do you think it's easier to live a raw food lifestyle in today's time, or was it easier back when you began?
To some extent, I think it is easier today. Fruits, vegetables and all healthful foods are probably more readily available today than they were years ago, unless one lived on a farm.

Do you think it is easier for a man or for a woman to follow this lifestyle, or does it make no difference?
I do not think it makes any difference today at all.

What is your current age?
Ninety.

How are your health and energy?
They are very good; I would even say excellent. Currently, I do not feel the vitality of a sixteen year old, but I know very few people my age who are able to run, play tennis, and things of that sort.

How much sleep do you usually get?
Generally, about six to seven hours per night.

How many hours of sleep do you think is necessary for most people?
What is necessary is for people to get enough hours of sleep to feel refreshed and awake in the morning. That is an adequate amount of sleep. Some people need eight hours, some need six hours, and some may even need nine or ten hours of sleep per night. It is a variable thing.

Have you noticed any mental changes in yourself or others when consuming a natural diet?
Yes, I have. I definitely feel that people who follow a normal, natural diet automatically think better and more clearly. There is no question about that, unless of course, they have reached

a stage of degeneration such as Alzheimer's disease or other illnesses.

Have you become more spiritual the longer you followed this lifestyle?
It has brought me closer to God.

What is your average daily diet like?
The typical, average day consists of two fruit meals and one vegetable meal. That is my own preference, but some people do very well with one fruit meal and two vegetable meals a day. I think it depends on their particular preferences, as long as variety is sure to be addressed. In other words, it is best to eat a changing variety of raw foods over time. Limiting ourselves to a few certain types of food is not in the best interest of good nutrition.

How many years have you been eating a raw diet?
I have been eating a raw food diet, to some degree, for the last fifty years. I eat mostly raw foods, but not always 100% raw. A few times a week, I eat a baked potato or something of that nature. Otherwise, I have been probably 95% to 98% raw over the years.

Knowing that cooked food is enzyme deficient, how do you justify eating cooked food occasionally?
I do not think it is of great consequence for me to consume an occasional baked potato or some other cooked food from time to time. I am not concerned about it, because I do not ordinarily do it. If I do eat one occasionally, it is not a poison. It is not something that is going to harm my health. When we realize the degree of poisoning that people do in their lives by drinking enormous amounts of coffee and taking drugs, we realize how resilient the body is. I am not pleading the cause or the case that we should be eating cooked foods, but I do not think that it is something that we need to make a tremendous

issue of, if it is done on occasion.

Do you take any supplements or super foods?
All of my food is super food because it comes from the trees and the soil and it is excellent. I do not take anything else other than nature's food.

Do you think people can become overweight while eating a raw diet?
People should not become overweight. If they do, it is harmful. They should deal with it by disciplining themselves or abstaining from food.

Do you think overeating is a problem for people in general?
I definitely think that overindulgence is the most prevalent error that people make, and it can shorten and alter the quality of life.

Does it make a difference what time of day people eat? How do you feel about eating late at night?
I think it preferable to go to bed with a stomach that is finished with its work. If it is not finished, the digestion of food will interfere with normal sleep and normal rest.

Are you familiar with the works of Hilton Hotema?
Yes.

He talked about living on very small amounts of food. How do you feel about that?
Luigi Cornaro, who lived from 1464 to 1566, found that a minimal diet was the most preferable. The body cannot deal with large amounts of food. This builds up toxemia because our bodies have to dispose of excesses in one way or another, especially if we overindulge.

Do you think it's possible to eat a diet consisting of 100% fruit?
Yes, as long as there is a wide variety of fruit available and we are

not limited to three to five types of fruit. Also, if we live in an area where we can obtain naturally grown fruits that are not shipped or stored for great lengths of time, I think it is fine.

Do you think eating greens is necessary in this type of diet?
Yes, I think it is excellent to eat greens. I say it is preferable to eat greens in addition to fruit.

Do you think it is important to eat seasonally and locally?
I do not think it is of great importance to eat seasonally. However, I feel it is best to eat foods that are local, especially if one can pick them from one's own trees. The highest degree of taste and nutrients are obtained this way. It is better to eat locally, but I do not think it is necessary to worry about whether a food has come from a distant place or not. I think we can use all foods to our advantage, those grown far away as well as the local ones.

Do you think climate is important, and should it be considered when making the change to an all raw diet?
It can be. Although, an individual who is eating proper foods and generally living a healthful life should be able to deal with any weather or climate. On the other hand, I think the less stress and exposure our bodies receive from extreme heat or cold, the better off we are.

Out of all natural foods, which do you think is most important?
I think all raw foods are important because each one supplies certain minerals and vitamins which complement the others. One type of food does not contain all the essential nutrients our bodies need. Also, all natural foods function as a large variety, not necessarily eaten at one meal; but over time, having a good variety is important.

Do you feel it is necessary to properly combine food

when eating a 100% raw food diet?

I think it is important to combine foods well, whether they are 100% raw or otherwise. It is important because things like concentrated proteins and concentrated starches should be eaten separately.

Is it necessary to drink large amounts of water?

It is important to replenish the fluids the body uses each day. It depends on the nature of food the individual is eating. If the foods are very juicy, one does not need to drink much water. If the foods are dry and concentrated, then more water is necessary. For the most part, it should be a matter of thirst.

Socially, what is the best suggestion you have for people making this change of lifestyle?

I think it is very important for people to read good material about eating naturally. Once they get the facts, they should automatically want to improve their health by changing their dietary habits. They need to have knowledge of why they should be eating this way, because if they do not, then they will fail to have the motivation.

Many people just beginning a raw diet have problems because their mates do not want to change. Do you have any comments or suggestions?

In this case, I feel it is an individual matter. Usually, it involves somebody who is not ready or not intelligent enough to make the change.

Many women on this diet stop bleeding during their menstrual cycle. Do you think it is healthy for a woman not to bleed when she is on a raw diet?

Ordinarily, if they are living a healthful life, yes, it is a healthy sign.

What is your opinion of nuts and seeds?

I think they are excellent.

What is your opinion of grains?
I do not think they are necessary.

What is your opinion of sprouts?
I think they are excellent.

What is your opinion of wild foods?
If the food has a good flavor and it is not very bitter, then I approve of it. If it tastes bitter, it should not be eaten.

What is your opinion of fasting?
Fasting is excellent, and it meets the needs of most people. There are some people who may be too old or too weak to fast beneficially. But for the most part, the average person can fast readily for two to three weeks. If they fast for that long, they should definitely be under professional supervision.

What is your opinion of physical exercise?
Absolutely, physical exercise is very important.

Where do you see the raw food movement heading in the future?
I think it will always be a struggle. There will be accepting people and people who are simply not interested. For example, some people, like myself, are interested in Natural Hygiene, but the vast majority of people today have moved towards a conventional way of life. The Vegetarian and Natural Hygiene Movements require discipline. Most people do not want discipline. Most people want to go the easy way or the way that appeals to their taste buds. They do not wish to discipline themselves to the point they need to.

Thank you for giving this interview. Is there anything else you would like to say to help people begin or stay on this diet?
In my point of view, the most important thing is for them to try the diet for a few months. Once they do that, they will no-

tice excellent, positive changes in their overall health and vitality. If they do not see positive changes, then it would be best for them to undergo a supervised fast. After the fast, it should change their lives. They will be living a more positive, healthful life. As time goes on, it should become so natural to them, they will never think about foods or anything else relating to health, because it will be automatic. Then they will involve themselves in more important things because healthful living will make them possible.

It is my wish that you've gained as much insight and raw knowledge from these interviews as I have.

Raw Knowledge, Part II: Interviews With Health Achievers

Here are some brief bio's of amazing people whose interviews appear in *Raw Knowledge, Part II: Interviews with Health Achievers*

Renée Loux Underkoffler

Renée Loux Underkoffler is a renowned proponent and example of the Live-Foods lifestyle. She is a celebrated chef and dedicates her focus and talents to health and live-foods nutritional education and the culinary arts of living foods. Renée lives on the island of Maui, Hawaii for much of the year and teaches all over the world. She works privately with health counseling, cleansing and rejuvenation and facilitates health retreats and workshops incorporating yoga, living-foods and balanced lifestyle.

Renée co-founded the Raw Experience Restaurant in Paia, Maui in 1996 and was illustrated and published by many media interests for her delight with healthy living and sumptuous culinary creations.Renée co-published and illustrated *The Raw Truth, the Art of Living Foods*, now in its fourth printing. An excellent guide to food, sprouting, information, *The Raw Truth* offers very approachable access to scrumptious raw and living foods recipes.

Renée has just written two new books, her second recipe book titled, *Euphoric Organics* and a volume in progress, *The Science of Spiritual Nutrition: Seeds for Change*, a guide to comprehensive living nutrition and fine gourmet food.

Renée has been an inspiration and example of the live-foods lifestyle for more than seven years. She has a profound yoga practice and nurturing approach for whole health. She teaches people through experience and compassion how to approach health and well-being, tailored to personal needs and challenges.

Dr. Ruth Heidrich

Dr. Ruth Heidrich, received her Ph.D. in Health Management in 1993. She is the author of *A Race For Life* and *The Race For Life Cookbook*.

A certified fitness trainer, holding the world record for fitness for her age group at the renowned Cooper Clinic in Dallas, Texas, she still actively competes in marathons and triathlons, having won more than 600 trophies and medals since her diagnosis of breast cancer in 1982 at the age of 47.

With Terry Shintani, M.D., she co-hosts the radio show "Nutrition & You" on KWAI-AM in Hawaii.

Ruth is president of the Vegetarian Society of Hawaii and the Mid Pacific Road Runners Club. She won four gold medals in the 1997 Senior Olympics, held in Las Vegas, Nevada.

Annie Jubb

Annie Jubb is the co-author of the *LifeFood Recipe Book, Colloidal Biology* and *Secrets of an Alkaline Body*, along with five other books on Whole Brain Functioning, her training program, co-created with her partner of fifteen years, David Jubb Ph.D. Whole Brain Functioning, (WBF), training is adventure based experiential learning to create deep resource states of consciousness through fire walking, sweat lodges and adventure ropes course. Annie is known to her clients as a shaman, healer, spiritual leader, amazing speaker, and an expert in the body-mind-spirit connection.

Katharine Clark

Katharine has worked in several areas related to the health field over the years. She is the CEO/President of Health Works Enterprises, Inc. and has built and currently enjoys a multi-million dollar network marketing company with Cell Tech organic whole food supplements.

Katharine was also a traveling holistic health consultant and trainer for many years during which she designed and delivered three-day business and health training workshops in more than forty cities in the United States and Canada. These activities helped people understand their physiology holistically and the simple changes needed to create a health promoting lifestyle, effecting a measurable behavior modification. She has also designed and conducted a one week residential retreat in Oregon for sixty to eighty women each year, before the annual corporate conference. The retreat included educational classes and recreational activities. She created a team to continue producing the event.

She was a holistic health consultant and practitioner with an extensive private practice, extending from one on one counseling and evening educational courses, to private nursing duty for the seriously ill.

Katharine is certificated in: Alchemical Hypnotherapy, Reflexology, Colon Hydrotherapy, Iridology Body Centered Psychoawareness, etc.

Educational background:
A.S. in Nursing, Indiana University, 1979
B.A. in Psychology, Indiana University, 1981
Certified Massage Therapist and Colon HydroTherapist, Florida School of Massage, Certified Iridologist, Rebirther, etc. She holds Florida licenses in R.N. and L.M.T.

Rhio

Rhio is a singer, actress and author, as well as an investigative reporter in the health field. As a performer, she has appeared on over fifty TV shows.

Currently she is completing her third CD album, entitled *Half and Half,* for the Latin and American markets. Rhio, of Hungarian-Cuban descent, is completely fluent in Spanish.

A syndicated radio show, the *Fruit and Veggie Lady* is currently in production and scheduled to begin airing early in 2002. The show is a two minute feature in which Rhio gives the power food "recipe of the day," along with other important information about eating to stay healthy.

CNN and American Journal have aired stories on the raw food lifestyle featuring Rhio. She is considered an expert in the area of raw and living foods.

About seven years ago, Rhio started *The Raw Energy Hotline* on one of her phone lines in New York City where she lives. While the NY hotline continues, Rhio has expanded to the Internet and now covers national and international information about the raw/live food lifestyle on her extensive website:

www.rawfoodinfo.com
The New York hotline number is **(212) 343-1152.**

Periodically, Rhio hosts living food potluck dinners at her spectacular Tribeca loft in downtown Manhattan. She also offers classes on how to prepare raw and living foods for students in both English and Spanish. Medical doctors, who believe in the raw lifestyle, regularly send her their patients to be trained in raw food preparation.

David Klein

David Klein is Publisher/Editor of *Living Nutrition Maga-*

zine, based in Sebastopol in Northern California. David is also a Healthful Living Consultant, giving nutrition and self-healing consultations. David also directs *Colitis and Crohn's Health Recovery Services* at **www.colitis-crohns.com**

His journey from chronic illness to superb health has given him uncommon intuitive and scientific insight into nutrition and healing, through which he is able to guide his clients from illness to complete rejuvenation with consistent success. David is a living example of what he teaches and I am proud to call him a good friend.

Books by David Klein:
The Fruits Of Healing - a Story about a Natural Healing of Ulcerative Colitis;

The Seven Essentials for Overcoming Illness and Creating Everlasting Wellness;

Self Healing Colitis and Crohn's;

Your Natural Diet: Alive Raw Foods by T. C. Fry and David Klein.

Arne Wingvist

Arne Wingqvist, was born 1919. He started with a vegetarian bill of fare in 1931. Ten years later he eliminated all milk-products from his diet. Since about 1985 he ate mostly fresh fruit, nuts, seeds and fresh, uncooked, vegetables, mostly green leafy ones, organic, if possible.

Arne lived in Sweden for many years. He moved to Belgium, living there from 1986 until August 1988, when he moved to the French Riviera. Recently, after I finished the first printing of this book Arne passed away. He was a great man and I am glad I had the pleasure of interviewing Arne. I have decided to leave Arne's interview in my book because there was so much helpful information that I know he was excited to share.

John Fielder

John Fielder has so much knowledge to share, I'm so glad I was able to get this interview with him. I've met many people in this field, but John's knowledge surpasses most of theirs. Now you, too, can learn from one of the luminaries through this interview. When you finish reading it, please make sure you check out John's web site for additional cogent information.

John Fielder has an extensive background in the raw food movement, surpassing most everyone alive today. His credentials speak for themselves. There is an extensive list of all his accomplishments in *Raw Knowledge, Part II*, plus a great interview.

Robert Sniadach

Dr. Sniadach is a musician, mango lover, and a big StarTrek fan. His educational background is unlike most others. He completed the Life Science Course back in 1985, has a Doctorate in Chiropractic and almost received his Bachelor of Science degree in electromechanical design engineering before that. Robert Sniadach completed a nine month internship on fasting with Dr. William Esser in 1994. (Dr. Esser's interview is in this book.) Dr. Sniadach is also a certified member of the International Association of Hygienic Physicians since 1994. Currently, he runs Transformation Institute, which offers comprehensive Home Study Courses in Natural Hygiene. He also works directly with Healthful Living International and the Healthful Living Consultants Group (HLC) overseeing the program of student education leading to qualification for membership in the HLC.

Arthur Andrews

Arthur Andrews ran a fasting retreat in California for many years, working with Dr. Herbert Shelton. They were also very close friends. Mr. Andrews, 80 at this writing, is living life to its fullest. When I bring up the subject of health, many people I interview talk mostly about food and eating. But in Mr. Andrews' interview, much of the information focuses not on eating, but on all the other important aspects of health: emotional control, environment, spirituality, etc. Because Arthur has worked side by side with Dr. Herbert Shelton for so many years, I don't think there is anyone alive except maybe Dr. Vetrano who knew him better. Read all about what Arthur has learned, and why he is a trail blazer in the health movement.

Dr. V. Virginia Vetrano

Dr. Vetrano was graduated with honors from Trinity University and then interned at the world famous Dr. Shelton's Health School, studying Natural Hygiene under both Dr. Shelton and Dr. Carl Correlle. They had chosen her to be the first graduate from the American College of Natural Hygiene, chartered by Mr. C.E. Doolin and Dr. Shelton. She then went on to study Chiropractic, receiving the "Keeler Plaque" award upon graduation.

Immediately upon graduation with a D.C. degree, Dr. Vetrano took over as manager and sole doctor practicing at Dr. Shelton's Health School for the following 18 years, guiding thousands through short and long fasts, teaching the principles of Natural Hygiene, editing, writing for and producing Dr. Shelton's *Hygienic Review*, and saving lives.

Wanting more knowledge, Dr. Vetrano enrolled in the Kansas City Naturopathic College, and later the United American Medical College in Canada, and received a further degree in Homeopathic Medicine. Her fluent French quickly opened the door for her to become an international speaker on the subject of Natural Hygiene. She has lectured extensively throughout the world. In the late 80's and early 90's Dr. Vetrano continued to lecture in the United States and abroad, making several films in California with the late T.C. Fry. She has been specially honored many times.

Dr. Vetrano was President of the American Natural Hygiene Society for two terms and served on its Board of Directors for several years. She had been a regular speaker for the ANHS from 1965 until 1987. She was also a certified member of the International Association of Professional Hygienists.

Paul Nison

I've interviewed so many great pioneers, hearing their opinions about health, life, the mind, body and soul. Also, I've received many requests to include an interview in which I am the subject. Through the years, I've often been interviewed and in my new book, I've decided to include one of my favorites. I feel it's one of my best because it covers many important aspects of health, including information about eating, weight control, detoxification, how to be happy in life, how to succeed at eating a 100% raw food diet and much more.

To order *Raw Knowledge, Part II: Interviews With Health Achievers* please contact me at:

Paul Nison
P.O. Box 443
Brooklyn, NY 11209
866-RAW-DIET
www.rawlife.com

**A note from the author: I'm constantly meeting new people with amazing stories to share. As this book, gets updated to future editions, even more great interviews will be added. Please make sure I have your most updated contact information, if you would like to be informed about future editions.

Also, if you feel you have an amazing story to share, or know of someone who might be a good subject for an interview, please contact me at the above address with the information.

Conclusion

In today's world, people are brainwashed and trained to do things that don't work. They do not understand that if you keep trying to do the same thing that doesn't work, you will end up with the same result every time you try to do "that same thing". That is why there is no cure for cancer, AIDS, or any of the other so-called "incurable diseases." As a good friend says, "There are few incurable diseases, but there are many incurable people." This is so true.

If you want to change the result, then you must change what you are doing. If you follow common society's ways of doing things, you will suffer from the same common illnesses that the common person suffers from. Medical doctors are not trained to cure; they're trained to control. Natural doctors are trained to cure and prevent. If followed correctly, a raw food diet will cure and prevent most disease known to man because it eliminates the cause. Quite simply, if you eliminate the cause, you can't get sick. "It's not what you add to your diet that will heal you but what you leave out. That is what I mean when I say it must be done correctly.

There is a cosmic law that will protect you better than many government laws ever could. It can't be seen, but it is out there. This cosmic law states: "What you give is what you get, and what you get is what you give." That is the cosmic cycle. If you give loving, free, happy, healthy thoughts, then that is what you will get in return. But in today's society, we are brought up to give fearful, scary, worrying thoughts and the things we suffer from most are the things we worry about most. We are trained to do things out of fear, when we should be taught to do things for pleasure. Government laws train us to do things with fear in mind. We always hear, "Pay your taxes, or else! Don't do this! Don't do that! Get shots for your kids, or else!" That is why we grow up as we do, suffering from the only true illness: "FEAR." Most people are in the habit of doing things to avoid a bigger fear. The only true cure is: "Knowledge." That is the only way to let go of the fear and obtain happiness. Government laws leave us with two choices: bad or worse. Either way, you can't win. When you have knowledge instead of habit, you are left with many choices: good, better, or even better than that. When you do things out of knowledge rather than fear, you can only have a positive outcome.

Once you clean your mind and body, you will experience the special power of the soul or the spirit. Start listening to cosmic law and you will be protected. Here is the main difference: government laws only look at the outcome, not at a person's intentions. Cosmic laws aren't concerned with the outcome; they look at intentions. That's why the cosmic law is: "Give good, and you will get good." This way, regardless of your results, you will be protected as long as you act with good intentions. Once you live by this law, you will realize what I am talking about. You'll never be put into a situation that will worry you. Live by the cosmic law and the universe will provide.

I named my first book *The Raw Life*, but many people

asked me why I didn't name it ***The Raw Diet***. It's not about diet alone; it's a lifestyle change. Yes, diet has much to do with it, but there is much more to it. It is not about being 100% perfect or 100% raw; it is about being 100% happy. If you're the type of person who is 100% happy with what you're doing, then there is no reason to change. You are either not ready or not in need of a change. But if you are anything less than 100% happy, then you must change if you want to be happier, healthier, wiser, and free. Chances are, if you try to eat a perfect diet of 100% raw foods and you are not ready for it, then you won't be happy eating it. But if you are ready to do it, you will be successful at it and you will find there is no easier way to become happy and live by the cosmic laws that will protect you from all bad things. I named this book ***Raw Knowledge*** because this is the knowledge that will set you free! It will tell you when your body is ready to eat raw foods, how to do so, and what the outcome will be. If you know the outcome, there can be no fear. With no fear, there is no doubt, worry, or illness.

Raw Knowledge will set you free!

The Bottom Line:
Summing it all up

The following is from Prof. Hilton Hotema's book, *Man's Higher Consciousness*. This book is a classic and I recommend it to everyone who wants to learn about true health, happiness and freedom. Read this book! Many of the ideas in *Raw Knowledge* have come to me from the body of Prof. Hilton Hotema's writings. He is the author of many books, but *Man's Higher Consciousness* is his most noted work and, in my opinion, his best. If you would like to order it or other books by Prof. Hilton Hotema, please contact me by email at paul@rawlife.com or call me at 866-RAW-DIET. I have several of Prof. Hilton Hotema's most popular books for sale on my web site: www.rawlife.com and I can tell you where to get all of his great books.

Prologue from Man's Higher Consciousness:

Life is Creation's greatest treasure for Man in the flesh, and most men should enjoy it much longer than they do. This can easily be done by learning the body's simple requirements and living in harmony with that knowledge, which is contained in Hotema's late work entitled, *Long Life in Florida.*

Some men are now living 120, 150 and 200 years and beyond. What is possible for one man is possible for millions more. Charlie Smith of Florida is vital and vigorous at the age of 119 and says he intends to live considerably longer. Much about him is contained in the book, *Long Life in Florida*, which everyone should read, because it's the greatest work ever written on longevity.

"In 1930, Santiago Surviate, an Indian, died in Arizona at the age of 135. In 1936, Zora Agha, a Turk, died in Turkey at the age of 162. In 1921, Jose Calverio died in Mexico at the age of 185. In 1795, Thomas Carn died in England at the age of 207. In 1933, Li Chung-Yun died in China at the age of 256. In 1566, Numes De Cugna died in India at the age of 370. He grew four new sets of teeth and his hair turned from black to gray four times.

In December 1888, when Mrs. Fred Miller was two years old, her mother found a little turtle nearly frozen in an alley near their home in Baltimore. She took the turtle home, named it Pete, nursed it back to health, and now at an age estimated to be more than 100 years, Pete is still the family pet and shows little signs of his age.

All Living creatures are ruled by the same laws of Creation, but they do not all live in harmony with those laws. Those that come the closest to it are those that live the longest in proportion to the length of time required for them to reach maturity of physical development.

There are many reasons, most of them preventable, why people die young and hospitals are filled with the sick, whereas others are seldom ill and live three to ten times longer.

It would logically seem that living creatures with the higher intelligence should be the ones to live the nearest to the requirements of the laws of Creation; but in action it seems to work the other way, the more intelligent creatures being those who appear to stray the farthest from the straight and narrow path with leads unto life (Mat. 7:13, 14).

The large majority of the so-called health writers are not

noted for longevity. They seem to die as early as those who read their writings. And some who live 120 years can't tell why they lived so long, as in the case of Diamond, who lived 120 years, wrote a book on long life in 1904 when he was 108, on page 43 of which he itemized "My Daily Menu", which is rather good, yet not one we would recommend.

To reduce longevity to a scientific basis means that we must learn the requirements of the body and supply them. The facts show that living is breathing. We can't die as long as we can breathe – and we stop living when we stop breathing.

Breathing is the primary function of the body. We can live for weeks without eating and for days without drinking, but, when we stop breathing for a few minutes, we stop living.

And right here is the most neglected spot in the entire health field. Why is that so? First, ignorance; second, the claim of science that man lives on what he eats; and third, no one has yet found a way to commercialize air and breathing.

This is the discouraging condition we found sixty years ago, when we set out to learn how to live healthfully and long. And so, we began almost alone to learn something about breathing and the Breath of Life.

The first valuable hint came when we found this: "If we maintain our blood in normal condition and circulation, sickness would be almost impossible. The blood is the life of the flesh. We are what we are by the influence of our blood flowing through our body" (Bernarr MacFadden, in Vitality Supreme, 1910).

Then there came another surprise when we discovered that blood is made of gas. The gases of the air constitute the total composition of the blood. We know that water is the product of the uniting of hydrogen and oxygen gases. When we drink water, we drink gases in fluid form. Blood is gases in fluid form. Everything can be transformed to gas by heat. The earth itself is constituted of condensed gas. There is the source and origin of all things.

We have heard of fire damp, ignis fatus, and will-o-the-wisp.

That fiery element is the Living Gas in what we eat and drink. That Living Gas is all the body uses of what we eat. Of that Living Gas the blood is made.

This is the first valuable lesson in dietetics. Scientists talk learnedly and foolishly about protein, carbohydrates, nucleic acids, fats, lipids, etc., ignoring the fact that the ox, elephant, horse and moose live in good health all their days on grass and green leaves.

The next lesson in dietetics is not to heat food and drive out of it the precious, volatile gases which the body uses in its laboratory to make its blood and the products it needs, which includes all the elements mentioned above.

Remember this one: Creation never uses second-hand material in its building work. The protein in the food we eat never becomes the protein of our body. That protein has served its purpose, is a used product, and is never used again by Creation in its constructive work.

The living gas in what we eat is all the body uses. The rest is useless waste, and cast off by the body as feces. Hence, most of what man eats goes down the sewer.

As gases are all the body uses in making blood and bone and building flesh, consider the condition of the blood, bone and flesh that are made of the poisonous gases that saturate the air of modern civilization, where health is the exception instead of the rule. If a chemist were to analyze the air we breathe and give us his report, we would be shocked to learn the great amount of poison the body must endure to live in our polluted environment.

This subject is so broad and vital, it would take a large book to discuss it adequately. But enough has been said to make a thinking person be more careful about the kind of air he breathes, the condition of the air in his home, and especially in his bedroom, where lack of activity during the night allows the air to stagnate and grow extra foul.

That's another reason why people die in their sleep. The polluted, stagnant air in their bedrooms paralyzes the breathing center of the brain, and they just stop breathing.

Stagnant air gets foul, like water in a stagnant pool. Keep the air in circulation in homes and bedrooms. Use electric fans for that purpose. Fewer people would die in their sleep if they had an electric fan in operation in their bedroom.

This writer (Hilton Hotema) is only fifteen years under the century mark, which he expects to pass by many years, as he feels as fit as he did forty years ago. Here he is telling the world in his work (*Man's Higher Consciousness*) some of the secrets of how he has done it.

To an intelligent, unprejudiced person who can and does think, the information contained in this work may seem simple. But it is the fundamental simplicities that are always difficult to accept, because they are so very simple, and, therefore, unbelievable on that account."

—Prof. Hilton Hotema

Many of Prof. Hilton Hotema's books are for sale on my website: www.rawlife.com or call 866-RAW-DIET.

*A special thanks to Health Research for permission to use this Prologue From *Man's Higher Consciousness*. Health Research has many excellent, rare and out-of-print books on Nutritional Research, Natural Healing, Health, Metaphysics, Religion and Esoterica. You may contact Health Research for more information about their long list of valuable books at:

Health Research
PO Box 850
Pomeroy, WA 99347
509 843-2385
888 844-2386
www.healthresearchbooks.com

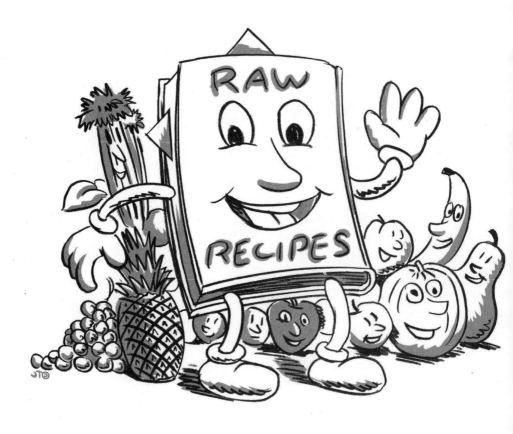

APPENDIX A:
Raw Food Recipes

The best diet is a simple one. When you start eating a raw food diet, you might feel a need for the taste of cooked food until your natural taste buds wake up. Here are some recipes to keep you going until your natural taste buds come alive. These recipes will help you during the transition to a simpler lifestyle. The length of transition time is different for everyone. You never want to say "never" and "I'll never eat this way again", but for best results, slowly but surely start cutting down on the number of raw recipes and start eating more raw mono meals (one food at a time). It's not easy to follow proper food combining rules when eating recipes, so over the long run, eating recipes every day can become a problem. But for now, if you're just starting out, enjoy these wonderful raw recipes. Keep moving forward. As time goes by, eat them with less and less frequency, until one day you're at a place where you only eat recipes on special occasions, if at all. Whatever you choose to do, enjoy your life, and smile!

When it comes to preparing raw food recipes, many people get discouraged because they are so difficult and time-consuming to prepare. Well, some of them are, but others are very simple and easy to make. Instead of breaking down the recipes into breakfast, lunch, dinner and desserts, I put them into sections called simple, intermediate and advanced. There is no such thing as "we need to eat three times a day - breakfast, lunch and dinner." Try to get out of the habit of eating by the clock and naming your meals. There is only one true meal, no matter what time you eat it: breakfast. When you are not eating, you are fasting; when you eat, you are breaking that fast. That's how we got the name "break-fast." Also, many recipe books include a section called snacks and desserts. Well, everything you put in your body is a meal, so I don't have a separate section for desserts or snacks.

**Always do your best to get your produce as fresh and organic as possible. The closer to the vine, the more divine. That is best, but don't make excuses; do the best you can!

Easy Recipes

For people who don't have much time to spare and want really healthy "Fast Food"

Mushroom Pizza
Serves 1

1 portabella mushroom
1 lemon
1/4 cup raw tahini or almond butter
1 tomato
1/2 avocado (optional)

Remove the mushroom stem and clean (rinse) the mushroom

cap. Turn cap upside down and squeeze the juice of the lemon on it, then pour in the nut butter, then layer thin slices of tomato. Add thin slices of avocado, if you like.
Recipe by Paul Nison

Sautéed Mushrooms
Serves 1

1 portabella mushroom
Nama Shoyu (raw soy sauce)

Remove the mushroom stem and clean (rinse) the mushroom cap. Chop up mushroom cap into squares or long strips and marinate in Nama Shoyu for two hours. *Recipe by Paul Nison*

Marinated Veggies
Serves 1

1 yellow squash
1 zucchini
2 lemons

Chop up veggies in a bowl. Add lemon juice and marinate for four to six hours. *Recipe by Paul Nison*

Avocado with Salsa
Serves 1

1 avocado
2 plum tomatoes - diced
1 tablespoon freshly squeezed lemon juice
1/2 clove garlic - chopped
1/2 tablespoon onion - minced
1 dash of cayenne pepper
1/2 tablespoon fresh cilantro - chopped

1 teaspoon olive oil
1/2 teaspoon Nama Shoyu (raw soy sauce) or soy sauce

Slice the avocado in half and remove the pit. Place all other ingredients in a food processor. Pulse until ingredients are combined yet still chunky. Pour salsa into the avocado where the pit used to be. *Recipe by Paul Nison*

Date Balls
Serves 1 (about 3 balls)

6 Medjool dates
3 pecans
2 tablespoons carob powder
shredded coconut or sesame seeds

Take the pits out of the dates. Put dates into a food processor with the carob powder. Mix well. Form into balls and stick a pecan in the middle. Roll in shredded coconut or sesame seeds. *Recipe by Paul Nison*

Paul Nison, Salad #1
Serves 1

spinach (as much as you like)
1/2 cucumber
1/2 stalk celery
1 avocado
1/2 red pepper (optional)
flax seeds – ground
juice of 1 lemon

Chop and mix all ingredients in a big bowl. Then sprinkle with juice of the lemon. *Recipe by Paul Nison*

Paul Nison, Salad #2
Serves 1

1/2 cucumber
1 stalk celery
1 avocado
1/2 red pepper (optional)
dulse - soaked for about 30 seconds
flax seeds - ground

Chop and mix all ingredients in a big bowl. *Recipe by Paul Nison*

Raw Sandwich

1 large eggplant
nut paté (refer to other recipes)
lettuce
tomato slices

Prepare nut paté, using a recipe from this book or another recipe book. Slice the eggplant into thin slices and use the slices as you would use bread. Place nut paté with lettuce and tomatoes between two slices of eggplant. *Recipe by Paul Nison*

Zucchini Pasta with Tomato Sauce or Pine Nut Sauce
Serves 2

3 large zucchinis
1 avocado (optional)

Tomato sauce:
3 tomatoes
1 handful sun-dried tomatoes
1 clove garlic
1/2 tablespoon fresh basil

1/2 tablespoon fresh oregano
1 small hot pepper

Pine nut sauce:
1 cup pine nuts
1/2 lemon
1/4 teaspoon nutmeg spice
1 small piece ginger
1 clove garlic
Nama Shoyu (raw soy sauce) or soy sauce to taste

Process zucchini in a saladacco. It will come out like angel hair pasta, very easy to use. To make either kind of sauce, mix well in a blender or food processor. Pour it over the zucchini (the "pasta"). Optional: I also like to cut up an avocado and mix it in with the sauce and the pasta. *Recipe by Paul Nison*

Avo-buttered Corn on the Cob

1 corn on the cob - freshly shucked
1 avocado - halved and pitted

With the corn in one hand and the avocado in the other, smear the avocado over the corn kernels and enjoy! Best eaten barefooted! *Recipe by David Klein*

Raw Muesli

2 cups raw oats
4 apples (red or yellow) - do not peel
1/2 cup macadamia nuts
1/4 cup raisins
dairy alternative OR fresh apple juice
OR two ripe mashed bananas moistened with water

Grate apples. Grate or chop nuts. Mix all ingredients together.

Add dairy alternative or fresh apple juice or two ripe mashed bananas moistened with purified water to make a milk. Eat immediately. *Recipe by Célène Bernstein*

Pineapple, Mango and Berry Salad

3 butter lettuce leaves
1 mango - sliced
1 cup finely diced pineapple or pureed pineapple
1 cup blueberries
1 cup strawberries

Arrange lettuce leaves on a plate. In the center, make a mound of cubed or pureed pineapple. Arrange blueberries, mango slices, and strawberries around the pineapple.
Recipe by Célène Bernstein

Sweet Waldorf Salad

4 golden delicious apples - diced
2 cups celery - chopped
1/4 cup macadamia nuts - chopped
1/4 cup raisins
2 tablespoons fresh apple juice

Combine apples, celery, raisins and nuts. Add apple juice to moisten. Toss ingredients well. Serve immediately.
Recipe by Célène Bernstein

Winter Fruit Salad

1 banana - sliced
1 apple (golden delicious or red) - sliced thinly
dates or figs
60 grams chopped macadamia nuts

Mix banana and apple in a bowl. Add dates or figs and nuts to the fruit. *Recipe by Celene Bernstein*

Kale Avocado Salad
Serves 2

This is a great way to prepare kale, which is difficult to eat raw for most people 'transitioning' to the raw foods diet. When Celtic sea salt is used and the kale massaged, the kale 'wilts' making it easier on digestion and definitely more palatable. This salad has grown to be a staple dish for the Tree of Life community and all who experience it.

1 head kale, any variety, shredded
1 cup tomato diced
1 cup avocado chopped
2 1/2 tablespoons olive oil
1 1/2 tablespoons lemon juice
1 teaspoon Celtic sea salt
1/3 teaspoon cayenne

In a mixing bowl toss all ingredients together, squeezing as you mix to 'wilt' the kale and creaming the avocado. Serve immediately. As a variation add chopped fresh herbs.
Recipe by Chad at The Tree of Life

Live Fries
Serves 5

Slice 1 lb. Jicama so it looks like French fries.
Combine in a bowl with:
1 tablespoon onion powder
2 tablespoons olive oil
sea salt to taste
1 tablespoon paprika

Recipe by Victoria Boutenko

Autumn Salad
with Orange Bavarian Cream Sauce

1 apple, diced
1 pear, diced
small bunch of Concord grapes (or other grapes)
squeeze of lemon

Dice the apple and pear and squeeze lemon juice over them. Take the grapes off the vine. Orange Bavaria cream sauce on page 361. Mix fruits together gently and put on a plate. *Recipe by Rhio*

Fruits & Roots
Serves 3-4

1 medium jicama
1/2 mango, chopped small
3 kiwi, chopped small
2 oranges or tangerines, chopped small
juice of 1/2 orange or tangerine
1/3 cup currants

Peel the jicama and shred, using a mandolin or grater. Set aside in a large bowl. Add the chopped fruit and currants to the bowl and toss with the orange or tangerine juice. Keeps for 2-3 days in the refrigerator. *Recipe by Rhio*

Intermediate Meals

For people who have a little bit more time, and want to further experiment with raw food recipes.

Carrocado Mash

6 to 10 large fresh carrots
1 large red or yellow bell pepper
1 ripe avocado
1 ounce whole dulse leaf
1 whole bell pepper (optional)

Soak the dulse leaf in water for a few minutes, then drain and thoroughly rinse, then squeeze out the water by hand.
Dice the bell pepper. Run the carrots through a Champion juicer with the blank plate installed, collecting the juicy pulp in a bowl. Remove the flesh from the avocado and, using a fork, mash the avocado into the carrot pulp. Add the dulse and bell pepper to the carrot-avocado mixture, and eat with a fork. Optional: Scoop out a whole bell pepper and stuff with the carrot-avocado mixture. *Recipe by David Klein*

Marinated Vegetables

You can use many vegetables for this, but those suggested here work particularly well. The vegetables can be used as a garnish for all sorts of meals and soups.

Choose from these vegetables:
purple sprouting broccoli
onions cut into thin rings
sliced mushrooms
asparagus
sliced aubergine (small eggplant)

Marinade:
1 medium red chili - de-seeded and chopped
2 cloves of garlic - chopped
1 inch of ginger - grated
1/2 cup olive oil or sesame oil

1/2 cup lemon juice
2 teaspoons soy sauce (optional)

Put the vegetables into a shallow dish. Mix all marinade ingredients together and pour over the vegetables, making sure they are completely covered. For best results, marinate for a day. Every so often, stir the vegetables to marinate them evenly.
Recipe by Sharon Holdstock

Coleslaw
This goes well with lighter main courses.

2 carrots
1 onion
1/2 of a small white cabbage
juice of 2 lemons
1 clove garlic
1 cup Brazil or macadamia nuts
6 dessert teaspoons of olive oil
1 pinch mustard powder
salt to taste (optional)

Thinly slice the carrots, cabbage, and onion (a manoline or food processor attachment works well for this), and mix them all together in a big bowl. Chop the garlic and put all the remaining ingredients in a blender and blend until smooth. Add water if necessary. Pour the mixture over the vegetables and mix until they are all coated. Add salt to taste, if desired.
Recipe by Sharon Holdstock

Frederic's Salad

Romaine lettuce
avocado
tomatoes

lime juice
raw corn
very little olive oil
red cabbage powder (or celery powder)

Dehydrate red cabbage in a dehydrator and then turn it into a powder using a coffee grinder. You can also do that with celery. It's my healthy seasoning, and it's colorful.
Recipe by Frederic Patenaude

Basic Nut Mixture

1 cup pecans
1 cup walnuts
1 cup almonds
1 cup pistachios
1 medium carrot - finely shredded
1/2 cup finely chopped white onions
1 tablespoon salt-free granulated garlic
1 1/2 teaspoons black pepper
2 tablespoons liquid aminos
or Nama Shoyu (raw soy sauce)

Grind each kind of nut separately in a food grinder, or use the S-blade in a food processor. Place all ingredients in a large bowl and mix well.
Variations: use the same measurements, same nuts, or nuts of your choice with the rest of the ingredients, adding grated ginger, garlic or seasoning of your choice. Form into balls, patties, a loaf or other desired shape. *Recipe by Annette Larkins*

Corn a Maize

3 cups fresh corn (6 medium sized ears)
3 tablespoons finely chopped green onions

3 tablespoons red bell pepper
3 tablespoons celery
1 tablespoon salt-free granulated garlic (or suit your taste)
1 tablespoon granulated onion (or suit your taste)
1 tablespoon lemon pepper (or suit your taste)
2 tablespoons Annette's Pesto (refer to recipe)

Wash and remove corn from cob; wash pepper and celery. Chop onions, pepper, and celery. Combine all ingredients with Annette's Pesto (see recipe below) and mix well.
*Recipe by Annette Larkins

Thick Herbal Paté

4 cups of sprouted grain with soaked seeds mix
4 tablespoons extra virgin olive oil
2 teaspoons Celtic sea salt
2 - 4 cloves of garlic chopped
2 sprigs of fresh rosemary leaves
12 large leaves basil
4 sprigs of sage

Blend in food processor, until reduced to a thick cream. Before serving, mix in a few leaves of wet dulse. Roll into a nori sheet with shredded carrots and soaked dulse. **Recipe by Viktoras Kulvinskas*

Live Hummus
Serves 5-7

Blend the following ingredients in a food processor:
2 cups garbanzo beans (sprouted for 1 day)
1/2 cup extra virgin olive oil
1 cup tomatoes (chopped)
1 cup celery (chopped)

salt to taste
1-2 tablespoons (dried), or 1 cup (fresh) dill or basil
1-2 tablespoons lime or lemon juice
hot peppers to taste
2-5 cloves garlic

Sprinkle with dried parsley flakes before serving.
Recipe by Victoria Boutenko

More Complicated Recipes

**For those who have the time, or for anyone to make
for that special occasion.**

Pizza
Serves 8

Pine Nut Sauce (see recipe above)
tomatoes - thinly sliced
Marinated Mushroom (see recipe above)
Marinated Veggies (see recipe above)
garlic - chopped
nuts – chopped

Crust:
2 cups carrot pulp
2 cups sunflower seeds
1/2 cup lemon juice
1 tablespoon onions

Mix all ingredients for the crust in a food processor and form
it into the shape of a big pizza crust. Put it into a dehydrator
and dehydrate overnight.

The next day, add Pine Nut Sauce (see recipe above), then, add thinly sliced tomatoes. Then, add marinated mushroom and marinated veggies (see recipes above). Then, add chopped garlic and thinly chopped nuts. *Recipe by Paul Nison*

Paul's Coconut Fruit Pie

1 banana - sliced thin
1 mango - sliced thin
shredded coconut and raisins
OR whole nuts

Crust:
2 cups walnuts
2 cups pecans
1/2 cup orange juice
7 medjool dates

Filling:
4 young coconuts
6 medjool dates - pitted
1 tablespoon psyllium powder
1 banana (optional)

To make the crust, mix all ingredients for the crust in a food processor until it has a doughy consistency. Press it into an 8-inch glass pie plate.

To make the filling, combine the meat of 4 young coconuts and the juice of one coconut with 6 medjool dates (pitted) and psyllium power in a blender or vita mix. (Optional: add one banana to mixture.)

Place thin slices of bananas and mangos at the bottom of the piecrust. Immediately pour the filling over the fruit.
Top the pie with shredded coconut and raisins or whole nuts around the edges. *Recipe by Paul Nison*

Ala Almond Paté

4 cups of almonds
2 cups finely ground carrots
1 cup chopped celery
1 cup chopped onion poultry seasoning mix
1 cup chopped pecans
sea salt to taste.
4 capsules of Super Blue Green Acidophilus
1 medium head cauliflower

Grind almonds very finely in food processor. Open the Super Blue Green Acidophilus capsules and sprinkle out the contents. Run chopped up cauliflower through food processor to chunky consistency - not mushy, for texture.

Mix all the ingredients well. Spread the mixture on a plate until one inch high. Let it sit overnight at room temperature to go through a microbe predigest phase. Can be refrigerated. Will keep up to four days. *Recipe by Viktoras Kulvinskas*

Chocolate Mousse Pie
with Whipped Vanilla Cream and Fresh Berries
Yields 8-10 servings from a ten inch pie.

The Chocolate Mousse Pie has been a well kept secret...until now. It is a dessert masterpiece of simple decadence, famed for pleasing even the most discriminating chocolate gourmet. The unsuspecting richness of the avocado lends the carob just the right oils for satiating indulgence.

1 ten inch pie crust
(see recipes below for Almond-Vanilla Crumble Crust
OR Pecan Graham Cracker Crust)
1 1/2 cups strawberries
1 cup fresh raspberries

(one berry may be substituted if both are not available)
2 1/2 cups avocado (3 medium avocados)
1 cup soft dates - pitted and soaked in water until soft
4-6 tablespoons maple syrup or as needed
1 tablespoon cold-pressed coconut butter (optional)
3/4 cup raw carob powder
4-6 tablespoons cocoa powder, or as needed
2 tablespoons non-alcohol vanilla extract
6 drops clear stevia (optional extra sweetener)
Vanilla Cream Frosting (refer to recipe below)
poppy seeds and fresh mint (for garnish)

Prepare pie crust according to recipe. Slice strawberries. Layer and press into the bottom of the crust. Spoon avocado into the food processor (without peel or pit). Blend until it begins to turn smooth.

Drain water from dates, if necessary. Add dates or maple syrup and vanilla. Blend until smooth. Spoon in carob and cocoa. Blend until smooth. Spoon in extra cocoa and carob for an even richer and thicker mousse.

Spread evenly on sliced strawberries. Prepare Vanilla Cream Frosting according to recipe below and spread on mousse filling. Cut into 8-10 slices. Carefully place raspberries or sliced strawberries, evenly covering the whipped cream. Garnish with poppy seeds and fresh mint. *Recipe by Renée Loux Underkoffler*

Almond-Vanilla Crumble Crust
Yields one 10-inch pie crust

1 1/4 cups soaked or sprouted almonds
3/4 cup almonds - dry or soaked and dehydrated
1/3 cup soft, pitted medjool or honey dates
OR 3-4 tablespoons maple syrup
1 finely chopped organic vanilla bean

OR 1 tablespoon non-alcohol vanilla extract
1 1/2 teaspoons cinnamon
1 pinch of good sea salt

In a food processor, grind either dry or soaked and dehydrated almonds into a fine meal. Set aside. Grind sprouted almonds into a fine meal. It might be necessary to scrape the walls of the food processor with a rubber spatula and continue grinding to obtain an even consistency.

Add dates or maple syrup to the sprouted almond meal and pulse-chop until well mixed. Scrape the walls of the food processor. Add in dry almond meal and chopped vanilla bean or vanilla extract. Pulse until well mixed. Press evenly into a glass 10-inch pie plate. If the dough is too moist, allow to stand, covered, in the refrigerator for a few hours or overnight until firm, or dehydrate at 108 degrees for one hour. *Recipe by Renée Loux Underkoffler*

Pecan Graham Cracker Crust
Yields one crumbly 10-inch pie crust

This graham-crackery crust is reminiscent of the traditional style.

2 cups soaked or sprouted pecans, dehydrated until dry
OR 1 cup soaked or sprouted pecans and 1 cup dry pecans
1/3 cup soft pitted dates OR 3-4 tablespoons maple syrup
2 tablespoon raw carob powder (optional)
1 tablespoon freshly ground cinnamon
1 tablespoon freshly ground nutmeg
1 tablespoon non-alcohol vanilla extract
1 pinch sea salt

Grind pecans into a fine meal in a food processor. It might be necessary to scrape the walls of the food processor and continue to grind until thoroughly mixed. Add dates or maple syrup to ground pecans and pulse-chop until well mixed. Scrape the walls of the food processor and add in ground cinnamon, nutmeg, vanilla extract and salt. Press evenly into a 10-inch glass pie plate. *Recipe by Renée Loux Underkoffler*

Vanilla Cream Frosting
Yields more than one cup of velveteen vanilla cream
The best basic cream frosting.

1 cup whole cashews - soaked half an hour in water
OR 1 cup macadamia nuts - soaked half an hour in water
1/4 cup soft dates - pitted and soaked in water until soft
OR 3-4 tablespoons maple syrup, or as needed
1 tablespoon cold-pressed coconut butter or olive oil
1-2 tablespoons non-alcohol vanilla extract
filtered water as needed

In a blender or Vita Mix, blend nuts, dates or maple, and vanilla, adding water one tablespoon at a time as needed to blend smooth. *Recipe by Renée Loux Underkoffler*

Ginger-Sesame Sushi Cone Rolls
with Miso Citrus Dipping Sauce
Serves 4-6

4 sheets Nori seaweed
1 yellow bell pepper - julienned thin
(red bell may be substituted)
1 Asian apple pear - julienned thin
green onion tops
Decorative greens: mizuna, radicchio or oak lettuce

Spread:
4 tablespoons raw tahini (ground sesame paste)

3 tablespoons white miso (salty soybean paste)
3-4 tablespoons lemon juice
2 tablespoons organic cane sugar or maple syrup
1 1/2 -2 tablespoons fresh ginger - peeled and minced
1/4 cup green onion - minced
4 tablespoons sesame seeds
sun-dried sea salt to taste

In a bowl, whip together tahini, miso and lemon juice. Add organic cane sugar or maple syrup and mix well. Mince green onion and ginger, and fold in with sesame seeds. Add sea salt only if necessary.

Use 4-5 tablespoons of the miso-tahini mixture for each nori sheet. Spread in a strip along one edge of a nori sheet. Layer sliced bell pepper, green onion tops and decorative greens on top, allowing well trimmed pieces to extend past the end of the sheet.

Roll tightly with the aid of a bamboo sushi roller. Gently wet the edge of the nori sheet with water to seal shut. Allow to stand several seconds to dry before slicing. A sharp, serrated knife works well. Wipe the knife between each cut to avoid sticking. Cut into different sized pieces and serve on a square plate.

Miso Citrus Dipping Sauce:
1 cup Nama Shoyu (raw soy sauce) or tamari
2 tablespoons lemon juice
1 tablespoon fresh orange juice
1 tablespoon maple syrup
sesame seeds for garnish

Mix together and serve in small dipping bowls.
Recipe by Renée Loux Underkoffler

Seasoned Asparagus Bundles with Shaved Hazelnuts and Marinated Pear

2 dozen tender asparagus stalks
4 cups hot water (not boiling)
1 generously sized pear, D'anjou or Bosc - peeled, cored, and sliced thinly
1 tablespoon Lemon Zest
1/2 cup lemon juice
1-2 tablespoons apple cider vinegar
2 tablespoons olive oil
1 tablespoon maple syrup (optional)
1/4 cup chopped fresh herbs: dill, parsley, cilantro and/or basil
1 teaspoon fresh coriander - lightly crushed (optional)
1-2 teaspoons good mineralized sea salt
black pepper to taste
4 hazelnuts per bundle - shaved on a fine grater
carrot or beet - peeled and "spiralized"

In a casserole dish, pour hot water over the asparagus and cover with a platter for 5-10 minutes, until softened and bright green. Drain off hot water.

Take asparagus stalks out of the casserole dish. Peel, core and slice pear. Place on the bottom of the casserole dish. Place asparagus on top of the sliced pears. Toss in remaining ingredients to marinate for 20 minutes or longer, leaving the pear slices on the bottom to absorb the marinade.

"Spiralize" carrot or beet into long threads. Use long threads to tie bundles of asparagus stalks.
Recipe by Renée Loux Underkoffler

Renée's Sunfired-Tomato Lasagna
Serves 4-6

Four young summer squash (zucchini) – thinly sliced lengthwise
Cut the tops and bottoms off the zucchinis. Small, younger
zucchini are more delicate, soft and desirable. Slice into flat
strips lengthwise. It may be easier to cut the zuchini in half to
yield even, thin strips. Layer evenly in a square or rectangle on
a platter or on individual servings on a plate.

Marinated Mushrooms:
4 portabella mushrooms - sliced thinly
4 cloves garlic - minced
3 green onions - chopped
4-6 tablespoons olive oil
2 tablespoons lemon juice or apple cider vinegar
1 tablespoon maple syrup or honey
Hand of fresh basil, julienne
Celtic sea salt
fresh ground black pepper

Slice mushrooms. Toss all ingredients well. Allow to stand for
at least thirty minutes or up to several hours. These mushrooms will keep like this for several days. Squeeze excess
marinade from mushrooms. Drape and layer over *Macadamia
Nut Ricotta.*

Macadamia Nut Ricotta:
1 1/2 cups macadamia nuts
1/4 cup pine nuts
1 clove garlic, chopped
4 tablespoons nutritional yeast
2 tablespoons olive oil (optional)
4-6 tablespoons filtered water, as necessary
Celtic sea salt

In a food processor, grind macadamia nuts, pine nuts, nutritional yeast and sea salt into a fine meal. Set aside a few tablespoons for garnish. Add in chopped garlic, olive oil and filtered water as necessary to blend into a thick sauce. Spoon and spread sauce over zucchini strips.

Sun-dried Tomato Marinara:
1 1/2 cups sun-dried tomatoes, soaked
in filtered water until softened
6 Roma tomatoes or 4 large tomatoes, sliced and seeded
2 cloves garlic
hand fresh basil
hand fresh Italian parsley
1 sprig oregano and rosemary
or dried Italian seasoning
2 tablespoons olive oil (optional)
1 tablespoon maple syrup or honey
1 teaspoon apple cider vinegar or lemon juice
Celtic sea salt to taste
fresh ground black pepper

Cover sun-dried tomatoes with water and allow to soak until soft, 10 minutes or more. Cut tomatoes in half and spoon out seeds. This will keep the sauce nice and thick. Roma tomatoes are smaller, oblong tomatoes, ideal for thick sauces as they tend to have more meat and fewer seeds.

Dice seeded tomatoes. Chop fresh herbs finely. In a food processor, grind softened sun-dried tomatoes, garlic, olive oil, maple or honey and vinegar or lemon.

In a bowl, fold in minced fresh tomatoes and fresh herbs. Season with sea salt and fresh pepper. Allow to stand a few moments. Generously spoon over marinated mushrooms
Recipe by Renée Loux Underkoffler

Apple Pie à la Mode
Serves 8
Can be topped with
Cinnamon Ice Cream
(see recipe)

1 Honey, Nut and Date Pie Crust (see recipe)
4 Granny Smith apples - peeled and cored
2 red apples - peeled and cored
1/4 cup raw honey
1 teaspoon Celtic sea salt
2 teaspoons cinnamon
3 Medjool dates - pitted, soaked one hour, and drained
1 teaspoon vanilla powder
1 cup raisins
2 tablespoons flaxseed - ground fine
chopped walnuts (optional)

Prepare pie crust according to recipe and press into a pie plate. Dehydrate, if desired.

Place 2 Granny Smith apples, 1 red apple, honey, salt, cinnamon, dates and vanilla into a food processor. Process until mixture is almost the consistency of applesauce.

Place mixture in a bowl. Chop the 2 remaining Granny Smith apples into small pieces the size of peas.

Take the remaining red apple and slice into thin slices that are sliced in half again.

Mix all of the apples together and add raisins. The raisins will soak up the juice from the apples.

Stir in flaxseeds and mix well. Let mixture stand at room temperature for half an hour. Place apple mixture on pie crust.

Optional: top with chopped walnuts. Top with cinnamon ice cream. *Recipe by Jackie Graff at the Living Food Feasts from Shinui Retreat*

Honey, Nut and Date Pie Crust
Serves 8

1 cup almonds - soaked for 12 hours, sprouted, and
dehydrated for 12 hours
1 cup pecans - soaked for 12 hours, drained, and dehydrated
for 12 hours
1 cup walnuts - soaked for 12 hours, drained, and dehydrated
for 12 hours
1 teaspoon Celtic sea salt
1 teaspoon vanilla powder
1/2 pound organic dates - seeds removed
1/4 cup raw honey

Place almonds in a food processor and process until nuts are
ground to flour. Add salt and vanilla, and pulse the food
processor. Add pecans and walnuts to the mixture in the food
processor and process until nuts are finely chopped. Add
dates and process well. Add honey and process well. Press
mixture into a pie plate until entire pie plate is covered. Place
in a plastic bag until ready to fill. Crust may be made ahead of
time and refrigerated or frozen. *Recipe by Jackie Graff at
the Living Food Feasts from Shinui Retreat*

Eggplant Rawvioli
With Spicy Red Pepper Marinara

*Because we've grown up in a society of rich and comforting
foods, it is very important while in transition to the raw
foods lifestyle not only to focus on just feeding our physical
bodies, but our emotional bodies as well. This is a key factor
when it comes to easing yourself into this diet, while keeping all levels of our being in balance. This dish is a great example of eating for optimum health and also being very
comforted while doing so.*

355

2 eggplants, sliced in thin rounds
1 teaspoon Celtic sea salt
2 cups cashews soaked in filtered water for 8-10 hours
1 cup pine nuts
2 1/2 tablespoons olive oil
2 tablespoons lemon juice
1 1/2 tablespoons Italian seasoning
1 tablespoon garlic minced
1/2 teaspoon Celtic sea salt
1/2 teaspoon black pepper, cracked
1/2 teaspoon cayenne, ground
1/2 cup water
1/2 cup sun-dried black olives pitted and diced
1 tablespoon thyme, fresh and minced
2 1/2 tablespoons basil, fresh and minced

The first step is to remove the bitterness from the eggplant, so a couple hours before the preparation of this dish, soak the sliced eggplant in warm water with the teaspoon of salt, then, set aside.

Next comes the ricotta filling. In a food processor, blend the cashews, pine nuts, olive oil, lemon, Italian seasoning, garlic, salt, pepper, cayenne and water until smooth. Mix in the chopped olives and fresh herbs by hand.

To put together, strain the salt water from the eggplants; on half of each eggplant round, place one to two tablespoons of ricotta, folding the eggplant into a half moon. Place on dehydrator sheet and dehydrate for 3-4 hours. Serve warm and with Spicy Red Pepper Marinara (see sauces). Garnish with basil leaf.
Recipe by Chad at The Tree of Life Rejuvenation Center

Pumpkin Pie
Serves 8

2 avocados, peeled and seeded
1 cup raw honey
4 dates soaked in 1 cup filtered water
2 teaspoons vanilla powder
1 teaspoon cinnamon
1 teaspoon nutmeg
1 teaspoon ginger
1 teaspoon Celtic sea salt
1 cup raw macadamias soaked 8 hours and drained
4 cups raw pumpkin, peeled
1 cup organic raisins
1 teaspoon psyllium
1 cup pumpkin seeds, washed, soaked for 8 hours, drained
and dehydrated for 6-8 hours
1 raw pie crust (see recipe in this book)

1. Place avocados, honey, vanilla, dates with soak water, cinnamon, nutmeg, ginger, salt, macadamias, and water into blender and blend until smooth.
2. Add pumpkin and blend until very smooth.
3. Add psyllium and blend well. Let this mixture sit for 15 minutes and blend well again.
4. Fold in raisins.
5. Pour into piecrust and top with 1 cup of pumpkin seeds. Refrigerate and enjoy.

Recipe by Jackie Graff at the Living Food Feasts from Shinui Retreat

Dressings & Sauces

Try these delicious dressings to add flavor to your salads or whenever you feel the need for some more flavor.

Tahini Dressing

4 ounces tahini
1/2 lemon - juiced
1 clove garlic
1 pinch of cayenne pepper
1 tablespoon of dulse or Nama Shoyu (raw soy sauce)

Combine all ingredients. Add water, blend or process, and serve.
*Recipe by Paul Nison

Tomato Basil Dressing

2 tomatoes
1 clove garlic
1/2 lemon - juiced
1 handful of basil

Blend or process and serve. **Recipe by Paul Nison*

Tahini Raisin Dressing

1/2 cup raisins - soaked
2 tablespoons tahini
1/2 lemon - juiced
1 tablespoon chopped onions
1/2 cup water

Blend and serve. **Recipe by Paul Nison*

Bright Red Dressing

1 cup almonds
1/2 cup sunflower seeds
1/2 cup beets, cut up
2 lemons juiced, or to taste
1 teaspoon sea salt
2 cloves garlic
1 teaspoon olive oil
1 teaspoon honey

Blend all ingredients to a creamy consistency at high speed.
Use a carrot to assist in the mixing.
*Recipe by Viktoras Kulvinskas

Classic Caesar Salad Dressing
An authentic, vegan version that will keep fresh for more than a week. Serve over freshly torn romaine lettuce. Excellent with crumbled Essene bread or Essene crackers.

1/4 cup tahini
1/4 cup pine nuts
1-2 cloves garlic
2 green onions (scallions) OR 1 medium onion
1 lemon - squeezed
2 - 3 tablespoons apple cider vinegar
1 - 2 tablespoons maple syrup or 2 soft dates
2 - 4 tablespoons nutritional yeast
1 teaspoon black pepper or to taste
1 teaspoon sea salt or to taste
2 tablespoons tamarind paste (optional)

Blend all ingredients until smooth.
*Recipe by Renée Loux Underkoffler

Annette's Pesto
Use as a sauce or dressing.

2 cups olive oil
5 cups fresh basil
1 cup pine nuts
1 cup walnuts
5 cloves garlic

Blend one cup of oil in blender with basil, adding pine nuts and garlic. Add second cup of oil and pulse into thick mixture.
*Recipe by Annette Larkins

Marinara Sauce
Serves 8
Serve with garlic bread sticks

2 cups basil
2 red and yellow bell peppers
2 tablespoons Nama Shoyu (raw soy sauce)
1/2 cup oregano
3 carrots
2 pints cherry tomatoes
1 teaspoon lemon juice
3 cloves garlic
1 cup sun-dried tomatoes - soaked 2 hours and drained
1 sweet onion
4 dates - seeded, soaked one hour, and drained
2 teaspoons Celtic sea salt
1/2 cup extra virgin olive oil

Place all ingredients except for olive oil in blender and blend well. Pour into a serving bowl and stir in olive oil.
*Recipe by Jackie Graff
Living Food Feasts from the Shinui Retreat

Spicy Red Pepper Marinara
Serves 4

2 cups red bell pepper chopped
1 cup tomatoes, chopped
1/2 cup sun-dried tomatoes, soaked for 2-3 hours
in filtered water
1/2 cup apple, cored and chopped
2 cloves garlic
2 tablespoons olive oil
1 teaspoon Celtic sea salt
1/2 teaspoon black pepper, cracked
1 teaspoon cayenne (optional)
1 tablespoon thyme, fresh and chopped
2 tablespoons basil, fresh and chopped
2 tablespoons chives, fresh and chopped

In blender, blend the red pepper, tomatoes, sun dried tomatoes, apple, garlic, olive oil, salt, pepper and cayenne until
smooth consistency. Pulse in the fresh thyme, basil and chives,
making sure not to blend fully, leaving small pieces of herbs in
sauce. Serve over Rawvioli or any raw vegetable pasta.
*Recipe by Chad at Tree of Life

Orange Bavarian Cream Sauce
Serves 1

4 oz. tangerine juice
2 oz. pine nuts, soaked
2 dates, chopped
1 tsp. agar-agar flakes
1/2 teaspoon fresh grated tangerine zest

Put all ingredients into a blender and blend well. Pour over
the fruit. Best when eaten freshly made. *Use Concord grapes

when in season. They have a unique flavor, like no other.
Recipe by Rhio

Liquid Meals

For quick healthy meals that will require very little digestion, conserve energy and leave you feeling full but not tired, try these great tasting liquid meals:

Blended Salad

1 handful of leafy greens (spinach or lettuce is best for this recipe)
1/2 cucumber
1 stalk celery
juice of 1/2 lemon
1 handful of sunflower sprouts (optional)
1/2 red pepper (optional)
1 avocado
1 teaspoon flaxseed or olive oil (optional)
1 tomato

Blend and serve. *Recipe by Paul Nison*

Coconut Shake

3 young coconuts

Blend the meat of 3 young coconuts with the water of one of them and serve.
Recipe by Paul Nison

Banana Drink

1 banana
2 dates
1/2 cup water

Blend and serve. Add more water if drink is too thick.
Recipe by Paul Nison

Apple Sauce

2 apples - peeled
1 banana
4 dates
water, as needed
nutmeg (for garnish)

Blend apples, banana and dates, adding enough water to
make an applesauce consistency. Sprinkle with nutmeg.
Recipe by Paul Nison

Nut Milk

1/2 cup soaked almonds or any other nut
4 medjool dates
1 cup water

Blend almonds with water, add dates, and blend again. Strain
through a sprout bag or cheesecloth. Use the liquid part;
that's your nut milk. Yum! *Recipe by Paul Nison

Pine Nut Pudding

1 cup pine nuts
1 cup medjool dates

1 cup water
Blend and serve.
Recipe by Paul Nison

Macadamia Pudding

1 cup macadamia nuts
1 cup medjool dates
1 cup water

Blend and serve.
Recipe by Paul Nison

Coconut Avocado Drink

1 young coconut
1 avocado
Blend the avocado with the meat and water of the coconut.
Recipe by Paul Nison

Coconut Water, Spinach and Avocado

1 young coconut
1 handful of greens
1 avocado

Blend the meat and water of the coconut, then add other
ingredients. *Recipe by Paul Nison*

Blended Mango

2 soft mangos
tahini or cashew butter (optional)

Blend the mangos and serve. You can add tahini or cashew butter, but it's also great by itself.
*Recipe by Paul Nison

Banana Tahini Drink

1 banana
2 tablespoons tahini
1 cup water

Blend and serve.
*Recipe by Paul Nison

Lemon Pudding
The best lemon pudding you will ever taste!

2 cups avocado, mashed
1 1/2 cups lemon flesh, without peel and seeds
juice of 1 lemon
2 cups pitted dates
4 tablespoons maple syrup or honey (optional)

Peel lemons with a knife. Cut them in half and slice them. Remove seeds as you encounter them. Blend the lemon flesh with the mashed avocado, dates and lemon juice. A food processor works well for this. If desired, add some maple syrup or honey. **Recipe by Frederic Patenaude*

Fig-Apple Sauce
Can be poured over sweet or sub-acid fruit. Absolutely delicious over mangos!

6 red or golden delicious apples
6 dried figs - soaked overnight in purified water

Drain figs and cut into slices. Slice and core apples. Blend apples and figs, adding a small amount of soaking water to make the consistency of a sauce. *Recipe by Célène Bernstein*

Fruit Sauce
Serve as a thick drink by itself or
as a sauce over sub-acid sweet fruit.

1 ripe mango, peeled
1 papaya, halved and seeded
2 peaches, peeled and pitted

Place peeled mango in a blender or food processor. Scoop out pulp of papaya. Add papaya and peaches to blender with mango. Blend until smooth. Use immediately.
Recipe by Célène Bernstein

Cashew-Apple Cream
Serve over sub-acid or acid fruit or pineapple.

2 golden delicious apples, peeled, cored and diced
1 cup cashew nuts
1/2 cup purified water

Blend apples with a little water. Add cashews and more water if needed. Blend well to make a smooth cream.
Recipe by Célène Bernstein

Creamy Miso Soup
Serves 2-4
Delicious served chilled or gently warmed,
this soup makes an excellent salad dressing
or dipping sauce.

1/2 cup avocado
1/2 cup tomato
2 cups coconut water or 1 cup fresh orange juice
and 1 cup water
1/2 cup water
2-4 tablespoon miso (a mix of dark and light is best)
1 teaspoon ginger, peeled
1/4 cup green onion, minced
4 teaspoons hulled hemp seeds or sesame seeds
2 teaspoons Orange Zest

Blend all ingredients except green onion, hemp or sesame
seeds and Orange Zest until smooth. Garnish with minced
green onion and a sprinkle of seeds and Orange Zest. *Recipe
by Renée Loux Underkoffler*

Live Chai Tea with Whipped Almond Milk
Serves 4-6
Made delicious with fresh spices.
Excellent iced or warmed .

1/2 cup almonds - soaked 2-8 hours in filtered water
5 cups filtered water
1/2 cup soft pitted dates OR 4-6 tablespoons maple syrup
1 tablespoon fresh ground cinnamon
1 1/2 teaspoons fresh ground nutmeg
1 inch fresh ginger, peeled and minced, or 1 tablespoon
ginger powder
1/2 teaspoon fresh crushed cardamon
1 teaspoon black pepper
1 tablespoon non-alcohol vanilla extract
1 tablespoon carob or cocoa powder (optional)
1 tablespoon slippery elm powder (thickener)

Blend almonds and water together until smooth. Strain almond

pulp from milk. This pulp may be saved and used again or in other recipes. Blend remaining ingredients until thoroughly mixed. Scoop off any almond "whip at the top" and set aside for garnish. Serve chilled or gently warmed in stout glasses with a fresh cinnamon stick and a drop of almond "whip".
*Recipe by Renée Loux Underkoffler

Superconscious Smoothie
If you long for morning or afternoon caffeine, this blend will more than make up for it! Get ready for a nutritious, instant energy-raising high!

Water of 1 large sweet organic coconut
or two small ones (use sweet yellow coconut
or young green coconut, including
the inside jelly, if possible) enough to
yield approximately 1 to 2 cups
2 cups organic frozen banana pieces
OR 3-5 room temperature organic bananas

Blend on "high" until desired consistency is achieved.
Drink immediately.
Variations:
Using the same ingredients as before, add one of the following: papaya, pear, mango, canistel (egg fruit), mamey sapote, black (chocolate) sapote, white (vanilla) sapote, raspberries, or blueberries!

*Recipe by Karen Fierro

Juices

The best way to conserve energy and still get the vitamins and nutrients you need is to juice. Here are some great tasting juices that you will enjoy.

Grape-Celery Cooler

Juice your favorite sweet grapes
After the grapes, juice 1 or 2 celery stalks per glass.

Stir and serve.
Garnish with mint leaves if desired.
Optional: add a small slice of fresh ginger root when juicing
the grapes or celery.
Recipe by David Klein

Green Drink

Juice any amount of leafy green vegetables with other
vegetables such as celery, cucumber, carrots, etc.
Example:

1 cucumber
2 stalks celery
4 carrots
Handful of spinach

Put vegetables through a juicer and serve
Recipe by Mother Nature

APPENDIX B:
The Answer to Ridding Your Body of All Known Diseases

There is only one true sign of illness, and it is unhappiness. However, many medical doctors like to give names to the discomfort people feel when they receive the body's warning signs. Doctors call this: disease. To follow is a list of some common diseases which can be cured by a simple raw food diet, if meals are kept small and if simple food combining rules are observed:

Cancer

Heart Disease

Arthritis

Candida Albicans

Diabetes

IBD: Colitis and Crohn's disease

Chronic Fatigue Syndrome

Mental diseases such as depression

Over and Underweight

APPENDIX C:
Your Daily Diet

The best way to make a simple and easy transition to a raw food diet is to be consistent and have fun. If you're not having fun, then it's just a matter of time before you'll give up. The way to have fun is to keep things simple and to go at your own pace. As long as you go at your own pace, you will have fun and never run into danger. It is very important to always remember that your health is not based on what you add to your diet. It is what you leave out that is important. Leave out the most harmful stuff and you will have a great raw life.

Once you clean your body of many of the toxins you have put into it during years past, you can go on a maintenance diet. But before you go on a maintenance diet, you have to know where you are, where you want to be, and how will you get there. You need a plan. Whether your goal is a 100% raw diet, a vegan diet, or just a vegetarian diet, getting there is just half the battle. You have to understand that there are three stages to it.

The Transitional Diet

You are on the Transition Diet when making the change from the diet you grew up with to the new diet you will be eating. This is the diet I speak of in my book, *The Raw Life*, and also in my talk, "How to make the transition to a raw food diet, or just improve your health." What kind of diet is it? It's a diet of removing the harmful foods you're used to eating, and replacing them with the best quality foods available. I've made a list of these foods in Appendix D to help.

During a transition diet, slight symptoms of discomfort may appear as part of the process. Many people who do not understand how the body works might take these symptoms as a negative sign. That is the biggest common mistake made by those on a transition diet and it is the reason many "give up." These symptoms are magnified to an even greater extent on a cleansing diet. You should not attempt a cleansing diet until you understand what these symptoms are and what they mean. If a transition diet is done at a moderate pace, then no danger can ever be met. If a person goes too fast, there is always some danger, but there is more danger during the cleansing diet. You should not worry about the danger during a transitional diet; just make sure you understand it. See the cleansing diet below to learn more about the symptoms of detoxification. Note that the more toxic a person is, the harder the time he will have and the more symptoms he will experience.

The Cleansing Diet

Technically, the *Transitional Diet* and the *Cleansing Diet* can be considered to be the same thing. They both cleanse the system. It is important not to go too fast when cleaning out in order to avoid any possible harm. If you go on a transitional diet first, slowly but surely in the right direction, your body will cleanse. The more bad stuff you leave out of your diet, the more your body will clean out. Once you have eliminated the bad foods and only good foods are left, and your body is stronger than when you started, it's a good time to begin a more cleansing diet. On this diet, you will rid yourself of the toxins that have built up in your system. Again, technically the two diets are the same, but the reason I differentiated them is for the understanding that if you clean out but don't change your diet, you are wasting your time. If you try cleaning the toxins out of your body and just change your eating habits for the time of the cleanse, then plan to return to eating a poor diet, that is not a good idea. That is why I say you should first change your diet to a transitional diet and then concentrate more on a cleansing diet. Then, once you are clean, you can go to more of a maintenance diet. It is important to clean out before you can rebuild. You have to understand what a detoxification is and what will happen during a detoxification. But most important, you have to understand the kind of diet that can help you detoxify. It's important to know the difference between the warning signs that you're in trouble due to overly rapid detoxification for your own good (this can happen), and the healing signs that you're doing fine.

The *Cleansing Diet* and period can consist of any of the following, or all of the following combined: fasting, juicing, blended diet, herbal cleanse, enemas and colonics.

What will you feel during a cleanse, and what is detoxification? It's different for everyone. Sometimes, but not always, during the first three to five days of giving up a food you are addicted to, it's common to experience headaches, toothaches, an old illness, rashes, flu signs or a cold, fever, chills, dizziness, or an uncomfortable feeling; or you might feel hyper or feel something that you think is hunger (it's not hunger, but just what we think hunger is). As time goes on, if you follow the diet correctly, a big weight loss is common during the first six

•

months. Even an underweight person can still experience a big weight loss. This is not to be feared, only understood. The body will lose weight because it is cleaning out. Many people get worried because in society, most people are overweight; being underweight scares people. They will look at you and try to convince you that you don't look good and you must stop this diet at once. They have no idea what they're talking about. If you let their comments get to you, you will fail. Understand what you're doing and don't listen to them. As long as you stick to your program, your weight will balance out once the body has cleaned out. It usually takes from six months to a year for that to happen. But remember, it may even take longer. The body has been filled with many toxins for many years, and you won't clean them out overnight. You must have patience. Eating more food or fatty food will keep your body dirty, and it will not speed up the process; it will only slow it down. Stay with the cleansing diet, and your weight will balance out. The cleaner the body becomes, the less food it will require to maintain life, and the less hunger you'll feel. Don't worry; even though you're eating less, if you make high food choices, your weight will balance out.

It's important not to try to stop any of the signs of detoxification with drugs. This will only slow the process down and make you more toxic. Also, once you're on a transitional diet and getting clean, the same drugs that never had an effect on you before can be harmful, because the cleaner you become, the more sensitive your body becomes to unnatural things. As long as you're going at your own pace, you won't be in any danger, so ride out the signs and you'll be fine.

What should you not feel, and when should you slow down or stop? You should not feel heart pain, extreme fever, nor unbearable pain. It's common to feel uncomfortable, but not unable to move. You shouldn't pass out or faint. The best thing would be to lie in bed and deal with what you will feel.

But if you feel any of the above, you need to slow down your cleansing diet. It helps to have a trained professional to help guide you.

The Maintenance diet

This is the diet you will follow on a normal daily basis:

The *Maintenance Diet* is the diet you will be on most of the time, once you have cleansed and detoxified. It is a personal diet that will be geared toward your lifestyle. What might be best for you and your schedule might not be good for someone else's schedule. It's very personal and you have to change and adjust it as much as necessary to go along with the changes and adjustments in life. Just understand that it should be different from the transitional diet and the cleansing diet. It should consist of the best sources of food available, hopefully food that is organic, whole, fresh and ripe. Just do the best you can.

Here are some guidelines:

Follow the rules of correct Food Combining.

Be careful not to overeat on sweet fruit, a very common problem with people who are eating a raw food diet. Do your best not to eat more sugar than you will burn throughout the day. Less is better. Sweet fruit is the best food for your body, but over-consuming it is very common and can cause problems to your health. It is very important to understand that the more sugar you consume, the more your body will crave it. The less you eat the fewer cravings you will have.

Keep your meals small. All your meals should be eaten to give you a satisfied feeling, but not a FULL feeling. You shouldn't feel like going to sleep after eating. You should feel light and great.

Don't eat late at night, if you can possibly avoid it.

Drink sufficient amounts of water. The more concentrated food you eat, the more water you need.

Don't eat anything for at least three hours before going to sleep.

Take an enzyme supplement unless you can get the food organically grown right out of the ground or off the tree.

Chew all of your food well.

Don't drink with your meals.

Do your best not too eat too many meals that consist of very high sugar foods or too many concentrated foods.

*Remember with these guidelines. It's not about being perfect, it's about being happy. So do the best you can, and don't get upset if you have a weak moment or a bad day. Learn from it and grow.

APPENDIX D

Fresh Vegetables

The biggest percentage of your daily diet should come from fresh vegetables such as these:

Salad Greens
arugula
bok choy
chicory
collard greens
dandelion
garlic greens
kale
lettuces
mustard greens
spinach
swiss chard
turnip greens
watercress
sunflower greens

Vegetables
asparagus
broccoli
cabbage
cauliflower
celery
corn
green beans

*Carrots, corn, parsnips, white potato, are all very high in sugars and should be eaten very sparingly. Because they are so high in sugar, they have a high glycemic index (for information about the glycemic index see fruits).

Fruits

Most people don't realize that any plant life containing a seed or seeds is a fruit. The more liquid a fruit has, the better it is for you. Other than melons, fruits that are commonly known as vegetables usually have the most liquid and are the best. Sweet fruits should be limited or eaten in small amounts.

cucumbers
zucchini
bell peppers
squash
apples
cherries
grapes
kiwi
lemons
papaya
pears
melons

berries
avocado
cantaloupe
grapefruit
persimmons
pineapple

It's best to select fruits that are organically grown, if available. It is just as important to make sure that the fruit is soft and ripe so that all the essential vitamins and minerals are present. Many fruits today are picked before they are fully ripe, which doesn't allow them to develop all of their essential vitamins and minerals. Be careful when choosing fruits. Make sure they are fully ripe. The fruit should be soft and have a sweet smell. Common fruits that are commonly picked unripe include:

mangos
oranges
peaches
plums

When you buy such fruits, make sure they are fully ripe!

High sugar fruits and other foods: the Glycemic Index.

Some fruits are sweeter than others. These fruits are higher on the glycemic index chart. The glycemic index indicates the rate at which sugar is absorbed into the blood. These high glycemic foods should be eaten sparingly because they can cause problems of elevated blood sugar leading to minor problems like drowsiness and fatigue, to more serious problems such as diabetes, hypoglycemia and heart disease. The higher the number, the greater the influx of sugar into the blood. Low glycemic foods are below 55, intermediate are between 55 and 70, and high are over 70. Because these high glycemic fruits are so sweet, they can be addicting. These fruits might taste good, but too many of them are not good for your body. There are many other high glycemic foods other than fruit, such as certain grains, vegetables and many processed foods, but I'm listing the fruits with which to be careful, that many on a raw food program tend to overeat. Among the common fruits to especially watch out for and limit are:

all dried fruit
watermelon
pineapple
raisins
bananas
apricots
cantaloupe
dates
kiwifruit
orange juice
grapefruit juice
mangos

*(Also very high are forms of sugar: glucose, honey, maltose and table sugar.)
**For more information about the glycemic index, I recommend reading: *The Glucose Revolution* by Jennie Brand-Miller, Thomas Wolever, Stephen Colagiuri and Kaye Foster- Powell. There are also many other useful and informative books. This one covers the issue well.

Exotic Fruits

We all know about the great-tasting fruit we see everyday: pineapples, avocados, oranges, bananas, etc. Those fruits are good, but there are many, many more fruits in the world that most people have never heard of. They are the exotic fruits that come from all over the world. There are so many fruits in the world that you could eat a different fruit everyday for the rest of your life and still not even come close to tasting them all. Let's learn about some of these great tasting fruits.

Here is a list of some fruits that are currently exotic. Someday, these fruits will become as common as apples and oranges.

Durian: If I had to describe it, I would say that it looks like an oversized deformed pineapple. Actually, it has a green to brown shell with spiky pine tree shaped thorns sticking out of it. On the inside, it has a sweet yellow flesh and large pits. The flesh is sweet and juicy with a custard-like consistency. It is known for its strong smell. Many people say it "tastes like heaven, but smells like hell." It is grown in Thailand and Malaysia and shipped frozen to Asian neighborhoods around the world. The durian is one of the most expensive fruits you will ever see, but since it tastes so good, it is well worth it.

Water coconut: These are big green coconuts with tender meat inside that you can eat with a spoon. They are the same as the coconuts you see in the stores with brown hair on them, but before they get that way. The water contained within the water coconut, also referred to as coconut milk, is the most nutritious liquid on earth. It is the one food that a person can live on exclusively without ever getting sick. It is also called a baby coconut or a young coconut. Sold in Latino or Asian markets, it comes from just about every tropical island or country.

Mangosteen: The small purple brown mangosteen cracks open to reveal tasty white segments with a very fine flavor. Known as the queen of fruits, they are grown in Southeast Asia.

Jack fruit: This is an enormous yellow-green fruit that can weigh over fifty pounds. Contained within are hundreds of individual bright yellow or orange segments. The Jack fruit has a slightly rubbery texture, tastes like tutti frutti bubble gum, and is grown in Florida, Hawaii, the Caribbean islands and Southeast Asia.

Star fruit: It tastes cool, crisp and watery. Shaped like a star, it is native to Asia, but also grows in Florida.

Mamey: On the outside, it looks like a big potato. On the inside, it has sweet orange flesh which, as in the avocado, surrounds a large pit. It is very filling.

Sapodilla: On the outside, it looks like a small potato. On the inside, it is brown with the texture of a non-crispy juicy pear, tasting like a mixture between caramel and honey. It is grown in the Caribbean where it is called Nispero, and also in Asia where it is known as *Chico.*

Cherimoya: Also known as a *custard apple*, it has a thick, creamy taste. The skin is green with many bumps. It grows in tropical climates.

White Sapote: On the outside, it is round and green. White inside, having the consistency of a soft apple, it tastes like vanilla pudding. Grown in tropical climates.

Black Sapote: Brown and soft when ripe, it is also known as chocolate pudding fruit because it tastes like chocolate pudding. Grown in tropical climates.

Nuts and Seeds

Nuts and seeds are best eaten after they have been soaked for several hours, which will add the water back to them, making them more digestible. Since it is very easy to overeat on nuts, be careful!

Best seeds:
flax
hemp
pumpkin
sesame
sunflower

Best nuts:
almonds
young coconuts
filberts
pecans
walnuts

Whole Grains and Legumes

It you can get truly good natural grains, they can be helpful during transition, but they are not recommend in the long run. Grains are not a natural food for the human body, and they are very hard for us to digest. For much more pertinent information about how grains are really bad for the body, please read: *Grain Damage* by Dr. Douglas Graham. You can order it from:

www.rawlife.com. Some people who eat a raw food diet decide to include sprouted grains in their diet. They feel grains are very helpful. If you do not want to exclude grains from your diet, then eat them sprouted. If you are going to eat grains, sprouted is the way to eat them. Don't worry about what other people will think of you if you continue to eat grains. Get the research and do what makes most sense to you.

Grains in order, starting
with the least harmful:

millet
quinoa
amaranth
teff
buckwheat (hulled)

Grains that are more harmful:

rye
spelt
basmati rice

Sea Vegetables

Eating sea vegetables is not easy at first. They are a food we were not brainwashed to love when growing up, but once you get used to them, you will love their different flavors and textures.

Sea vegetables have an abundance of minerals and trace elements. They are high in calcium, iodine, potassium, magnesium, phosphorous, iron, and Vitamins A, B1, B2, B6, B12, C and niacin. Ounce for ounce, sea vegetables are higher in vitamins and minerals than any other food group. They are one of nature's richest sources of vegetable protein and Vitamin B12. They also provide carotene, chlorophyll, enzymes and fiber. Sea vegetables are a rich source of minerals that are essential to maintaining and improving one's health.

There are many different types of sea vegetables. Here are a few of the most popular with their main benefits:

Alaria
- Delicious raw in salads, either pre-soaked or marinated.
- Comparable to whole sesame seeds in calcium content (1100mg/100g).
- Very high Vitamin A content, comparable to parsley, spinach, or turnip greens.
- Very high in B vitamins.

Arame
- Nutty sea vegetable taste.
- Very high in calcium, phosphorous, iodine, iron, potassium, and vitamins A and B.

Dulse
- Delicious as a raw snack, with distinctive strong sea flavor.
- Great in salads.
- 22% protein: more than chickpeas, almonds, or whole sesame seeds.
- A handful gives a whole day's supply of iron and fluoride.
- The same handful will provide more than 100% of the RDA for Vitamin B6 and 66% of the RDA for Vitamin B12.
- Relatively low in sodium (1740mg/100g), high in potassium (7820mg/100g).

Hijiki
- Very high in calcium, Vitamins A, B1, and B2, and phosphorous.

Kelp
- Tastes great marinated.
- Exceptionally high in all major minerals, particularly calcium, potassium, magnesium and iron.

- Rich in important trace minerals such as manganese, copper, and zinc.
- One ounce of kelp provides the recommended daily dose of chromium, instrumental in blood sugar regulation.
- That same ounce provides many times the RDA for iodine, essential to the thyroid gland.

Nori
- Distinctive mild, nutty, salty-sweet taste.
- Great in salads and can be used to make vegetable nori rolls.
- 28% protein: more than sunflower seeds, lentils, or wheat germ.
- An excellent source of naturally occurring manganese, fluoride, copper and zinc.
- Of all the sea vegetables, Nori is the highest in Vitamins B1, B2, B6, and B12, Vitamin C and Vitamin E.

Fermented Food

Fermented foods have undergone the introduction of a friendly culture: *Acidophilus, Koji, Bifodis,* to name just a few.

Some examples of fermented foods are:

miso
amazake
seed cheese
kim chee
sauerkraut
yogurt

I don't recommend fermented foods for one's diet. If something is not needed and can possibly cause a problem, then why take the chance? Yes, there are some good things about fermented foods. Certain important and friendly bacteria grow during the fermentation process. These bacilli encourage healthy intestinal flora and regular bowel movements. The problem is, whenever you deal with a fermented food, you risk the chance of also harboring unfriendly bacteria. Many people today suffer from fungal, mold, yeast, or bacterial infections. Eating fermented foods could irritate this condition and make it worse. Many people eat a healthy diet without including any fermented foods, and they are in perfect health. That is proof that fermented foods are not needed to achieve perfect health. That is why I say, if it's not needed and there is a chance that something could go wrong, then you're better off not eating it at all.

Dehydrated Food

Dehydrated food is any type of food that has had its water removed. Some foods are dried naturally in the sun, but many are dried in a machine called a dehydrator. Some examples are *dried fruits*, *Essene Bread* and *dried herbs.*

Two of the many problems with cooked food are: **a:** you remove the water and **b:** you kill all the enzymes. When you dehydrate a food, you just remove the water, but you still leave most of the enzymes in tact, as long as you didn't use temperatures above 110 degrees.

Dehydrated food can be good, but it can also be harmful, depending on who is eating the food. If someone has been eating a very poor diet for many years consisting of cooked, fried, baked and steamed food, dehydrated foods can be a big step forward. But if you've been eating an all raw diet for many years and then start eating a lot of dehydrated foods, it can do major harm. The problem with dehydrated food is that when it's eaten, you too will be dehydrated. It's like swallowing a dry sponge. It will soak up all the liquid in your body. One of the biggest causes of illness today is dehydration. You're either hydrating yourself or dehydrating yourself. If you do eat dehydrated foods, make sure you drink a lot of water throughout the day. If you are new to a raw food diet, it's okay to enjoy dehydrated foods to help you overcome the cravings for the tastes that you are so used to. But the longer you eat a healthy diet, the more you should avoid eating dehydrated foods if possible. It is also helpful when eating dehydrated foods to soak them in water before eating; this will help return some of their lost liquid.

Sprouted Food

Sprouted food is any type of seed, nut, grain, or bean that has been soaked in water, exposed to air and indirect sunlight, and if rinsed daily, has started to form a new plant, beginning with a sprout. Some examples include: almond sprouts, buckwheat sprouts, sunflower sprouts and mung bean sprouts.

Sprouted foods are one of the highest forms of food you can put into your body. They are very helpful for the building of new cells, providing the cells with additional oxygen. Sprouts are often very high in chlorophyll.

Sprouted foods are good, but are not necessary to living a healthy lifestyle. There are studies showing the positive effects of eating sprouts in cases of people suffering from certain illnesses, but it is not proven anywhere that a healthy person needs to eat sprouts. Enjoy sprouts if you like the taste, but there is no reason to feel you have to rely on them.

Juicing

Fiber is very important to the system. It acts like a broom that sweeps away all the unneeded stuff you've put in your body. When we eat fresh fruits and vegetables, our bodies extract as liquid what they need from the fiber, which then passes on to the lower digestive tract. As I've said in this book, the body is the best juicer in the world. When you juice in your kitchen with a juicer, the extracted liquid is juice, containing the same elements as the juice you would have gotten from eating the fruits or vegetables in their whole state. By drinking only the juice, you're eliminating a digestive process, extracting the liquid from the fiber and efficiently supplying the body with nutrients. If the juice you make in your juicer is from fresh, ripe, raw, organic produce, you'll be delivering the maximum amount of nutrients to your body in minutes. That is the popular reason people today choose to juice. But juicing is advantageous for another reason. It gives the body a well-needed rest, thus saving the body's stored energy.

It is important to have the sweeping effect of fiber, so completely cutting out fiber from the diet is not recommended. But, giving the body the rest it needs to heal is also important. A good balance of fresh whole foods and fresh juices will ensure that you are giving the body both the sweeping, cleaning effect plus rest.

Food Combining

There are many different types of raw foods, and each type will take a different length of time to digest. Your body will have to work harder to digest foods if you eat them in poor combinations. Ideally, you want your body to waste as little energy as possible. For this reason, it's important to combine your foods properly. I suggest you read some of the many books written about food combining to learn as much as you can. (Refer to the recommended reading list in the back of this book.) I've added a food combining chart to help you follow the rules of proper food combining for best digestion.

To help your understanding of proper food combinations and to make it simpler for you, always remember to eat high liquid foods with other high liquid foods and more dense foods with other dense foods.

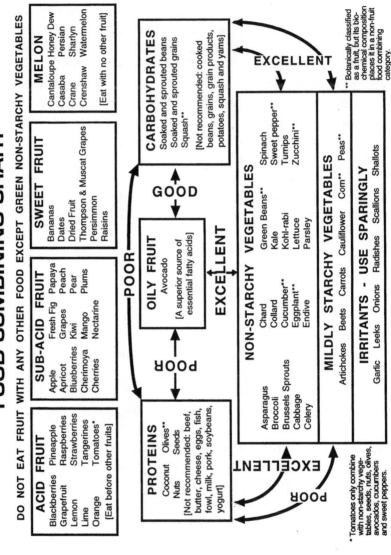

FOOD COMBINING CHART

DO NOT EAT FRUIT WITH ANY OTHER FOOD EXCEPT GREEN NON-STARCHY VEGETABLES

(Chart courtesy of Dave Klein)

An All Fruit Diet?
Are green foods necessary in the diet?
Too much fruit?

It is not up to me to say if one can live for a long time on only fruits and no green foods, BUT... up until the time this book was written, I have not met anyone who can live exclusively on only fruits with no greens. Yes, maybe they can (or have) for a certain length of time, but everyone I have met or heard of who has tried to do it has experienced problems in the long run.

There is no doubt in my mind about it: fruits are the best food for man, if eaten fresh, ripe and not overeaten. A part of our diet should consist of fruits, but I see too many people eating too much sweet fruit and the result is sickness and disease. Many people who condone overeating on sweet fruit will tell people that as long as they balance out their sugars with fats and greens they'll be fine. I disagree. Less is more, and the answer is not to eat more of something else, but to eat less of what you're overdoing. The best way to go would be to not eat more sugar than you will burn. There are people who try to justify eating large amount of sugar rich meals throughout the day by over-exercising. Once again, the answer is not to do more, but to do less. If exercising a few hours once a day, not much sugar is needed to supply the body with fuel for that exercise. Sugar in any form, if abused, can cause problems to your health. People will be better off, the more they realize this.

At the beginning of time, the body was most likely equipped to thrive on an all-fruit diet. But over the years, our fruit has gotten worse, and so have our environments and bodies. Today, I feel that our bodies need the important benefits of chlorophyll. Chlorophyll, found mostly in green foods, is the pigment in plants within which photosynthesis takes place.

Why is chlorophyll so important to the body? Chlorophyll is the blood of plants, just as hemoglobin is the blood of humans. The only difference between the two molecules is that chloro-

393

phyll is centered on magnesium, while hemoglobin is centered on iron. Both chlorophyll and human blood are forms of liquid oxygen. When you eat foods rich in chlorophyll, you add oxygen to the bloodstream. Everyone could benefit from adding more greens to the diet. As I've said in this book, oxygen is very important for maintaining good health and thriving. Eating greens is the way to oxygenate the bloodstream.

On a high fat / high protein diet, the body's oxygen supply is substantially reduced. Many people think that their oxygen supply is not reduced at all on a raw food diet. That is not true, especially if one is overeating. If one is only eating fruit, there is a good chance that he is overeating, and it's likely that he is eating fruits that are very high in sugar. This can reduce the oxygen supply in the bloodstream just as much as a high fat / high protein diet can.

Without sufficient oxygen in our blood, we develop symptoms of low energy and sluggish digestion and metabolism. When that happens, we are unable to oxidize or burn up food efficiently. When we are unable to digest, assimilate and eliminate thoroughly, we reduce the blood oxygen level even further. When that happens, the body becomes ripe for cancer and many other diseases.

There are many ways to bring oxygen into our bloodstreams, but unless we first eliminate the causes of oxygen deprivation (such as smoking, high-fat / high-protein cooked foods, alcohol, drugs, poor breathing, overeating and sedentary habits), any attempt to oxygenate the blood will fail.

Excellent sources of chlorophyll are all leafy green vegetables, wheatgrass, green leaf sprouts, sea vegetables, algae, and E-3Live.

E-3Live Super Green Food

I recommend adding E3Live to your diet. I have met many

people who don't particularly like the taste of leafy greens. Because of this, they don't eat them in sufficient quantities to get enough vital chlorophyll. The solution is E3Live. When it comes to chlorophyll, you need it in your diet and there's no better source then E-3Live. One tablespoon has more chlorophyll than several green salads put together. In fact, E3Live contains more chlorophyll than any other natural food – even five times more than wheatgrass!

E3Live also has a plentiful supply of pre-digested amino acids, the building blocks of protein, and a purely vegan source of hard-to-find human-active Vitamin B-12.

So if you're eating a raw food or vegan diet, adding *E3Live* is like having nutritional insurance against hidden nutritional deficiencies.

Here are some of the reported benefits. Eating *E3Live* can:
* increase energy, stamina and feelings of well-being;
* increase mental focus and concentration;
* stabilize mood swings;
* purify and nourish the blood through the power of chlorophyll;
* help maintain normal blood sugar levels;
* help normalize weight;
* stimulate and enhance the immune system;
* normalize the appetite, naturally;
* promote intestinal regularity;
* promote the growth of stronger nails, smoother skin and silkier hair.

The benefits go on and on.

*E-3Live is available at www.rawlife.com

APPENDIX E

Protect your body, mind and spirit while at the same time protecting the environment, the planet, the universe.

It is important to take care of your mind, body and spirit, but it is just as important to take care of your home and your environment for future generations. You might not think this is very important, but just think about where we would be today, had past generations polluted and damaged the environment. We don't want our kids to inherit poor living conditions, so we must do the best we can do to preserve what is left.

We must protect our rainforests and treat our environment with kindness, love and understanding. Remember, you give what you get. If you kill the environment, you are giving death. If you kill the important plants on the planet, you are giving death. Instead, let's recycle as much as we can and use our heads. Some great books to help you do this are noted in the recommended reading section in the back of this book. Read them, understand them, and take action!

One of the best ways to help preserve our environment, and at the same time help our bodies, is to use hemp products. The following information about hemp was written by my friend **Tiffany Cole**, and is one of the most powerful lessons I would like everyone to understand. Don't believe what people say without investigating it yourself. The information below should help you do that.

HEMP KNOWLEDGE FOR A HEALTHY PLANET

M any of us are learning the importance of organic farming. We are choosing to turn away from the denatured, chemically treated, genetically engineered "foods" that are offered to us by the major supermarket chains and their suppliers in agri-business. The number of natural health food stores that offer fresh, organic produce is growing daily.

As we educate ourselves about the natural lifestyle, we realize that what we put into our bodies and our children's bodies will affect our own health, the health of future generations, and the health of this beautiful planet Earth.

But, how often do we think about what we put on our bodies? Did you ever stop to wonder, "How are my jeans and T-shirt affecting my health?" What about the paper I use? Have you asked yourself what effect the paper in your printer has on your health? When you jump in your car to drive to work, is your health the first thing that comes to your mind?

Probably not! It makes so much sense that what we put into our bodies will make us sick. But, as we get deeper into the causes of dis-ease, we find that almost all of our daily choices will have a great impact on our health.

Almost half of all the agricultural chemicals used on U.S. crops are applied *not* to the many commercially grown fruits and vegetables you have heard about. One half of all these chemicals being dumped onto the soil are used to treat only one crop: cotton.

Eighty percent of solid and airborne pollution in our environment results from fossil fuel energy sources such as petroleum used to fuel automobiles.

Eight thousand years ago, half of the earth's land area was covered by ancient forests. Today, only one fifth of these original forests remain as they were.

The Current Global Rates of Rainforest Destruction:

- **2.4 acres (1 hectare) per second: equivalent to two U.S. football fields**
- **149 acres (60 hectares) per minute;**
- **214,000 acres (86,000 hectares) per day: an area larger than New York City;**
- **78 million acres (31 million hectares) per year: an area larger than Poland.**

These facts and figures can seem overwhelming. What can we do to solve these problems? And besides, what does all this have to do with the raw food diet?

When we eat organic raw fruits and vegetables, we are moving forward in a positive direction. Our choices at the supermarket are affecting the world economy and moving agriculture towards a more healthy way of growing food. But is there more we can do?

IMPORTANT CHANGES

As you become more natural, you will want to create the cleanest, most healthy environment for yourself as possible. As your diet becomes pure and refined, you will notice other changes. You may yearn for nature. Maybe you will want to visit Hawaii or move to the country. As you become more sensitive, you may feel more compassionate towards animals. Perhaps, you will realize that wearing them seems as strange and inhumane as eating them. These changes may be as subtle as an irritable or nauseous reaction to the noxious smell of a diesel truck driving by. Your natural lifestyle begins to encompass more than food. This is a major step forward.

Our health and happiness will increase in proportion to the positive choices we make. Beyond food choice, what can we do to make our lives more happy and healthful? We can find alternatives to the unnatural products filling up our homes and lives.

HEMP

The hemp plant is one of the most useful plants on earth. It is harvested for its fibers, seed, seed meal and oil. Hemp is a distinct variety of the plant species cannabis sativa L. Due to the similar leaf shape, hemp is frequently confused with marijuana. Cannabis is the only plant genus that contains the class of molecular compounds known as *cannabinoids*. Two major cannabinoids are THC, a psychoactive ingredient and CBD, and antipsychoactive cannabinoid. One type of Cannabis is high in the psychoactive THC, and low in CBD, the antipsychoactive cannabinoid. This is known as marijuana. Another type is high in CBD, but low in THC. This type is known as industrial hemp.

Humans have been using hemp for thousands of years. The oldest relic of human industry is a scrap of hemp fabric that dates back to approximately 8000 B.C. Hemp grows well without using herbicides, fungicides or pesticides. It grows fast and attracts few pests and is easy to grow in temperate as well as tropical climates. Because it leaves the soil rich in nitrogen deposits, it suppresses weeds and can actually help regenerate depleted soil.

HEMP CLOTHING

Hemp is the most versatile fiber for making textiles. Hemp produces 250% more fiber than cotton. Hemp is used to make socks, shoes, jackets, dresses, and purses, home furnishings, carpets, rope, and more. Hemp is nature's longest fiber, which means it lasts longer, compared to the shorter fibers of other plants. It is four times stronger than cotton. The first Levi's jeans were made from 100% hemp.

Today, you can find quality hemp clothing in retail stores around the country and on the Internet. You can wear hemp shoes instead of leather. Most companies making hemp clothes are environmentally aware, so their clothes are un-dyed, or they use low impact or vegetable dyes. When you wear hemp clothes, you feel the difference on your skin. It can be manufactured into a soft, luxurious fiber similar to linen. As you continue to wear natural, chemical free clothing, your body will begin to reject unnatural manmade or chemically treated fabrics, just as it would reject denatured foods.

HEMP PAPER AND TREE ALTERNATIVES

Hemp can be made into fine quality paper. The long fibers in hemp allow such paper to be recycled several times more than wood-based paper. Because of its natural brightness, it needs no chlorine bleach, which means no extremely toxic dioxin being dumped into streams.

Hemp can be used to replace wood fiber, saving forests for oxygen production, watershed and homes for wildlife. It can yield 3-8 dry tons of fiber per acre. This is *four times* what an average forest can yield.

You can build a house with hemp. Fiberboard made from hemp is twice as strong and three times more elastic than fiberboard made from wood. Its strength and flexibility make it resistant to cracking and breaking. And, one acre of hemp provides the same amount of material as four acres of trees.

HEMP FUEL

Hemp is also used as fuel for cars. It can be converted in to bio-diesel. ***Bio-diesel*** is the name for a variety of ester-based oxygenated fuels made from hemp oil, other vegetable oils or animal fats. The concept of using vegetable oil as an engine fuel dates back to 1895 when Dr. Rudolph Diesel developed the first diesel engine to run on vegetable oil. He demonstrated his engine at the World Exhibition in Paris in 1900 using peanut oil as fuel. Hemp is the number one producer of biomass on earth, which can be converted to methane, methanol, or gasoline at a cost comparable to petroleum, and hemp is much better for the environment. Hemp can produce ten-times more methanol than corn, and it burns clean. Hemp fuel does not contribute to acid rain or global warming.

If we implemented hemp in only these three areas: clothing, wood and fuel, we could begin to heal the destruction already done to the environment and prevent more destruction in the future.

HEMP NUTRITION

Hemp can also help heal our bodies. The Hemp seed is the highest natural source of essential fatty acids (EFAs) in the plant kingdom. EFAs are responsible for generating life energy (from foods) and transporting that energy throughout our systems.

It's also high in some essential amino acids, including gamma linolenic acid (GLA), a very rare nutrient also found in mother's milk. Amino acids are the building blocks of protein. We know that eating complete proteins such as animal protein is the most inefficient way to get our protein, while eating raw nuts, fruits and vegetables supplies our bodies with the amino acids needed to create the right protein, in the right amounts for the human body.

Hemp seed oil is a delicious compliment to the raw food diet. It can be used in any recipe as you would olive oil. Also, it is usually found in dark bottles, in the refrigerated section of the health food store, which guarantees it is not rancid.

Hemp nut butter or "Hempini" is also delicious. Renowned nutritionist Dr. Fred Bisci says that hemp nut butter is extremely healthy and is actually a better source of protein than many other nut butters. It's great with celery sticks, bananas or medjool dates.

The raw hemp seed itself can be eaten as a snack or sprinkled on salads. Ground in the Vita Mix or blender, it makes a delicious, buttery hemp meal that can be used in raw cookies, candies, cakes, burgers, pesto, nut loaf or other recipes.

Hemp is a precious gift from the planet earth. Entire books have been written about the uses and benefits of hemp.

So, where can I get more hemp?

HEMP MYTHS

If you ask the average person, you may get a chuckle or a sly grin, "What are you going to do with your hemp shirt, roll it up and smoke it?" This is the attitude of most people who have been inundated with propaganda from the federal government. It is illegal to grow hemp in the United States for political and ultimately financial reasons. What would happen to the oil, cotton, timber and plastic corporations if hemp were widely available? In the early part of this century, hemp was a threat to these industries, so they used their influence to make it illegal. This was easy because of its close relationship to marijuana.

But, hemp was once a thriving industry. Both Presidents Washington and Jefferson grew hemp. The federal government subsidized hemp during the Second World War for its many uses. U.S. farmers grew about a million acres of hemp as part of that program. Since then, however, many wealthy corporations have used their political and financial influence to give hemp a bad name.

Like the foolish man who built his house on sand, the picture of the world painted for us by the government, media, medical and corporate establishments is an illusion.

The wise man built his house on the rock. Educated people paint their own picture. Use your knowledge to change the world. Vote with your dollars. Buy hemp. Encourage the stores you frequent to carry hemp products. Write letters to your representatives and to the media.

As you use more natural and environmentally friendly products such as hemp, your life will become more meaningful. You will see how your health and the health of the planet are interconnected. Every tree we destroy means a little less oxygen for us to breathe. Every stream we pollute means a little less water for us to drink. Our choices make an impact.

Health does not end with our own bodies. A healthy planet is health for everyone, a growing tree, a singing bird, a rippling stream. When we eat natural food, we choose life for ourselves. When we strive for a natural world, we choose life for us all.

RESOURCES/ BIBLIOGRAPHY

Hemp and Marijuana: Myths and Realities
By David P. West, Ph.D.

www.naihc.org

www.worldrevolution.org

www.greenpeace.org

www.hempcar.org.

www.thehia.org

www.abouthemp.com

www.atlascor.com

Fred Bisci, Ph.D.

MORE INFORMATION

The North American Industrial Hemp Council
www.naihc.org

The Hemp Industries Association
www.thehia.org

Hemp Car
www.hempcar.org

DEA Attempting Legislation to Ban Hemp Food
www.votehemp.com

HEMP PRODUCTS

Women's Organic Fashion
www.earthspeaks.com

Men's & Women's
www.hemphousemaui.com
www.sativahempwear.com

FOOD & OIL
www.thehempnut.com

ALL THINGS HEMP
www.panworldtraders.com
www.rawganique.com
www.hempstores.com

Dr. Bronner's Magic Soaps
www.drbronner.com

APPENDIX F
Natural Child
Birthing

I believe in everything being done in its most natural environment to achieve optimum results. Regarding the issue of birthing a child into this world, the average person would have you believe it's natural to give birth to a baby in a hospital. However, if you look at the animals in nature, how many go to a hospital to deliver their babies? Of all harmful places, you would think hospitals are safe, but that is not so. In truth, hospitals are very unsafe, not only for newborns, for everyone. As I stated many times in my first book, with the exception of the emergency room, the hospital's only valuable part, if you are sick and want to heal quickly and remain healthy, stay as far way from a hospital as possible. Many people believe hospitals are needed, especially expecting parents. This is not true at all. It's unnatural to have a baby in a hospital. There is much proof to support my statement. Many books and articles have been written about natural childbirth (away from a hospital).

To follow are two excellent articles, the first by my friend, **Michele Barber**, who has overcome the crazy myth that the only safe way to bring your child into this world is to go to a hospital; the second article, entitled "Natural Childbirth and Raw Food" is by my Canadian friend, **Jinjee**.

407

Birthing in the Raw: Rebellion Against Modern Medical Myth

When I told my birthing class instructor that I believed childbirth could be painless, she laughed. She, like many others, was against the negative effect of drugs, and believed pain management was the only alternative. All my life I'd had excruciating periods, but when I started eating 100% raw foods, within months I had forgotten cramps and what they felt like. Why should contractions be different? On June 11, 2001, I felt this incredibly powerful force rhythmically pulling me open, an intense, yet not uncomfortable feeling. I arrived at the birthing center almost completely dilated, jumped into the Jacuzzi, took a bunch of pictures - grinning like a loon, mid-contraction - and had my baby. In those first moments, all I could see was him.

Two years before the birth of my son, I was a completely different person. I suffered from severe asthma, allergies, hypoglycemia, eczema, bladder infections, migraines, and insomnia. I couldn't touch a dog or walk outside in the winter without puffing away on my inhaler. I virtually lived on over the counter medications, popping pills daily to ease my symptoms. On June 2, 1999, my friend Layla let me read the first chapter of *Nature's First Law: the Raw Food Diet*. The writers' passion captured me instantly, and we nearly had an argument when she took back her book. That evening, I purchased my own copy. I read it twice in a row. The next day, I stopped eating cooked food. By New Year's, I'd lost over sixty unwanted pounds, and all signs of my ailments had vanished without a trace.

Having learned firsthand the amazing potential of the human body, I saw my pregnancy as a delightful challenge. I studied the different stages of labor and common hospital procedures. It soon became apparent many of the practices considered normal are harmful and unnecessary. The sterile environment, bright lighting, and surrounding illness and death cause tension in the mother and her birth partner. Birth is seen as an emergency, resulting in invasive pelvic exams, bothersome fetal monitoring, and strict guidelines to control the expectant woman's choice of positions for both laboring and delivery. The surgical precision of episiotomies, being easier to stitch than potential jagged tears, is preferred by doctors, nurses and some midwives. Epidurals are offered freely, with no care to inform the mothers of possible damaging side effects. Evidence that the lack of cervical and vaginal stimulation from local anesthesia during birth decreases neurotransmitters' facilitation of the mother - child connection. Furthermore, their babies will be less responsive, cry more, and five times more likely to be addicted to amphetamines as adults. Synthetic hormones like Pitocin are given to speed cervical dilation, causing contractions to become unbearably ineffective muscle spasms. Mothers are told not to push when they feel the urge, and made to strain when they don't. This exhausts her, increases stress on the fetus and causes vaginal tearing. It is no surprise to discover the rate of caesarians in this country is over 20%. Outraged, I avoided hospitals like the plague for the entirety of my pregnancy.

Natural childbirth was plainly the only option for me. Friends and strangers told me I was very brave to endure such torture. I decided to deliver my baby in a birthing center, since I had a very small bathtub and wanted a water birth. I investigated the effects of hypnotherapy, breath control, hydrotherapy, aromatherapy, affirmations, visualization, and doulas [trained labor assistants] during labor. These methods work by relaxing the mother. In my birth education class, I realized I was the only person, male or female, not afraid of childbirth. I stubbornly refused to believe something so beautiful should be feared. Gradually I found more and more stories of painless, even sensual birthing experiences. I concluded my perception of birth would shape my reality. I was right.

Media, patriarchal dogma, medical institutions, family and friends portray to society contractions are agonizing. The truth is, during birth, the brain produces endorphins to counteract the magnitude of those tremendous sensations with pleasure. When the body is given proper fuel: raw organic fruits, vegetables, seeds, nuts, and clean water, it can perform all its functions optimally. Thoughts and emotions regarding childbirth also play a big part. It is important to research the physical aspects of delivery in order to unlearn negative concepts about labor pains. Therefore, becoming aware of pain management techniques mentioned above can help build confidence. However, familiarity with pain management techniques is not a necessity. It is more helpful to talk with or read about women who had enjoyable birth experiences with little or no medical assistance.

Birth is intended by nature to bridge the gap between creation and existence, and construct an unbreakable bond between mother and child. Trust your body's knowledge, believe in its ability to create new life, delivering it safely into your arms. Only in the absence of fear will truly natural birth be experienced.

Natural Childbirth and Raw Food

One of the most rewarding experiences we have been through is the natural home births of our children. There were many reasons that we opted for home births. I have studied with midwives and have delivered all five of my children. When each of them was in the womb, I was a raw foodist. The first two when I ate 80% to 90% raw food, and the last three when I was 100% raw. The births when I was a 100% raw foodist were the easiest, the labors lasting under two hours. The babies just slipped into the world. The prenatal preparation started about four months before they were conceived. All through the pregnancy, walking in nature was the main form of exercise. Stretching and breathing were also important factors in the process.

We feel a major concept behind the labor is that a child in the womb can already hear and see. But the sounds and lights are muted because the fetus is surrounded by water. Therefore, we wanted to create an environment that was as close to natural light and sound as possible. My studies had also led me to believe that many mothers tear because they're lying on their backs when they deliver. This also means they're lying on their tailbones. The tailbone is a hinge which should be free to swing open to allow the baby more room to pass through. But by lying on this hinge, more pressure is put on the frontal hinging systems, causing tearing. But, by having the mother squat, with someone supporting her from behind, the whole hinging system is allowed to move freely. Supported squatting also reduces the stress and pain of the passage through the birth canal. We also massaged olive oil into the perineum which also helped prevent tearing because it made the tissue more elastic. Olive oil is also a natural antiseptic.

Often babies whose mothers are raw foodists don't gain as much weight and size in the womb, which also makes for easier births. All of my children were born breathing with clear airways. They all had full heads of hair. As soon as they came out, they opened their eyes, looked around and were very alert.

They all weighed between six and seven pounds, which I think is a perfect weight for a newborn baby. As soon as they were born, I placed them on their mother's nipple and allowed them to nurse, because the first milk contains a clear substance that clears any mucus from the airways. At this time we rubbed the thick cream like substance covering them at birth into their skin. This substance is designed to protect them from the air. I then waited about ten to twenty minutes for the cord to stop pulsating while there was still a transfer of blood taking place between the child and the mother. After the cord stopped pulsating, I tied it off in two places, about an inch from the baby, and cut the cord in between the two knots. All of my children were born on the full moon, most in the early morning around sunrise. They were all born into a room of natural light, quiet sounds and lots of plants. All of them were fed only mother's milk for at least the first six months, and then mashed up bananas and avocados for the first year. After which, other fresh foods and juices, both vegetables and fruit were introduced into their diet.

As of this writing, none of our kids have had anything more than a stuffy nose for two days at a time. None of them have had any of the common childhood diseases. Their energy levels are through the roof and their immune systems are robust. Even though I delivered all of my own children without the help of a midwife, I would in no way recommend this to anyone else. Even though I did an intense amount of studying, in the end, I don't think that I can claim any of the credit. I feel that we were just very, very blessed.

Jinjee and Nutman run a nonprofit organization through which they have created a campaign called "Take a Fruit Break", a national TV ad campaign to get kids to eat more fruit in place of junk food.
For more information see *http://www.takeafruitbreak.com*

To contact Jinjee or NutMan write to:

15-180 Central Rd.
Duncan, BC
Canada V9L 5X7

You may also call them or visit their wonderful website which has excellent information about the raw food diet and lifestyle.

Phone: 250 715-0133
Website: www.thegardendiet.com

E-mail: info@thegardendiet.com

Recommended websites for empowering information and birth stories:

www.geocities.com/rawbabymama/—Visit Michele Barber

www.mothering.com —Mothering magazine's site, wonderful articles on home birthing

www.birthpower.com

www.unassistedbirth.com—Inspiring birth stories, informative articles pertaining to home birthing.

www.naturalchildbirth.org

www.bestfed.com—breastfeeding, natural birth.

http://www.ravensperch.com/homebirth/research/
This one has great links, studies and statistics.

APPENDIX G
Home Schooling

Natural Education, Also Known as Homeschool

I believe very strongly that one of the most unnatural habits is today's practice of parents sending their children to be trained by strangers in a room with many other strangers. Today public schools are in the business of training kids to do what everyone else is doing. This is why so many people think the way they do. If you want your kids to grow up and suffer from the same unhappiness, sickness and poverty so many people suffer from today, then have them trained the same way many kids are trained (public schools). But, if you want your kids to thrive in everything they do, and most importantly, if you want your kids to learn to think for themselves and do what makes sense to them and not to everyone else in society, then "teach" them yourselves. I believe dogs should be trained to do tricks, but children should be taught, not trained. Many people make excuses for not homeschooling their kids, but, as I've said, there's action and there are excuses. You have to do whatever you decide. Visualize it, and it will happen. If you really believe in something, and want to do it badly enough, make it happen no matter what, and it will happen. Where there's a will there's a way! Many people today are home-schooling their children. Talk with them, ask questions, get answers, get the knowledge. Most importantly, take action!

Since I don't have any children of my own, many people ask me how I know homeschooling is best. In my travels, I've met many homeschooled children, and after seeing first hand how great all these kids are, especially when compared with public school kids, there is no question in my mind that teaching your children by yourself is best. Just to note: even though it's called homeschooling, many of the lessons are given outdoors in nature. Therefore, natural education would be more appropriate.

To follow are a few articles written by people detailing their experience in homeschooling their children. The first is by my friend, **Karen Ranzi**. Karen has two beautiful children who eat healthfully and are homeschooled.

Homeschooling: An Option That Makes Sense

After enjoying our lives together during their early years, I sent my two children to public school to sit in classes with many other children of the same age. Something inside me felt great despair and loss at leaving my children in a large, cold building to be raised by someone who is not their mother for a good part of their daily lives. But at the time, I had been ignorant of any other options other than expensive, private schools with a smaller teacher/student ratio. I had breastfed each of my two children for four to five years and raised them on a vegan diet. It was my natural maternal instinct to remain with my children, but at the time, I did not realize or understand that I could keep them with me when they became school age. When my first child, Gabriela, was in third grade, and my younger child, Marco, was in kindergarten, both in public school, I was first exposed to homeschooling through some mothers I met at an Attachment Parenting Group, also called a Continuum Group after a book entitled "The Continuum Concept." The belief they held so dear to them was that young children require their mothers to nurture them as they grow and mature through various stages of their lives, and that to force separation so prematurely would be harmful to their development.

At the time I began attending this Continuum Parenting Group, my children were still in public school, and I was frequently a volunteer there so that I could be near them. However, once I became more aware that I had an alternative, and began reading books about homeschooling, I started to observe incidences in school which I felt were detrimental to emotional and educational growth. My daughter, Gabriela, sat at a desk for many hours of the day listening to her teacher lecture. She was compliant with doing all the work, but she appeared unhappy and unmotivated when in the classroom setting. My son, Marco, was bored in kindergarten and was reprimanded for trying to leave the room. He was also scolded when he tried to get off of a single file class line to hug me when I was volunteering in the library. In addition to these disappointments in the system, I observed junk food being used numerous times as a reward for completion of academic work. This totally upset me because I believe that rewards, and food rewards in particular, are an obstacle to increasing motivation, and only work temporarily.

I began to feel instinctively that public school was a place where my children's spirits were not being nurtured, and where health and nutrition messages totally conflicted with our values at home.

At this time (1995), I had already become a 100% raw foodist, and I knew that my children were being bombarded with toxic foods as well as toxic substances and pesticides in

417

school cleaning materials.

My son, Marco, was never interested in school, and when he met children who were being homeschooled, he expressed strong resistance to attending public school; and so after careful consideration, my husband and I withdrew him that year. Gabriela continued in school for another half year. It was at a parent-teacher conference with her third grade teacher that I made the decision to take her out of school as well. The teacher explained to me that Gabriela was doing extremely well at school, but that she liked writing so much that she didn't want to switch to other subjects. She felt that this was hindering her from learning in other areas. I knew that Gabriela loved writing and liked to see her projects to completion, but this continued to be a source of conflict between her and the teacher. Gabriela pleaded with us to take her out of school, so after the holidays she did not return to third grade.

We have been homeschooling now for six years. One of the main questions continually confronting us is about socialization with other children. I feel that when children are placed into a situation with 20-30 children of their own age with only one adult, this is extremely limited socialization. These children most often learn to socialize only with children of their own age. And they don't have the individualized attention from a loving, caring adult which is so necessary as they grow. I believe that my two children are very well socialized. They interact with children of all ages and spend a lot of time with adults in their lives as well. My fourteen year old daughter Gabriela has friends as young as five and as old as sixteen. She also considers some of my adult friends to be close friends of hers.

One very valuable thing that I have noticed with Gabriela over the homeschooling years is that she has maintained her imaginative and playful ways. Most children her age are involved with who is popular at school, while she is still involved in creative, imaginative play, such as dressing up and acting out a variety of characters she had read or heard about.

If you have strong questions about the desirability of compulsory schooling, then homeschooling is an excellent alternative. Homeschooling is legal in all 50 states. Thousands of people have been homeschooled and have gone on to lead happy, productive lives, and to actualize their potential.

Karen Ranzi
New Jersey

The next article is by **Andy**. I met Andy and her family on one of my book tours. There was something special about Andy's children. When I asked how the kids turned out so wonderfully, she said homeschooling; then we got into a big talk about it. Please read Andy's experience:

We made the decision to homeschool when our firstborn child was only one year old. A friend had loaned me the book, "Teach Your Own," by John Holt. Neither my husband nor I had ever heard of homeschooling before reading this book, but the author's words caused us to reexamine all of our conceptions about education and our own personal school experiences. I think that giving birth at home had empowered me and broadened my sense both of my own capability and of the power of choice.

We wanted our son to retain his curiosity and his passion for learning. We knew that these qualities would remain intact only if he could be allowed to follow his own interests. We didn't want his self-esteem messed with by being pressured to learn something before it was right for him, before he was ready. We have since had two more children. Today they are 14, 12 and 8.

None of them have ever been to school. They have wonderfully rich, enjoyable, low-stress and socially active lives. They are bright and passionate young people with unique personalities and interests. Through our network of homeschooling families they participate in a multitude of activities: theater, history through films, classic literature for teens, writer's groups, hands on math groups, Ultimate Frisbee.

Destination Imagination, and an annual Craft Fair are just a few examples of the activities that they have chosen to participate in and which homeschooling parents are freely sponsoring. Two of my children are practicing musicians, all three of them are active in sports. "Unschooling" (or interest-led learning) as the branch of homeschooling that we have adopted is called, has also rubbed off on my husband and me. Dormant interests in us have been unearthed, and we are both pursuing new interests and trying new things. Our decision to homeschool has been one of the most fruitful choices we have made, for our children, for us and for our family.

Andy Migner
Boxborough, Ma.

To follow is a touching poem that Andy wrote about her and her husband's homeschooling experience:

When you reached Kindergarten age
Homeschooling was not yet the rage,
But John Holt's writings seemed quite sage.

He urged us to keep you out of school,
Away from mindless deskwork and senseless rules,
From social cliques and pressures to be cool.

You had learned so much already,
Your course was sure and steady,
As long as you could learn when you were ready.

We wanted you to go at your own pace,
Not be ensnared in a vicious and unnecessary race
That separates children in time and place.

We also wanted time with you
To bond, to laugh, to work things through.
We knew these years at home were precious few.

The early years were really sweet.
We slept in late, no bus to meet,
Read chapters, books, still in pajama'd feet.

With friends and groups, we hung around
At Crane Beach and Walden Pond,
Ever curious and observant, you did astound.

You learned so much without even trying.
There's absolutely no denying
A mind that's free from others' prying

Will develop enormous powers of acuity,
Tremendous keenness and agility,
Great problem solving ability.

As you have grown older, our lifestyle has changed.
More scheduled activities have been arranged,
Pursuing your interests in a manner that is "free-range."

When we made the choice to set you free,
We were rewarded, both you and me,

For now life long learners we will always be.

Our contributions, whether great or small,
As heartfelt answerings to a deep inner call
Are certain to be a gift to all.

RESOURCES ON HOMESCHOOLING

Home Education Magazine at 800-236-3278
or 907-746-1336

HEM-Info@home-ed-magazine.com

http://www.home-ed-magazine.com

APPENDIX H
Vaccinations Healthy or Unhealthy?

I strongly believe that one of the unhealthiest, most unnatural things done today is the vaccination of our children. People are putting sickness into their own kids at a very young age. They are led to believe that vaccinations are good, healthful and necessary, however that is false as you will see when you read the following article about the dangers of vaccination.

The information for this article was obtained from a variety of sources, including books, lecturers, and organizations. The author of the article to follow prefers to remain anonymous. The information might seem very shocking to you at first, but please don't get scared and understand its meaning. Use the knowledge and take action!

Are You A Victim of Vaccination?

Vaccination of children was accepted for decades with few questions asked, but during more recent years it has become a great source of concern. Acute symptoms from shots, such as high fevers, inflammations, and physical and neurological problems have been observed in a number of children following the administration of vaccinations. The long-term effects of these vaccines on children's developing bodies are just beginning to be investigated and understood. It is highly possible that immune system dysfunction, chronic fatigue syndrome, allergies, nervous system disorders, cancer, and other illnesses are connected to earlier vaccinations and medications.

Thousands of children who were administered the routine DPT (diphtheria, pertussis [whooping cough], tetanus), MMR (measles, mumps, rubella), or OPV (oral polio) vaccine died or were struck with debilitating seizure disorders, mental retardation, physical handicaps, learning disabilities, or other chronic illnesses following a reaction to the routine vaccination.

The National Vaccine Information Center (NVIC) in Virginia reported that one large U.S. study found that "1 in 875 DPT shots produces a convulsion or collapse/shock reaction, which means that some 18,000 DPT shots cause American children to suffer one of these neurological reactions every year." The MMR (measles, mumps, rubella) vaccine can cause encephalitis (brain inflammation) and death. The NVIC reported another U.S. government study which found a relationship between rubella vaccine and chronic arthritis, and some nervous system and blood disorders are also believed to be reactions to the rubella vaccine.

Vaccines, once injected, go straight to the DNA. In addition to causing auto-immune disease, cancer, and seizures in children, it is now thought that autism and sterility may also be the results of vaccination. Smallpox, polio and hepatitis B vaccines may be accountable for AIDS.

The vaccines contain many different toxic substances, including formaldehyde and aluminum.

There is evidence that many of the diseases we are being vaccinated against were actually on their way out before the vaccines were even invented. You have the right to protect your children, and to interpret God's law in your own way. If you believe that God and nature are one and that it is wrong to ingest any foreign materials of unhealthy or unnatural composition into the body, then you have the right to protect yourself and your family. The first step is to read and acquire as much information as you can, then get in touch with an organization such as NVIC or Vaccination Alternatives, and contact individuals knowledgeable in this area. Below is a list of the organizations, books, and websites involved with vaccinations. It would also be helpful to find a support group of people opposing vaccination.

RESOURCES WITH INFORMATION ABOUT VACCINATION:

Websites

http://www.909shot.com (NVIC)

http://www.garynull.com/

http://www.access1.net/vial
(vaccine information and awareness)

Organizations

The National Vaccine Information Center (NVIC)
512 W. Maple Avenue, #206
Vienna, VA. 22180
1-800-909-SHOT

Raw Food Diet Testimonials

Since I woke up to the message about the raw food diet, hundreds of people have written to me and told me incredible stories about their own wake-up calls. Many of them are just beginning, but have come to the realization that the raw life is the answer. Many have found levels of health and energy they never dreamed could exist. Many more of them have found a deep spiritual connection and realize that there's much more to life than what meets the eye.

When I read these testimonials, I save them, thinking that one day they will help inspire other people. Now, I would like to share with you some of the more interesting and inspiring testimonials I've received. Enjoy!

E.S of Seattle Washington writes:

I ordered your audio tape, and I listen to it every day for motivation to keep me raw... I've been raw for two years, but I need help:

Please make another audio cassette for more motivation.

When there are no other raw fooders around, your cassette is the only thing to keep me going raw.

My cooked food cravings are so bad, the only way I can stay raw is to fast one day a week for cravings-management purposes. Fasting kills all the cravings for a few days. I can't be raw at this time without fasting as a cravings-abatement tool. The cooked-food cravings are monstrous. What do you think about this?

I am seriously addicted to the HEAVY feeling after a meal - I go nuts if I just eat a greens salad and a fruit salad for a meal. So I end up eating lots of bananas and nuts. Sometimes I just try to stay with the light feeling after a meal of greens and fruit, but the absence of a heavy feeling drives me to gorge on nuts, bananas, etc. I know you say to speak positive, but in this area I feel hopeless. But at least I'm raw!

Thank you so much for your help and motivation, you have been my angel!

N.T. of San Diego, California writes:

I started reading your book today. I will admit that the first time I glanced through the chapters, I thought it would not do much for me. Now I truly in all sincerity believe it to be the best book on raw foods there is. I have a lot of studying to do, but I think I will put it off so I can keep reading your book. Your book is awesome. It truly is. Finally, the best information is available. And that is the people who are most successful in eating raw foods.

Finally, it is not information about eating what tastes good by having so many recipes and stupid combinations and de-hydrator recipes and just JUNK! None of it is natural, and who can heal like that? It is about simplicity and mono diets are the best, but up until your book that information was not

MADE TO FINALLY STAND OUT in your book about eating the most natural. Keep speaking the truth and thank you. Just get it out there at all cost. I know you are doing it anyhow regardless of what I say, but thank you nonetheless.

N.D. from Atlanta writes:

I really enjoyed your talk, and I have since bought your book. I love it! It's so humorous. I sit there chuckling at all the different "punches" of egg man, milk man, meat man, and the lot. I'm learning a lot, and I find myself looking forward to reading the book. I've read books on health issues in the past, but I don't think I've ever had such a swell time. It really motivates me, and my "opponents" seem so foolish after I read about their pitiful punches and imagine them in their cartoon form.

Yesterday I was reading *The Raw Life*, and then I decided to go to the gym. I got on one of the stepping machines, and from my vantage point I could see there was a boxing ring down below on the first floor! I've never thought much of or about boxing, but I decided to take note of it this time. A lone man was practicing in the ring for about twenty minutes. I watched him with his various punches and stances and tried imagining him taking out chicken man or coffee man. It was some funny stuff.

Yesterday after church, I was invited by some people to go to a restaurant to celebrate someone's birthday. I decided to go, but I was determined not to eat anything cooked, even if that meant not eating anything and just getting water. At home it's a lot easier to just eat raw, but when I go out with friends and such, I usually use it as an excuse to eat cooked food. The menu at the place where we went was not even inclined for "cooked" vegetarians, but they had fresh squeezed orange juice, and I got some of that.

Then I thought of a plan. I asked the waitress if I could buy a whole orange. She agreed. I also got a small salad of lettuce and carrots. I know it wasn't the perfect meal because of wrong combinations and the food wasn't organic, but for me it was a big step. I resisted all the cooked food I could have tried, such as a baked potato, rolls, croutons, or maybe a side of steamed veggies. The other people thought my meal seemed odd and asked me a lot of questions. I just told them I only felt like eating raw foods. They told me I needed some grains to help balance my meal, but I said I didn't care for any. They told me I was skinny enough and needed fattening up if anything. I just chuckled to myself.

Anyway, I'm really going to do this. I'm going to eat only raw foods. I'm going to be really truly healthy. I'm going to be a champion.

M.D. of Kansas, Missouri writes:

I am really new to the raw food idea. I haven't eaten pork or beef for over ten years, I don't drink anything but water and fresh juices, I won't touch anything with artificial sweetener, and I avoid hydrogenated oils and most dairy products, but the raw food thing is pretty new. I met a lady in Colorado last summer who introduced me to the concept. I'm really interested in health, so I was fascinated by the information she shared, but it seemed really radical at the time... especially since I'm around a lot of bodybuilding types who are avid believers in a contest diet of chicken, tuna, rice, and green vegetables.

Since December, I've been studying a lot about detoxification, energy fasts, and other health related issues, so I was primed to hear your message. Ever since hearing you speak on Saturday, I'm amazed at how my thoughts about different foods have changed. Thank you for your message and help.

K.L. of Los Angeles, California writes:

I don't think I have ever been so inspired in my life! I got The Raw Life in the mail yesterday, and this morning I decided to dive right in. Well, I have just spent the last five hours reading it from cover to cover! I didn't have a clue as to how much time had passed; that's how absorbed I was. I've read many other raw-food, natural hygiene, enzyme books, etc., but none of them has ever set off such a spark in me as your book has. You were the perfect person to set me on the right path. Thank you so much for helping me to decide to change my life for the better!

T.B. of England writes:

I bought your book and enjoyed it very much. Good fun and very informative reading. I am endeavoring to change to 100% raw. It's early days so far, but I am very determined. It can be very hard when you are surrounded by cooked food and your only choice is salads - and sometimes not even that - if you want to go out and socialize. I think that England is very behind in this way of living - and it's diabolical outside of London! Although there is always a good supply of fruit and veg, which is the main thing. However, I'm awe-inspired by this revelation of eating raw; I never imagined the benefits to be gained by doing it or indeed that it is our natural way. Keep up the good work!

A.B. of Las Vegas, Nevada writes:

Was 280 pounds! Now 118 pounds and dress size 3! Yeah! Without The Raw Life I would be dead!!!!!!!!!!!! I am only 31 years old!!! Paul Nison saved my life!!! What can he do for you?!!! Thanks Paul!!!

S.B. of Tempe Arizona writes:

You're a gem. Thanks tons! I want to tell you that since your presentation, I've been on a wonderful roll. No, no, no, not a jelly roll or a Kaiser roll, but a roll of enthusiasm that is contagious only to me. The more I'm inspired, the more I inspire myself. It's so cool! Again, thanks.

R.C. of Prescott, Arizona writes:

Hello, Paul. I attended a talk you gave at a natural foods store in Prescott, Arizona last fall. I was inspired. I had read about raw foods eight years earlier but had not adopted the diet. I gave up all meat except seafood in '93 and had gone dairy-free with great results on and off for years since that time. I have always sensed that there is an ideal, pure way to eat, and I have been searching for it for many years, making small changes along the way, but always challenged with addictions to unhealthy foods.

Then I heard your message.

Hearing about your experience and actually meeting someone who was 100% raw changed my life. I bought your book and spent every last minute of my spare time over the next few days reading and re-reading about raw foods. Between last fall and this May, I went 100% raw for periods of a week or two while scouring other raw food books and experimenting with raw recipes. I have been raw now for over one month straight! In fact, my one-year-old daughter Ruby (my first) has been 100% raw her entire life! I continue to read books about raw food and read articles on the Internet as well. All the time I am learning more and am more motivated as a result.

I want to say thank you for going out and spreading the word. Your inspiration has started something for me that has been nothing short of transformational. I trace my whole experience with raw foods back to the day I met you. You are making a big difference. Keep up the great work.

B.D. of Canada writes:

I have just finished reading your book. You did a good job. Your efforts deserve to be congratulated. Besides being very positive, inspiring, and convincing, your words give suffering humanity more than hope; they also give people the assurance that perfect health is within everyone's reach (if they were willing to change their eating habits). Because what you say is substantiated by the experiences of so many living examples, including yours, no one should doubt the statements you make.

If everybody followed the guidelines of your book, there would be hardly any need for hospitals and doctors, and the economies of all countries would benefit immensely from the astronomical sums of money they would save in medical care. Unfortunately, such a thing is a utopian dream, because the majority of humanity has to continue suffering, due to divine design (the Law of Karma), and nothing will ever change that. But that doesn't mean we shouldn't try to improve the lot of as many people as possible; and your book does just that. The people that are meant to follow those principles will follow them and benefit from it; all others will continue to suffer, but that cannot be helped.

C.D. of Livonia, MI writes:

Dear Mr. Nison,

I have just read your book. It was incredible. I wish I had written it. My personal experiences have included five years of vegetarianism and one experience with a tremendous 10-day raw juice "fast." After the fast, I truly felt many years younger. It was a fantastic feeling. Now, I am trying to imagine how awesome I will feel after being a raw foodist!

Just this week, I began your suggested transitional diet, where I eat only fresh fruits for breakfast. Things are changing already.

Thank you for writing the book that is sure to improve the lives of anyone who reads it and applies it.

K.G. from Portland, Oregon writes:

Dear Paul,

I just read your book *The Raw Life* for the third time. It is so excellent, so inspiring. Thank you for the lifeline to health and wholeness that you offer to the world through your example and your work.

I have been following a raw food diet for a year and a half now. My diet is pretty much "all over the map", with considerable trial and error. The Natural Hygiene system, which I have felt resistant to, is now the direction my body and heart clearly are asking to go...and the direction I believe I need to go in order to heal.

Heartfelt thanks and blessings.

T.M. of Michigan writes:

Hi, Paul. I have to tell you what happened after I wrote you yesterday. I went to a local health food store that serves living foods in their café, and while I was waiting, I looked at their books. The second one I saw was YOUR book, *The Raw Life*. How awesome! (I didn't know people carried it around here.) I read it almost all the way through last night. Even though

I've been in and out of raw foods for the last 13 years and have read T.C Fry, Ann Wigmore extensively (grown sprouts), and David Wolfe's great book *The Sunfood Success System*, Gabriel Cousins books, etc., for some reason, your book hit me, and I GET IT!!! I thought I had gotten it before, but this time I REALLY get it! The desire to eat cooked foods is COM-PLETELY emotional. Also, I can relate to the fact that you recovered from a serious illness. Again, thank you so very much, and many blessings.

ORGANIZATIONS AND RESOURCES

Raw-Food Products, Information, Contacts and Organizations

When I was writing this book, I had a big list of organizations and resources, but I have decided not to include them in this book. People are always moving, companies are always opening and closing or relocating, and I don't want to fill up pages with information about a group or resource in Seattle if one of my readers is living in Florida. It is very important for people to know what support is close to them, but since it's always changing, I have thought of a better way to give you the most updated information you need to help you. If you contact me by email or by phone and let me know exactly what you are looking for, I will put you in touch with the right organization or contact. This way, I can give you the most up to date information and put you in touch with the exact person you need to contact. There are many raw food organizations and contacts in every one of the United States and all over the world. You would be surprised! Get in touch with me wherever you live and I will send you the appropriate information. I have included in the following pages, healing retreats, raw restaurants and raw publications

The Raw Life
c/o Paul Nison
P.O. Box 443
Brooklyn, NY 11209
866-RAW-DIET
(866-729-3438)
Web Site: www.rawlife.com
Email: Paul@rawlife.com
This is the World's Premier Source of the best
raw food books, videos, and audio products about
the raw food diet and health available. Sign up
for the free email list on the contact page of this
web site to get updates on raw events in your area.

HEALING RETREATS

Ann Wigmore Foundation
P.O. Box 399
San Sidel, NM 87049
505-552-0595
The Ann Wigmore Foundation is a retreat and
healing center that advocates enzyme-rich plant-foods
to heal the body. Educational classes are offered.
Call or write for more information.

Ann Wigmore Institute
P.O. Box 429
Rincon, Puerto Rico 00677
USA

787-868-6307
Email: wigmore@caribe.net
The Ann Wigmore Foundation is a retreat and
healing center that advocates enzyme-rich
plant-foods to heal the body. Educational classes
are offered. Call or write for more information.

Creative Health Institute (CHI)
918 Union City Road
Union City, MI 49094
517-278-6260
CHI is a healing center offering 1-3 week cleansing
and detoxification programs using wheatgrass
and raw plant foods.

Hippocrates Health Institute
1443 Palmdale Court
West Palm Beach, FL 33411
800-842-2125
Hippocrates is a healing retreat emphasizing
the use of raw plant foods. Write or call for
more information.

L.O.V.I.N.G.
(Longevity from Organic Vegetarian Enzymatic
Indigenous/Indoor Nutriceutical Garden)
P.O. Box 2853
Hot Springs, AR 71913
1-800-WHEAT-GRASS
www.naturalusa.com/viktor/sanctuary.html
Contacts: Viktoras Kulvinskas and Youkta
This resort/school is situated on 90 acres within
Ouchita National Forest. Each year in the spring,
L.O.V.I.N.G. hosts an "International Women's

Festival of The Healing Arts."
L.O.V.I.N.G. promotes the following themes:
Micro-agriculture and live-food preparation;
Divine Life-Style Consultant Self-Healing Training;
Spiritualized Guidance Applied to the 21st Century.
(How to know, before Earth changes visit your area,
what to do, how to enjoy the now, and grow
spiritually under all conditions.)
Write for a detailed brochure.

Optimum Health Institute (OHI)
6970 Central Avenue
Lemon Grove, CA 91945
OHI is a detoxification institute. They have 1, 2, 3
and 4 week programs. 100% raw plant-foods are
served on the premises. OHI offers very affordable rates.
Write or call for a free brochure.

Optimum Health Institute (OHI)
Rural Route 1
Box 339-J
Cedar Creek, TX 98612
512-303-4817
The new OHI in Texas operates a similar program
to that found at OHI in San Diego. Write or call
for a free brochure.

Tree Of Life Rejuvenation Center
P.O. Box 778
Patagonia, AZ 85624
520-394-0067
Tree Of Life was founded by raw-foodist,
Dr. Gabriel Cousens. This center now features
residential rooms for guests, a raw-food restaurant

open to the public, beautiful gardens, training sessions and meditations. Write or call for more information.

Rest Of Your Life Health Retreat
P.O. Box 102
Barksdale, TX 78828
830-234-3488
e-mail: vvvetrano@hilconet.com
Nestled on a crystal clear river in the Texas Hill Country away from the noise, smog, and maddening crowds, this Natural Hygiene center provides a peaceful, restful, and relaxing environment. This retreat is run by two medical doctors: Gregory and Tosca Haag. Tosca is Dr. Vetrano's daughter; Dr. Vetrano is Dr. Herbert Shelton's greatest student.

The Himalayan Institute
RR1, Box 1127
Honesdale, PA 18431
www.himalayanInstitute.org
800-822-4547
570-253-5551
The Himalayan Institute is dedicated to helping individuals develop themselves physically, mentally and spiritually, as well as contributing to the transformation of society. All the Institute programs - educational, therapeutic, research - emphasize holistic health, yoga, and meditation as tools to help achieve modern science of Eastern teachings and Western technologies.
*Fresh fruits and salads are served daily.
Call for more information.

Kwatamani Private Organic Gardens
and Spiritual Retreat
PO Box 706
Chipley FL 32428
941-850-258-9684
E-mail: kwatamani@hotmail.com
Web Site: www.livefoodsunchild.com
The Kwatamani Private Organic Gardens
and Spiritual Retreat TM & The Kwatamani Holistic Institute
are committed to advancing the spiritual message of divine
consumption of raw and living foods - fresh and natural
fruits, vegetables, seeds, nuts, and grains - as the first
divine step to a holistic living way of life.

Raw Food Restaurants

I always say, "Why make things harder for yourself, if you don't
have to?" What I recommend is that you keep your food very
simple. **Simple = fun = consistent**. You should make easy
recipes at home, but if you want to treat yourself to the best
raw food recipes, there are many great restaurants all over the
world that either have some raw recipes on their menu or are
100% raw. Visit them to taste some great recipes and also to fit
in socially with others. Take your friends or family out to dinner
at one of these fine places. These restaurants are wonderful for
the holidays or just a night out. More and more places are opening all the time and, unfortunately, closing all the time. This is
the most current list as of the printing of this book. I will do my
best to update the list with each new printing. Enjoy!

Arnold's Way
Raw & Vegetarian Café and Education center
319 West Main Street (in rear of Dressher Arcade)
Landsdale, PA 19440
215-483-2266
www.arnoldsway.com

Caravan of Dreams
405 East 6th Street
New York, NY 10009
212-254-1613
www.caravanofdreams.net

Delights Of The Garden
2616 Georgia Avenue NW
Washington, D.C. 20001
202-319-8747

Eco-politan Organic Bar & Eatery
2409 Lyndale Avenue South
Minneapolis, Minnesota 55405
www.ecopolitan.net
info@ecopolitan.net
617-874-7336

Enzyme Express
1330 East Huffman Road
Anchorage, Alaska 99515
907-345-1330

Karyn's Fresh Corner
3351 North Lincoln Avenue
Chicago, IL 60657
773-296-6990

Living Community Center
330 East Seventh Street
Tucson, Arizona
520-623-0913
www.livingcommunitycenter.com

Organic Garden Restaurant & Juice Bar
294 Cabot Street
(near the Cabot Cinema-Rte. 62 off Rte. 128)
Beverly, Massachusetts 01915
978-922-0004
www.organicgardencafe.com

Quintessence
263 East 10th Street
New York, NY 10009
646-654-1823
www.quintessencerestaurant.com

Quintessence
566 Amsterdam Avenue
New York, NY 10024
212-501-9700
www.quintessencerestaurant.com

The Raw Truth Café,
Healing Center, and Eco-Shop
3620 East Flamingo Road
Las Vegas, NV 89121
702-450-9007

Source Of Life Juice Bar
@Everlasting Life Health Food Supermarket
2928 Georgia Avenue, NW

Washington, D.C. 2001
www.everlastinglife.net
202-232-1700

The Sprout Café
Shinui living food learning center
1475 Holcomb Bridge Road
Roswell, GA 30075
770-992-9218
www.sproutcafe.com
www.shinui.biz

Super Sprouts
720 Bathurst Street
Toronto, Ontario
M5S 2R4
Canada

www.supersprouts.com
416-977-7796

Tree of Life
771 Harshaw Road
Patagonia, AZ 85624
520-394-2589

Well Springs Garden Café
2253 Highway 99
@Jackson Hot Springs
Ashland, OR 97520
541-488-6486

Roxanne's
320 Magnolia Avenue

Larkspur, CA
415-924-5004

*Non restaurants but great places
to get raw and live foods:*

High Vibe Health & Healing
85 East 3rd Street
New York, NY 10003
888-554-645
www.highvibe.com

Jubbs Longevity LifeFood Store,
Organic Juice Bar & Patisserie
508 East 12th Street
New York NY 10009
212-353-5000
www.lifefood.com

Please note that all the lists in this book are up to date at the time of print-ing, but people move and stores open, close, and relocate, so these contacts can change.

Publications

Just Eat An Apple Magazine
P.O. Box 1704
Hurst, TX 76053
Web site: www.sunfood.net
E-mail: fred@sunfood.net

Living Nutrition Magazine
P.O. Box 256
Sebastopol, California 95473-256
707-829-0362
Web site: www.livingnutrition.com
E-mail: dave@livingnutrition.com

Fresh Network
P.O. Box 71
Ely, CAMBS, CB7 4GU, UK
+44-0-8708-00-7070
Web site: www.fresh-network.com
E-mail: info@fresh-network.com

RECOMMENDED READING

.

K nowledge will make your transition to the raw food diet and lifestyle much easier. Why make it hard when you don't have to? The books I sell on this website and the information will make everything easier for you.

Remember, knowledge and fear are two different things. They are opposites. You can't have both in your life. If you have any fear, then you just don't have the knowledge. If you want the knowledge to replace the fear, check out these great books below. I have a choice to endorse many and all raw food books on the market, but I've been very selective and have picked the books that I feel will help you the most. These books are easy and fun. You will enjoy them. That is the secret to consistency: enjoyment. Now get the knowledge, and start living your life to its fullest and have a great RAW LIFE!

Raw Foods

A Doctor's Raw Food Cure by Dr. O.L.M. Abramowski

The Seven Essentials for Overcoming Illness by David Klein

Nature's First Law: The Raw Food Diet by Stephen Arlin, Fouad Dini and David Wolfe

The Sunfood Diet Success System by David Wolfe

Blatant Raw-Foodist Propaganda by Joe Alexander

Conscious Eating by Dr. Gabriel Cousens

Feel-good Food: A Guide To Intuitive Eating by Susie Miller and Karen Knowler

Mucusless Diet Healing System by Arnold Ehret

Nature the Healer by John and Vera Richter

Survival into the 21st Century by Viktoras Kulvinskas

Journey to Health by Annette Larkins

The Hippocrates Diet by Ann Wigmore

The Sunfood Way to Health by Dugald Semple

Your Natural Diet: Alive Raw Foods by David Klein and T.C. Fry

Spiritual Nutrition and the Rainbow Diet by Gabriel Cousens

Living Foods for Optimum Health by Brian Clement

The Cure is in The Cause by Dr. Ruza Bogdonovich

Fasting

Fasting Can Save Your Life by Herbert Shelton

Golden Path to Rejuvenation by Morris Krok

Rational Fasting by Arnold Ehert

The Miracle Of Fasting by Paul Bragg

Fasting For Health and Long Life
by Dr. Hereward Carrington

Amazing New Health System - The Inner Clean Way
by Morris Krok

Food Combining

Food Combining Made Easy by Herbert Shelton

Food Combining Simplified by Dennis Nelson

Fruitarianism

Fruit the Food and Medicine for Man by Morris Krok

Glimpses of Reality by Benito DeDonno

Perfect Body by Roe Gallo

Juicing

Juiceman's Power of Juicing by Jay Kordich

Longevity and Immortality

Become Younger by Dr. Norman Walker

Live Longer by Hilton Hotema

Why Do We Age? by Hilton Hotema

Man's Higher Consciousness by Hilton Hotema

Diet Health and Living on Air by Morris Krok

How to Live to be 90 by Hilton Hotema

Natural Hygiene

Fit for Life books number 1 and 2 by Harvey and Marilyn Diamond

Maximizing Your Nutrition by Dennis Nelson

Parenting and Children

The Children's Health Food Book by Ron Seaborn

Raw Kids by Cheryl Stoycoff

Raw Family: A True Story of Awakening by Victoria, Igor, Sergei, and Valya Boutenko

Natural Childbirth

Spiritual Midwifery by Ina May Gaskin

The Continuum Concept by Jean Liedloff

Primal Mothering in a Modern World by Hygeia Halfmoon

Unassisted Childbirth by Laura Kaplan Shanley

Raw Food Recipe Books

Dining in the Raw by Rita Romano

Living in the Raw by Rose Lee Calabro

Hooked on Raw by Rhio

Not Milk...Nut Milks! by Candia Lea Cole

The Raw Gourmet by Nomi Shannon

The Raw Truth: The Art of Loving Foods
by Jeremy Safron and Renée Loux Underkoffler

Raw - The Uncook Book by Juliano

The Sunfood Cuisine:
A Practical Guide to Raw Vegetarian Cuisine
by Frederic Patenaude

The Vegetarian Guide to Diet & Salad
by Dr. Norman Walker

The High Energy Recipe Guide by Dr. Douglas Graham

Shazzie's Detox Delights by Sharon Holdstock

Resource Guides

Dictionary of Natural Foods by William Esser

The Great Exotic Fruit Book by Norman Van Aken

Self Help and Personal Development

As You Think by James Allen

Diary of a Health and Truth Seeker by Morris Krok

Kindred Soul by Morris Krok

The Wisdom of James Allen by James Allen

To Be, or Not to Be! by Richard Schnackenberg

Creative Use of Emotion by Swami Rama and Swami Ajaya (Many of the ideas in the MIND room came from this book.)

How I Found Freedom in an Unfree World by Harry Browne

Peace Pilgrim: Her Life and Work in Her Own Words by Friends of Peace Pilgrim

Home Schooling

The Homeschooling Book Of Answers by Linda Dobson

The Unschooling Handbook by Mary Griffith

The Teenage Liberation Handbook by Grace Llewellyn

Dumbing Us Down: The Hidden Curriculum of Compulsory Schooling by John Taylor Gatto

Teach Your Own by John Holt

How Children Learn by John Holt

Family Matters by David Gutterson

Homeschooling for Excellence
by Micki and David Colfax

Vaccination

Immunization Theory vs. Reality
by Neil Miller

The Immunization Resource Guide
by Diane Rozairo

Immunizations: The People Speak
by Neil Miller

What About Immunization?
Exposing the Vaccine Philosophy
by Cynthia Cournoyer

What You Don't Know About Vaccines
Could Hurt Your Child
edited by Jesse Noguera

What Every Parent Should Know
About Childhood Immunization
by Jamie Murphy

A Shot in the Dark
by Harris Coulter and Barbara Loe Fisher

Vaccination, Social Violence and Criminality,
the Assault on the American Brain
by Harris Coulter

Vaccines: Are They Really Safe and Effective?
by Neil Miller.

Immunization: The Reality Behind the Myth
by Walene James.

Vegetarian and Vegan Diet

Mad Cowboy by Howard Lyman

Diet for a New America by John Robbins

Vegan Nutrition: Pure and Simple
by Michael Klaper

Beyond Beef by Jeremy Rifkin

Water

Your Body's Many Cries For Water by F. Batmanghelidj

Fitness and health:

Nutrition and Athletic Performance
by Dr. Douglas Graham

Raw Power! Building Strength & Muscle Naturally
by Stephen Arlin

Yoga

Yoga Gave Me Superior Health
by Theos Bernard

110 Years of Youth Through Yoga
by Charles Arnold

Pet Care

Reigning Cats & Dogs by Pat McKay

Cleansing and healing

Toxemia Explained by John Tilden

The Fruits of Healing by David Klein

Be Your Own Doctor by Ann Wigmore

Why Suffer? by Ann Wigmore

The Cure is in the Cause
by Dr. Ruza Bogdanovich

Why grains are harmful

Grain Damage by Dr. Douglas Graham

Against the Grain by Jax Peters Lowell

Many of these titles are available on my website at:
www.rawlife.com or call **866-RAW-DIET** (866-729-3438)
to see if books are in stock. If I don't have them, I can
get them or tell you where to get them.

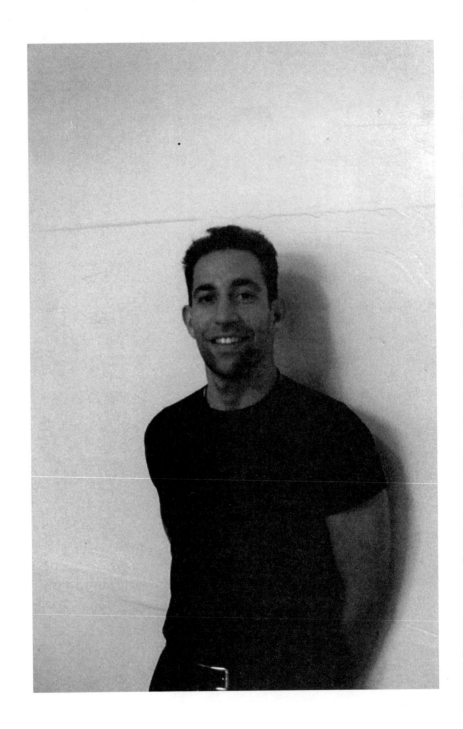

ABOUT
THE AUTHOR

Until the age of nineteen, I ate the Standard American Diet (SAD) and never suffered from any problems other than the common upset stomach or headache. Sometimes I would get a cold, but I thought that was normal. But then, the stomachaches started to get worse. I would get colds more often, and I started to worry. I decided to go to the hospital and get checked to see what the problem was. After running many tests, the doctors told me I had food poisoning. They gave me some medication and sent me home. I thought the drugs the doctors gave me would cure me, but during the following three weeks the pains kept coming back worse and worse. They got so bad that I wasn't even able to walk five feet without having to go to the bathroom, whether I had eaten or not. I was wasting away. My weight dropped to 125 pounds, and everyone I knew told me I looked terrible. I tried everything I could think of that would put weight on my body. I ate big portions of fatty foods with increasing frequency. Plus, I stopped doing all exercise in order not to burn too many calories. Nothing I tried worked; my condition just kept getting worse. I was willing to deal with the intense pain, but then one night, I saw blood in my stool. Now, I was really scared. I went to the doctor and the lab ran many tests on me. I felt like some scientific experiment. But, I would have done anything to find out what the problem was, so I could cure it. Up until then, I thought everyone had the common pain I was having. But once I saw blood, I knew the problem was much more serious than I had ever imagined.

Finally, from the doctor, I received my wake-up call. I was diagnosed with ulcerative colitis. Although most people would consider this a tragedy, I consider it one of the best things that ever happened to me. When I found out what I had, I remember thinking to myself, "Now I can stop trying to figure out what the problem is, and let the doctors cure me." What a big mistake that was.

First, let me explain what ulcerative colitis is. If you've ever had an ulcer, you know how painful that can be; well, my whole intestinal tract was lined with many ulcers. Ohhhhh! The worst pain in the world, and the only relief was to go to the bathroom many times and sit there for about thirty minutes to an hour. I remember, no matter where the bathroom was, people would knock on the door and ask me if I was okay. I would think, "NO, I'm not okay, I'm very sick," but I never said anything, because who would understand? How many people ever heard of ulcerative colitis or knew what it was? In brief, for those of you who still don't understand what it is, ulcerative colitis is not an easy illness to live with. The colon is achy and inflamed with ulcerations, sometimes with bleeding. It is accompanied by spasmodic and frequent bowel movements. The typical poor diet, increased bowel movements, decreased assimilation of swallowed food, along with drug therapies, all add up to malnutrition and decreased vitality, not to mention misery and a ruined life.

I would get colitis flare-ups about six times a year. Every time I went to the doctor, she told me to stay away from dairy foods until I felt better. Then, she increased the dosage of steroids she was giving me. After a few weeks, when I would feel better, she said it was okay to eat dairy foods again. I then ate foods that contained huge amounts of dairy. Sometimes this would be a whole big pizza. Then the flare-ups came back. Finally, I recognized the pattern and cut out dairy products altogether. I was very pleased with the results. I became sick less often. After that, I began to eliminate whatever the doctors told me it was okay to eat: eggs, meat and sugar to name just a few. I told my doctor, "I feel better without these foods."

She told me, "Food has nothing to do with your condition." After hearing that from her, I knew I was on the right track. I said to myself, "If she's such a good doctor, why do I keep seeing the same people in the waiting room every time I come for a visit? She doesn't heal them, that's why. If she did, they wouldn't need to come back."

At age twenty-three, I left my stressful job as an office manager for a big Wall Street firm in New York's financial district, and moved to West Palm Beach, Florida. I was still having colitis flare-ups, but not as often or severe. By seemingly sheer coincidence, I moved near a place called the Hippocrates Health Institute. I would visit the Institute often during my daily walks around the neighborhood. It was there that I learned about the raw-food lifestyle and about live foods. I immediately put myself on an 80% raw-food diet. What a difference it made! I told my doctor in New York about my improvement and she said, "Raw foods are no good for your condition." Once again, I knew I was on the right track!

Feeling much better, but not totally cured, when I was 25, I moved back to New York and resumed working at the stressful job I had left. In New York, I met many people who had adopted a raw-food diet. I began reading books on the raw-food diet and lifestyle. In a Manhattan bookstore, I picked up a book by David Klein called, *The Fruits of Healing, - A Story about a Natural Healing of Ulcerative Colitis.* It was exactly what I needed to read. I then heard David Wolfe, of *Nature's First Law*, speaking on a local radio show about the raw-food diet. *Nature's First Law* is an organization dedicated to spreading the word about the raw food movement. David Wolfe is one of the authors of *Nature's First Law: The Raw Food Diet,* a book he and his co-authors wrote. After speaking to Dave Klein and hearing David Wolfe on the radio, I decided to switch to a 100% raw-food diet. I also decided to join a raw-food support group. At that support group, I met raw foodists, Matt Grace and Tom Coviello, and later, at a fantastic lecture she gave, I met Roe Gallo. The more I got involved with the raw-food lifestyle, the more positive my outlook on life became. Speaking to all of these people, and seeing what great health they enjoyed, influenced me to enjoy a diet consisting mostly of fruit. That was the final piece in my health puzzle.

Since going 100% raw, I have completely overcome ulcerative colitis. I feel better than ever, and have become increasingly inspired about life. I quit my stressful job and began working as a raw-food chef in a vegetarian restaurant. I organize raw-food potlucks every month. I've started a raw-food support group, and I give lectures on the raw-food lifestyle to help others who have gotten their wake-up calls.

I've been traveling the world to experience the pleasures of new cultures and exotic fruits. Since adopting the raw-food diet, I've gone through several "healing crises." I'm happy for these episodes of elimination, as they are clearly my body's way of cleaning, healing and rejuvenating. At one time, my weight went all the way down to 118 pounds, but by then I had gained an understanding of how the body works, and I didn't panic. Now my weight remains at a healthy looking 145 pounds, and I know the raw-food diet is the best way for me to go. The people I knew before I was sick, when I was growing up and overweight, look at me now and tell me I'm too skinny or I'm underweight. But everyone meeting me now, and not knowing me then, tells me how great I look. Either way, I go by how I feel, and I feel great. I think I look great too, and I no longer worry about what other people think. That is another advantage of the raw food diet: I stopped trying to please everyone else, and now I please myself first.

Anyone can overcome any dis-ease or sickness the way I did. My books, videos, tapes, CDs and lectures will help you accomplish that. All I can do is tell you about it, the rest is up to you. I encourage you to learn from my experiences and the experiences of others. With a healthy mind, you can over-come anything.

For more information about me, please visit my website at: **www.paulnison.com**

I give lectures all over the world about health and empower-ment. To see an updated list of where I will be speaking, go to my web site: **www.rawlife.com**. If you would like to have me speak to your group or if you know someone who might be interested in having me speak, please contact me at the e-mail address or telephone number below.

I'm looking forward to meeting everyone interested in en-hancing the powers of his or her mind, body and soul.

You may contact me by e-mail: **paul@rawlife.com** or telephone: **866-raw-diet** (866-729-3438).

I would like to thank you for reading this book and for all your support. Keep up the great work.
Keep seeking raw knowledge.
It is your life.
You are in control.
You can do it.
You will do it.
Have a great raw life!

PICTURES

The following pages contain pictures of my transition from a diseased, unhappy life, to a life of health, happiness and freedom. I have seen transitions like mine in thousands of people. It's never too late. Keep moving forward and you'll get there!

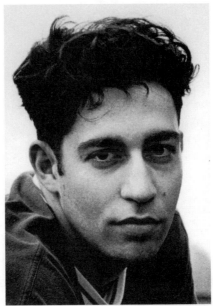

Paul Nison before the raw life.
Notice dark circles under the eyes and no smile.

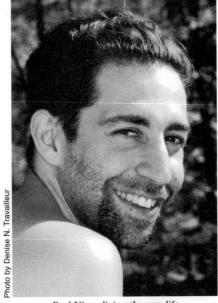

Photo by Denise N. Travailleur

Paul Nison living the raw life.
Notice twinkle in the eyes and big smile.

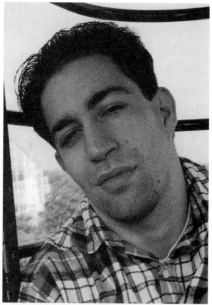

Paul Nison before the raw life.
Overweight and unhappy. Barely surviving.

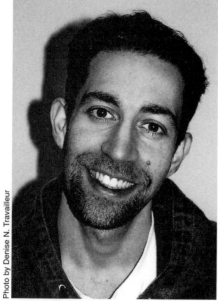

Photo by Denise N. Travailleur

Paul Nison living the raw life.
Happy, healthy and thriving.

467

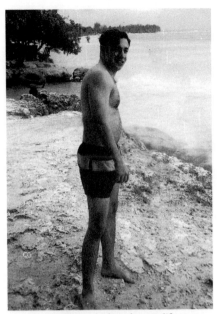

Paul Nison before the raw life.
Out of shape and with ulcerative colitis.

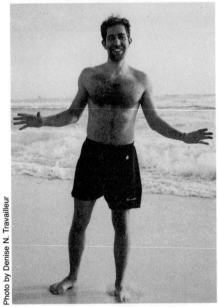

Photo by Denise N. Travailleur

Paul Nison living the raw life.
Slim and fit and cured.

Words are powerful,
But nothing speaks louder than action.
Say what you do,
Then do as you say!

Take your life to the next level:
STEP UP, KEEP MOVING FORWARD, NO LIMITS.

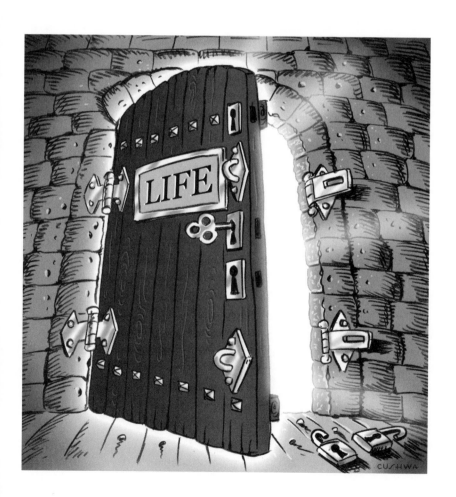

INDEX

A

B

C

ORDER FORM

RAW KNOWLEDGE: ENHANCE THE POWERS OF YOUR MIND, BODY AND SOUL
PLEASE SEND ME ___ COPIES AT **US$ 24.95 PER COPY**

RAW KNOWLEDGE PART II: INTERVIEWS WITH HEALTH ACHIEVERS
PLEASE SEND ME ___ COPIES AT **US$ 19.95 PER COPY**

THE RAW LIFE: BECOMING NATURAL IN AN UNNATURAL WORLD
PLEASE SEND ME ___ COPIES AT **US$ 19.95 PER COPY**

US Shipping and Handling:
$3.50 per first item, $1.00 for each additional item.
Canada and Mexico Shipping and Handling:
$15.00 per first item, $6.00 for each additional item
Outside North America Shipping and Handling:
$25.00 per first item, $6.00 for each additional item

TOTAL AMOUNT ENCLOSED $_____

SHIP TO:
(Please print)

NAME _____

ADDRESS_____

CITY_____STATE_____

ZIP CODE_____COUNTRY_____

EMAIL ADDRESS_____

PHONE NUMBER_____

Please copy or cut out this form and mail with a check, money order or bank draft
in US currency payable to:

Paul Nison
P.O. Box 443
Brooklyn, NY 11209

To contact the author e-mail: paul@rawlife.com
Or go to the website: www.rawlife.com
You may also call 866-RAW-DIET (866-729-3438)

***As time goes by the mailing address may change several times. Please
check website or call for most updated contact information.**